OTOLARYNGOLOGY RESEARCH ADVANCES

SENSORINEURAL HEARING LOSS

PATHOPHYSIOLOGY, DIAGNOSIS AND TREATMENT

OTOLARYNGOLOGY RESEARCH ADVANCES

Additional books and e-books in this series can be found on Nova's website under the Series tab.

OTOLARYNGOLOGY RESEARCH ADVANCES

SENSORINEURAL HEARING LOSS

PATHOPHYSIOLOGY, DIAGNOSIS AND TREATMENT

FRANCESCO DISPENZA
AND
FRANCESCO MARTINES
EDITORS

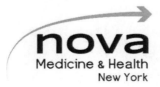

Copyright © 2019 by Nova Science Publishers, Inc.

All rights reserved. No part of this book may be reproduced, stored in a retrieval system or transmitted in any form or by any means: electronic, electrostatic, magnetic, tape, mechanical photocopying, recording or otherwise without the written permission of the Publisher.

We have partnered with Copyright Clearance Center to make it easy for you to obtain permissions to reuse content from this publication. Simply navigate to this publication's page on Nova's website and locate the "Get Permission" button below the title description. This button is linked directly to the title's permission page on copyright.com. Alternatively, you can visit copyright.com and search by title, ISBN, or ISSN.

For further questions about using the service on copyright.com, please contact:
Copyright Clearance Center
Phone: +1-(978) 750-8400   Fax: +1-(978) 750-4470   E-mail: info@copyright.com.

NOTICE TO THE READER

The Publisher has taken reasonable care in the preparation of this book, but makes no expressed or implied warranty of any kind and assumes no responsibility for any errors or omissions. No liability is assumed for incidental or consequential damages in connection with or arising out of information contained in this book. The Publisher shall not be liable for any special, consequential, or exemplary damages resulting, in whole or in part, from the readers' use of, or reliance upon, this material. Any parts of this book based on government reports are so indicated and copyright is claimed for those parts to the extent applicable to compilations of such works.

Independent verification should be sought for any data, advice or recommendations contained in this book. In addition, no responsibility is assumed by the Publisher for any injury and/or damage to persons or property arising from any methods, products, instructions, ideas or otherwise contained in this publication.

This publication is designed to provide accurate and authoritative information with regard to the subject matter covered herein. It is sold with the clear understanding that the Publisher is not engaged in rendering legal or any other professional services. If legal or any other expert assistance is required, the services of a competent person should be sought. FROM A DECLARATION OF PARTICIPANTS JOINTLY ADOPTED BY A COMMITTEE OF THE AMERICAN BAR ASSOCIATION AND A COMMITTEE OF PUBLISHERS.

Additional color graphics may be available in the e-book version of this book.

Library of Congress Cataloging-in-Publication Data

ISBN: 978-1-53615-048-3

Published by Nova Science Publishers, Inc. † New York

CONTENTS

Preface		ix
Section 1. Pathophysiology of Sensorineural Hearing Loss		1
Chapter 1	Anatomy and Physiology of the Peripheral and Central Auditory System *Fabio Bucchieri, Fabio Carletti, Sabrina David, Francesco Cappello, Giuseppe Ferraro and Pierangelo Sardo*	3
Chapter 2	Genetics in Sensorineural Hearing Loss *Alessandro Castiglione*	25
Chapter 3	Congenital Sensorineural Hearing Loss *Sara Ghiselli, Bruno Galletti, Francesco Freni, Rocco Bruno and Francesco Galletti*	37
Chapter 4	Neuroplasticity and Sensorineural Hearing Loss *Francesco Dispenza, Alessia Maria Battaglia, Gabriele Ebbreo, Alessia Ceraso, Vito Pontillo and Antonina Mistretta*	55
Chapter 5	Neuroradiology of the Hearing System *Cesare Gagliardo, Silvia Piccinini and Paola Feraco*	67
Section 2. Sensorineural Hearing Loss: Pathology		145
Chapter 6	Age-Related Hearing Loss *Rocco Bruno, Bruno Galletti, Pietro Abita, Giuseppe Impalà, Francesco Freni and Francesco Galletti*	147
Chapter 7	Traumatic Sensorineural Hearing Loss *Michele Cassano, Valeria Tarantini, Eleonora M. C. Trecca, Antonio Moffa and Gianluigi Grilli*	169

Chapter 8	Advanced Otosclerosis Nicola Quaranta, Vito Pontillo and Francesco Dispenza	189
Chapter 9	Sudden Sensorineural Hearing Loss Valerio Giustino, Francesco Lorusso, Serena Rizzo, Pietro Salvago and Francesco Martines	207
Chapter 10	Cause, Pathogenesis, Clinical Manifestations and Treatment of Meniere's Disease and Endolymphatic Hydrops Sergio Ferrara and Francesco Dispenza	217
Chapter 11	Autoimmune Inner Ear Disease Francesco Dispenza, Alessia Ceraso, Antonina Mistretta, Gabriele Ebbreo, Francesco Barbara and Alessia Maria Battaglia	233
Chapter 12	Occupational Hearing Loss Giampietro Ricci, Egisto Molini, Mario Faralli, Lucia Calzolaro and Luca D'Ascanio	251
Chapter 13	Single Side Deafness in Children Antonio della Volpe, Arianna Di Stadio, Antonietta De Lucia, Valentina Ippolito and Vincenzo Pastore	267
Section 3. Treatment of Sensorineural Hearing Loss		**279**
Chapter 14	Pharmacological Treatment of Sensorineural Hearing Loss Angela Cavallaro, Carla Cannizzaro, Francesco Martines, Gianluca Lavanco, Pietro Salvago, Fabiana Plescia, Anna Brancato and Fulvio Plescia	281
Chapter 15	Management of Sensorineural Hearing Loss with Hearing Aids Pasquale Marsella, Alessandro Scorpecci and Sara Giannantonio	299
Chapter 16	Cochlear Implant of SNHL Patients Pasquale Marsella, Sara Giannantonio and Alessandro Scorpecci	311
Chapter 17	Presbyastasis: From Diagnosis to Management Serena Rizzo, Valeria Sanfilippo, Pietro Terrana, Lorenza Lauricella, Dalila Scaturro, Francesco Martines and Giulia Letizia Mauro	355

Editors' Contact Information   **365**

Index   **367**

Related Nova Publications   **373**

Preface

Hearing loss is one the commonest disabling disease affecting worldwide the population of all age. The impairment of hearing may be the cause of retard of language development in children, the cause of scholar issues in adolescent, the cause of worsening in quality of life in the adults, and the cause of isolation of aged people. In our opinion the knowledge of genetics and congenital disorders is mandatory for those physician that work in the field of hearing disorders, for this reason a section was dedicated to genetics in hearing loss.

In this book we present the hearing loss in all its facets, starting from the basis of pathophysiology and anatomy, passing through the clinical and instrumental diagnosis and, finally, describing the most important diseases causing hearing loss with a reasoned treatment options. A section was dedicated to the imaging of the ear that often helps the clinicians to reach a correct diagnosis and lead the surgeon to the best treatment option.

The prompt identification of patients with hearing loss is the key of management of that disease, in all kind of presentations; consequently it is necessary that the physician (specialist or not) must keep in mind the most important features of the hearing impairment to address the patients to the most appropriate treatment. All the pathology leading to hearing loss were described in a section in which the readers will find all information needed to make diagnosis and therapy.

The treatment of the hearing loss is continuously evolving with the progress of technology and we gave a wide space to describe all treatment options available for the patients and providing all information useful to manage correctly the hearing diseases.

We thank all contributors of this Edited Book for their competence and professional work.

Francesco Dispenza, MD, PhD
Francesco Martines, MD, PhD

Section 1. Pathophysiology of Sensorineural Hearing Loss

In: Sensorineural Hearing Loss
Editors: F. Dispenza and F. Martines

ISBN: 978-1-53615-048-3
© 2019 Nova Science Publishers, Inc.

Chapter 1

ANATOMY AND PHYSIOLOGY OF THE PERIPHERAL AND CENTRAL AUDITORY SYSTEM

Fabio Bucchieri, Fabio Carletti, Sabrina David[*],
Francesco Cappello, Giuseppe Ferraro and Pierangelo Sardo

Department of Experimental Biomedicine and Clinical Neuroscience,
University of Palermo, Palermo, Italy

ABSTRACT

The auditory system is responsible for the hearing sense and it consists of the peripheral auditory system (outer, middle and inner ear) and of the central auditory system (vestibular and cochlear nuclei, auditory and vestibular pathways and vestibular and auditory cortices). The outer ear comprises the auricle and the auditory canal and its function is to guide air pressure waves to the middle ear. The middle ear consists of the tympanic membrane, connected to the inner ear by three ossicles (malleus, incus and stapes), which vibrations allow the transmission of originally airborne sound waves to the perilymph of the inner ear. The middle ear provides a pressure gain as well as enhanced quality of the sound waves transmitted to the inner ear and protects it from high pressure levels produced by loud sounds. The stapes footplate of the middle ear connects to the oval window of the cochlea, an inner ear spiral-shaped bony canal. The stapes of the middle ear connects to the oval window in the cochlea. The vibrations of a flexible membrane (basilar membrane) on which sensory cells (hair cells) reside are responsible for the transduction of the sound waves into electrical impulses.

The vestibulocochlear nerve (CN VIII) transmits both hearing and balance information from the inner ear to the brain. The vestibular (balance) and cochlear (hearing) components of the vestibulocochlear nerve target different nuclei. The vestibular component reaches the vestibular nuclei in the pons and medulla oblongata. The cochlear component instead reaches the ventral and dorsal cochlear nuclei, located

---

[*] Corresponding Author's Email: sabrina.david@unipa.it.

laterally at the junction between the pons and medulla, in close proximity to the inferior cerebellar peduncle. CN VIII emerges from the brainstem at the cerebellopontine angle and exits the posterior cranial fossa of the neurocranium through the internal acoustic meatus of the temporal bone. Here the vestibulocochlear nerve splits, thus forming the vestibular nerve and the cochlear nerve. The vestibular nerve innervates the vestibular system of the inner ear, which is responsible for detecting balance. The cochlear nerve travels to the cochlea, forming the spiral ganglia of Corti, involved in the sense of hearing.

The hearing pathway originates in the cochlear nuclei which receive first-order auditory input from the organ of Corti in the cochlea. The second neuron of this pathway is located in the superior olivary nuclei of the pons where the majority of the auditory fibers synapse, crossing the midline. The fibers ascend, forming the lateral lemnisc and proceed towards the inferior colliculus in the mesencephalus. The last relay, prior to the primary auditory cortex, occurs in the medial geniculate body of the thalamus. A tonotopic organization is evident throughout the hearing pathway, from cochlea to auditory cortices.

In the balance pathway, neurons synapsing on the hair cells of maculae and cristae ampullares of the semicircular canals converge in the vestibular ganglion. The sensory fibers originating from here join the sensory fibers from the cochlear ganglion to form the vestibulocochlear nerve and terminate in the vestibular nuclei of the pons and medulla. The axons originated in these nuclei reach different areas of Central Nervous System (CNS), such as the spinal cord, the cerebral cortex, the cerebellum and the nuclei controlling extrinsic eyes muscles. The vestibular nuclei also receive input from proprioceptive neurons, as well as the visual system.

1. INTRODUCTION

1.1. Anatomical Bases of Hearing: An Overview

In this paragraph, we describe briefly the main anatomical structures involved in hearing, i.e., the ear, the vestibulocochlear nerve, the cochlear nuclei and the auditory cortex.

1.2. The Ear

From an anatomical point of view, the ear consists in three parts; the external, the middle and the internal ear. In the next paragraph, the morphology of each part will be briefly summarized.

External Ear

The external ear includes the auricle (pinna) and the external auditory canal (meatus). The *auricle* is composed of a thin plate of elastic cartilage, covered by a layer of skin. It is attached in place by ligaments, and has two groups of muscles, extrinsic and intrinsic ones. There is a deep depression (concha) that leads into the external auditory meatus and is covered by two small protrusions: the tragus, in front, and the antitragus, behind. The funnel-like curves of the auricle collect sound waves and direct them toward the middle ear.

The *external auditory meatus* is a slightly curved canal, about 2.5 cm in length, that extends from the floor of the concha to the tympanic membrane. The meatus contains two types of glands: sebaceous glands and ceruminous glands (modified sweat glands that secrete cerumen).

Between the external and the middle ear there is the *tympanic membrane*. It is a membranous structure located on the medial part of the auditory meatus. The tympanic membrane is comprised of three layers of tissue: an outer cutaneous layer, a fibrous middle layer, and a layer of mucous membrane on its innermost surface. The membrane is held in place by a thick ring of cartilage. It has the capacity to vibrate and to receive sound waves that are amplified to an appropriate magnitude. The membrane vibrates as the sound waves strike it, and transmits the vibrations towards the small bones of the middle ear.

Middle Ear

The middle ear, or tympanic cavity, is connected to the epitympanic recess, the antrum and the cells within the mastoid portion of the temporal bone. Medially, the auditory (or Eustachian) tube links the tympanic cavity with the nasopharynx. The tympanic cavity is an air-filled space, covered by a columnar epithelium, that contains 3 tiny bones (known as *ossicles*), called the malleus (hammer), incus and stapes (stirrup). Sound waves that reach the tympanic membrane cause it to vibrate. This vibration is then transmitted to the ossicles, which amplify the sound and pass the vibration to the oval window (a thin membrane between the middle and the inner ear). Hammer and stirrup movements are limited by two small muscles, the tensor tympani and the stapedius, respectively.

Inner Ear

The inner ear consists of 1) the otic labyrinth (membranous labyrinth), 2) the periotic labyrinth (osseous labyrinth), and 3) the otic capsule (part of the petrous portion of the temporal bone which surrounds the internal ear).

The *otic labyrinth* is a closed system of endolymph-filled ducts and sacs contained within the inner ear. It has the same general shape as the osseous labyrinth and consists of structures surrounded by perilymph.

In particular, it includes the cochlea, which is involved in hearing, and the vestibular system (consisting of three semicircular canals, as well as a saccule and an utricle), which is responsible for maintaining balance. The cochlea is filled with fluid and contains the organ of Corti — a structure that contains thousands of specialized sensory hair cells with projections called cilia. The vibrations transmitted from the middle ear produce tiny waves which make the cilia vibrate. The hair cells then convert these vibrations into nerve impulses, or signals, which are sent to the brain via the auditory nerve.

The semicircular canals also contain fluid and hair cells, but these hair cells are responsible for detecting movement rather than sound. When you move your head, the fluid within the semicircular canals (which are oriented vertically at right angles to each other) also moves. This fluid motion is detected by the hair cells, which send nerve impulses about the position of the head and body to the brain to allow maintaining the balance.

The utricle and the saccule work in a similar way to the semicircular canals, providing information on the body position in relation to gravity, allowing postural adjustments as required.

The *periotic labyrinth* consists in the vestibule, the periotic semicircular canals, the scala vestibule and the scala tympani. The vestibule is the largest portion of the periotic labyrinth. It surrounds the utriculus and the sacculus. The periotic semicircular canals surround the otic semicircular ducts. They contain a great amount of periotic trabecular tissue. The scala vestibule or vestibular duct is a perilymph-filled cavity inside the cochlea of the inner ear that conducts sound vibrations to the cochlear duct. It is separated from the cochlear duct by Reissner's membrane and extends from the vestibule of the ear to the helicotrema, where it joins the tympanic duct.

The tympanic duct or scala tympani is one of the perilymph-filled cavities separated from the cochlear duct by the basilar membrane, and it extends from the round window to the helicotrema, where it continues as the vestibular duct.

The purpose of the perilymph-filled tympanic duct and vestibular duct is to transduce the movement of air that permits to the tympanic membrane and the ossicles to vibrate, into a movement of the liquid and of the basilar membrane. The latter stimulates the organ of Corti inside the cochlear duct, composed of hair cells attached to the basilar membrane and their stereocilia embedded in the tectorial membrane. Indeed, the organ of Corti is located in the scala media of the cochlea, between the vestibular duct and the tympanic duct and is composed of mechanosensory cells, known as hair cells. These cells lie on the basilar membrane of the organ of Corti and are organized in three rows of outer hair cells (OHCs) and one row of inner hair cells (IHCs). These hair cells are supported by Deiters' cells, also called phalangeal cells. Above them is the tectoral membrane which moves in response to pressure variations in the fluid-filled tympanic and vestibular canals. The movement of the basilar membrane in relation to the tectorial membrane causes the stereocilia to bend. They then depolarize and send impulses to the brain via the cochlear nerve. This produces the sensation of sound.

The *otic capsule* is the portion of the petrous part on the temporal bone which surrounds the internal ear, derived from the embryotic mesenchyme which surrounded the early otic vescicle. A part of this mesenchymal tissue passes through the precartilaginous and cartilaginous stages prior to ossification. Therefore, the bony otic capsule is known as cartilage bone.

1.3. The Vestibulocochlear Nerve

The vestibulocochlear nerve (CN VIII) transmits both hearing and balance information from the inner ear to the brain. It consists mostly of bipolar neurons and forms two branches: the cochlear nerve and the vestibular nerve.

The vestibulocochlear nerve reaches the middle portion of the brainstem called the pons (which also contains fibers leading to the cerebellum). It runs between the base of the pons (and medulla oblongata, the lower portion of the brainstem) in the cerebellopontine angle. The vestibulocochlear nerve is accompanied by the labyrinthine artery, which usually branches off from the anterior inferior cerebellar artery (AICA) and then continues along the VIII nerve through the internal acoustic meatus to the internal ear.

The cochlear nerve, responsible of hearing, travels away from the cochlea of the inner ear where it starts as the spiral ganglion of the organ of Corti. The inner hair cells of the organ of Corti are responsible for the activation of afferent receptors in response to pressure waves reaching the basilar membrane through sound transduction.

The vestibular nerve originates from the vestibular system of the inner ear. The vestibular ganglion (Scarpa's ganglion) extends processes to five sensory organs. Three of these are the cristae located in the ampullae of the semicircular canals. Hair cells of the cristae activate afferent receptors in response to rotational acceleration. The other two sensory organs are the maculae of the saccule and the utricle. Hair cells of the maculae in the utricle activate afferent receptors in response to linear acceleration, while hair cells of the maculae in the saccule respond to vertically directed linear force.

CN VIII emerges from the brainstem at the cerebellopontine angle and exits the posterior cranial fossa of the neurocranium through the internal acoustic meatus of the temporal bone. Here the vestibulocochlear nerve splits, thus forming the vestibular nerve and the cochlear nerve.

1.4. The Cochlear Nuclei

The vestibular (balance) and cochlear (hearing) components of the vestibulocochlear nerve target different nuclei. The vestibular component reaches the vestibular nuclei in the pons and medulla oblongata. The cochlear component instead reaches the ventral and dorsal cochlear nuclei, located laterally at the junction between the pons and medulla, near the inferior cerebellar peduncle.

The hearing pathway originates in the cochlear nuclei which receive first-order auditory input from the organ of Corti in the cochlea. The second neuron of this pathway is located in the superior olivary nuclei of the pons where the majority of the auditory fibers synapse, crossing the midline. The fibers ascend, forming the lateral lemnisc, and proceed towards the inferior colliculus in the mesencephalus. The last relay, prior to the primary auditory cortex, occurs in the medial geniculate body of the thalamus.

In the balance pathway, neurons synapsing on the hair cells of the maculae and cristae ampullares of the semicircular canals converge in the vestibular ganglion. The sensory fibers originating here join the sensory fibers from the cochlear ganglion to form the vestibulocochlear nerve, and terminate in the vestibular nuclei of the pons and the medulla. The axons originated in these nuclei reach different areas of the Central Nervous System (CNS), spinal cord, the cerebellum, the nuclei controlling extrinsic eyes muscles, thalamus, and the cerebral cortex.

1.5. The Auditory Cortex

The human auditory cortex is the part of the temporal lobe that processes auditory information.

It is located bilaterally, at the upper sides of the temporal lobes, on the superior temporal plane, within the lateral fissure and comprises parts of Heschl's gyrus and the superior temporal gyrus.

The auditory cortex was previously subdivided into primary and secondary projection areas and further association areas. The primary auditory cortex (AI) is situated in the posterior third of the superior temporal gyrus (also known as Brodmann area 41), next to Wernicke's area. The secondary auditory cortex (AII) is located more rostrally in the temporal lobe and contains Brodmann area 42. The modern divisions of the auditory cortex are the core (which includes AI), the belt, and the parabelt. The belt is the area immediately surrounding the core; the parabelt is adjacent to the lateral side of the belt. These latest areas help to integrate hearing with other sensory systems.

Studies indicate that auditory fields of the primary auditory cortex (AI) receive ascending input from the auditory thalamus, and point-to-point input from the ventral division of the medial geniculate complex; thus, it contains a precise tonotopic map. The primary auditory cortex (AI) has a topographical map of the cochlea.

Neurons in the auditory cortex are organized according to the frequency of sound to which they respond best. Neurons at one end of the auditory cortex respond best to low frequencies; neurons at the other respond best to high frequencies.

Studies have revealed the presence of six cell layers. The pyramidal cells correspond to 85% of AI. The remaining 15% are multipolar or stellate cells. Inverted stellate cells also exist (Martinotti cells), as well as cells with candelabra-shaped dendritic configurations. Most ascending fibers originate in synapse with the pyramidal cells of layer IV, but this is not always the case. However, these contacts represent only 20% of the excitatory fibers that project to cortical neurons: the other 80% comes from other neurons in the ipsilateral cortex.

The primary auditory cortex is subject to modulation by numerous neurotransmitters, including norepinephrine, which has been shown to decrease cellular excitability in all layers of the temporal cortex. Alpha-1 adrenergic receptor activation, by norepinephrine, decreases glutamatergic excitatory postsynaptic potentials at AMPA receptors.

2. PHYSIOLOGY OF THE AUDITORY SYSTEM

The auditory system detects sounds and uses acoustic cues to both identify them and locate their origin in the environment. The perceptual phenomenon called *sound* is produced in the brain by stimulating the ear with periodic longitudinal waves of alternating low and high pressure (rarefactions and compressions, respectively). These waves propagate at different speed depending on the properties of the elastic medium through which they travel (330 - 340 m/s through air). The absolute intensity of sound, measured in pascals (Pa), is related to the amplitude of the longitudinal wave; however, the intensity of audible sounds is usually measured in decibel sound pressure level (dB SPL): this logarithmic scale relates the absolute sound intensity (*PT*) to a 20 µPa reference pressure (*Pref*), roughly corresponding to the average human threshold at 2000 Hz. Due to its logarithmic nature, in this scale intensities of sounds are compressed, in such a way that a tenfold increase in absolute sound intensity just corresponds to a 20 dB SPL increase.

$$\text{dB SPL} = 10 \times \log_{10} \frac{(P_T)^2}{(P_{ref})^2} = 20 \times \log_{10} \frac{P_T}{P_{ref}}$$

Sounds with amplitudes from 0 to 120 dB SPL can be comfortably heard, whereas higher sound pressure levels cause pain and can damage the ear. Acoustic waves have typically an amplitude of about 60 dB in a normal conversation.

The subjective experience of tonal discrimination (*pitch*) of a sound depends on wave frequency, measured in hertz (Hz, waves per second). Humans can hear sounds in the frequency interval from ~20 to 20,000 Hz; perception of speech encompasses frequencies between 60 and 12,000 Hz.

On the basis of both temporal pattern and regularity of acoustic waves we can distinguish pure tones (characterized by a single frequency), sounds (characterized by a perceived fundamental frequency, or *pitch*, and overtones) or noises, with no recognizable periodic elements.

Sounds characterized by the same SPL but different frequencies are not perceived as equally loud; these differences in perception are accounted for by the phon scale, developed by adjusting the intensities of test tones to be equal in loudness to reference tones of 1000 Hz (normal hearing threshold is ~4 phon, whereas discomfort and pain are perceived at 110 and 130 phon, respectively).

2.1. Outer and Middle Ear Actions: Funneling and Conduction of Sound

The auditory system is specialized to discriminate frequency, amplitude, and direction of acoustic waves, as well as to interpret temporal patterns of sound amplitude and frequency of words and music.

In the outer ear the pinna and the tragus together funnel sound waves into the external auditory canal, focusing sound waves on the tympanic membrane (or eardrum). Depending on the angle of incidence, the same sound is reflected differently off the pinna and tragus: on this basis, these structures are able to emphasize some sound frequencies over others, inducing peaks and *notches* in the sound spectrum. The positions of peaks and notches depend on (and provide information about) location of the sound source, even when using only one ear (monaural sound localization); such information is important for localizing sounds in the vertical plane (elevation). Then, each heard sound is a combination of both a direct component and a reflected one (by pinna and tragus), and causes the tympanic membrane to vibrate.

The middle ear, represented by the air-filled chamber between the tympanic membrane on one side and the oval window on the other, ensures efficient transmission of sound from air into the fluid-filled inner ear, by transferring vibrations of the tympanic membrane to the oval window through a chain of three delicate bones called ossicles: the malleus (or hammer), incus (anvil), and stapes (stirrup). Since water is highly incompressible and dense, it has very higher acoustic impedance (defined as the ratio of sound pressure to volume velocity) than air (about 10,000 times higher) and sound traveling directly from air to water has insufficient pressure to move the dense water molecules: then, transferring sound vibrations from air to cochlear fluid needs an *impedance-matching device* that saves most of sound's energy, which would be otherwise largely (>97%) reflected back to air when encountering a watery medium exerting a stronger opposition to movement brought about by a pressure wave. Impedance matching, and successful transferring of most energy to inner ear fluids, is obtained through amplification (gain of about 25 to 30 dB in the middle frequencies), due to both a larger area of eardrum than the footplate of the stapes (~ 20:1 ratio) and, to a lesser extent, a lever action exerted by malleus and incus, increasing the pressure applied to the footplate (the combined action of eardrum/footplate ratio and ossicles lever causes a ~ 55 times pressure increase over the oval window). For lower and higher frequencies, however, more energy is lost. Equalization of air pressure on opposite sides of the tympanic membrane is realized through the eustachian tube, which connects the middle ear to the nasopharynx.

2.2. Inner Ear Function: Transduction of Sound

Movements of the stapes against the oval window create traveling pressure waves within the cochlear fluids. Each movement of the oval window induce changes in pressure of scala vestibuli (inward = increase, outward = decrease) and opposite movements of round window and changes in scala tympani. The different pressure between scala tympani and scala vestibuli causes the basilar membrane (and the organ of Corti) to bow upward (when pressure in scala vestibuli > scala tympani) or downward.

The contraction of muscles of the middle ear, tensor tympani (inserted onto the malleus) and the stapedius (inserted onto the stapes), reflexively activated by high sound levels, dampen the transfer of sound to the inner ear by controlling the stiffness of the ossicular chain, in this way exerting a protective action and a suppression of self-produced sounds (e.g., voice, chewing).

Sound frequency and amplitude are encoded in the cochlea and further analyzed in the CNS. In fact, the cochlea performs as a spectral analyzer, evaluating complex sounds according to their pure tonal components, in such a way that each pure tone stimulates a specific region; in fact, different regions of the basilar membrane are tuned to particular frequencies. The *frequency* of the sound determines which region of basilar membrane vibrates most along the cochlea, high frequencies generating maximal vibrations in the basal region, whereas lower frequencies generate their maximal amplitudes near the cochlear apex, thus determining which hair cells of the organ of Corti are stimulated. In the auditory system, a *place coding* is based on this selectivity. Such low-apical to high-basal gradient of resonance is underlain by mechanical characteristics (stiffness and taper) of the basilar membrane. In fact, whereas the cochlea tapers from base to apex, the basilar membrane tapers in the opposite direction, being wider at the apex; moreover, the narrow basal end is stiffer (~100 times) than the apical end. However, the intrinsic frequency selectivity afforded by basilar membrane tuning is not great enough to account for the very selective responses observed in hair cells and auditory nerve fibers; in fact, active mechanisms are necessary to achieve this high frequency selectivity (see below).

2.3. Hair Cells Functions

The vibration of basilar membrane is transduced by hair cells of organ of Corti, mechanoreceptors specialized to detect very small movement along one particular axis, located at the junction between endolymph and perilymph; these polarized epithelial cells are characterized by an apical end specialized to transduce mechanical energy into receptor currents, whereas the basal end is in contact with perilymph and synaptically drives the activity of primary afferent neurons of the acoustic nerve (Hudspeth and Corey, 1977). In the apical end, the stereovilli of *inner* hair cells float freely in the endolymph, whereas the stereovilli of the *outer* hair cells project into the cantilevered tectorial membrane, free to tilt up and down since it is attached only along one edge. Inner hair cells transduce mechanical energy of sound into electrical energy, whereas the active movements of outer hair cells modulate the amplification of the signal. Due to a K^+ gradient, auditory endolymph has a positive voltage relative to the perilymph (+80 to + 90 mV), being this endocochlear potential the driving force for sensory transduction in both inner and outer auditory hair cells. The composition of endolymph increases the K^+ transduction current flowing from endolymph into the hair cells, due to both the concentration gradient and the large electrical gradient. Once a sound stimulates the cochlea, K^+ flows into the hair cells with little energy expenditure by the hair cells, as K^+ is flowing down its electrochemical gradient; that is why hair cells do not require a high blood flow, that would bring noise and interfere with sound reception.

In hair cells, receptor potentials are evoked by mechanically gated ion channels: in fact, specialized elastic filaments called *tip links* (or *gating springs*) are present at the tips of stereocilia, mechanically attaching (like a spring) the top of each stereocilium to the upper side of the adjacent taller one, in line with the axis of maximal bundle sensitivity (Brownell et al, 1985; Pickles et al, 1984). Destruction of the tip links by enzymatic (elastase) or chemical (calcium chelators) treatments can abolish mechanical transduction. Deflection of stereocilia in the excitatory direction stretches the tip links and increases their tension, in this way pulling on the channel gate and increasing the probability of channel opening. Deflection in the opposite direction release the tip link and let the channels close. Maximum compliance of stereocilia bundle occurs when roughly half the transduction channels are open. As a consequence of direct gating of transduction channels, hair cell transduction occurs much faster than in other sensory modalities: the delay between bundle deflection and the onset of receptor current is about 10 ms at 37°C, being such speed essential in order to detect sound frequencies in auditory range of Humans.

When the hair bundle is in resting position a standing inward cations (mainly potassium and small amount of calcium) current flows through 15-20% of mechanically activated channels, located near the tips of the stereocilia (one or two channels per stereocilium), and this inward positive current tends to depolarize the hair cells. Maximal transducer conductance changes up to about 10 nS have been observed. The proportion of open channels, and consequently the inward current, are increased when the hair bundle is displaced toward the tallest stereocilium; the current flowing across the basolateral membrane depolarizes the membrane, activating some voltage-dependent conductances.

On the contrary, movement of the stereocilia bundle away from the tallest stereocilium hyperpolarizes the basolateral membrane of hair cells by reducing the inward current: remarkably, displacements in depolarizing direction produce larger responses than equal deflections in the opposite direction, describing a sigmoidal displacement–response function, shifted from its midpoint; because of such relationship, changes in membrane potential due to acoustic stimuli inducing symmetrical sinusoidal deflections of the bundle will produce both sinusoidal (AC) and superimposed depolarizing steady-state (DC) changes, the system being saturated by 300 nm deflections.

It must be noted that, whereas receptor currents are induced without attenuation across frequency, receptor potentials are susceptible to filter characteristics of the basolateral membrane depending on the time constant, ranging from sub- millisecond to a few milliseconds duration at the resting potential; this passive property lets the membrane act as a low-pass filter with a dynamic cutoff frequency ranging from tens of hertz to about 1 kHz. Furthermore, receptor potentials may activate voltage-dependent channels in the basolateral membrane, in this way modifying the resistive component of the time constant. Moreover, the capacitance of the basolateral membrane is also highly voltage dependent in outer hair cells: in these cells the membrane filter could therefore be influenced by changes in both resistive and capacitive components. Due to the filtering of the basolateral membrane, the AC component of receptor potential is halved for every octave increase in frequency above the cutoff, becoming negligible at very high frequencies; on the contrary, the DC component of receptor potential is not affected (this effect is called *rectification*). A fundamental difference is observed between main responses to electrical changes in inner versus outer hair cells: inner cells modify the amount of neurotransmitter released at the level of synapses with afferent neurons, outer cells change their length and thereby amplify the movement of the basilar membrane.

In the inner hair cells synapse, the release of neurotransmitter depends on membrane receptor potential. In resting position the depolarizing inward cation current induces a basal neurotransmitter release: further depolarization increases the number of released vesicles, whereas hyperpolarization decreases it.

On the other side, outer hair cells express an integral membrane motor protein termed prestin along their lateral wall and are able to respond to electrical stimulation by altering their length in a voltage dependent manner: depolarization shortens the cell, whereas hyperpolarization induces elongations (Liberman et al, 2002; Zheng et al, 2000). When basilar membrane moves upward, a shear force between stereocilia of outer hair cells and the tectorial membrane develops, forcing hair bundles to tilt toward longer stereocilia: this movement opens transduction channels in outer hair cells, through which K^+ flows inward, further depolarizing the cells (the voltage change is termed receptor potential). This process is called mechanical to electrical transduction, and the consequent depolarization contracts the motor protein prestin, a member of the SLC26 family, which outer cells express at very high levels: the contraction of reciprocally linked prestin molecules shorten the outer cells (the process is called electromotility or electrical to mechanical transduction). This voltage dependent mechanical response, only limited to outer hair cells, is not evoked by activation of voltage-dependent ionic conductance.

On the contrary, *downward* movements of the basilar membrane induce hyperpolarization of outer cells and their elongation. This motor activity is restricted to the lateral membrane of the outer cell. Length changes up to 5% are observed: they are not dependent on ATP, microtubule or actin systems, extracellular Ca^{2+}, or changes in cell volume. The maximum sensitivity of the response is about 30 nm/mV, observed at a depolarized voltage with respect to the resting potential of the cell. This motor activity is maintained and modulated through the intervention of a stretch-activated chloride conductance, and intracellular chloride is required for the activity of the voltage sensor. *In vivo*, the motor action of outer hair cells is probably responsible for otoacoustic emissions.

Remarkably, the voltage-dependent mechanical response of outer cells could be influenced by the time constant of the cell, mainly because transmembrane AC receptor potentials will be greatly attenuated at high frequencies: this effect could theoretically limit the motor response, if this is only driven by receptor potential. Nonetheless, some mechanisms let the inner ear overcome the limiting effects of the membrane filter encountered for acoustic stimulation at high frequency: in fact, a role of a mechanically activated flux of chloride through the lateral plasma membrane is evident in the function of prestin *in vivo* (Rybalchenko et al, 2003), which could underlie a voltage independence; moreover, active mechanical responses of the stereocilia bundle may be driven by calcium influx through mechanically activated calcium-sensitive channels, not limited by the membrane filter. The motor properties make the outer hair cells act as a cochlear amplifier: acting as both receptors and effectors, they are able to sense and enhance movements of the basilar membrane; in fact, contraction of outer hair cells enhances upward movement, whereas hair cell *elongation* accentuates the *downward* movement of the basilar membrane. Therefore, outer hair cells electromotility is necessary for sensitive hearing and sharp frequency discrimination. Hearing sensitivity and frequency selectivity are impaired by mutation of the gene for prestin or if outer cells are damaged (e.g., by some antibiotics) or absent.

The mechanical events originated in outer hair cells boost basilar membrane movements and enhance stimulus to the inner hair cells. The amplified upward movement of the basilar membrane forces endolymph to flow out from beneath the tectorial membrane, toward its tip; this flow causes the hair bundles of the inner hair cells to bend toward longer stereovilli, consequently opening transduction channels and depolarizing the cell. This depolarization opens voltage-gated Ca2+ channels, and the consequent rise of $[Ca^{2+}]_i$ induces synaptic vesicles fusion and glutamate release, depolarizing afferent neurons.

When the stapes moves inward, all described processes reverse as well: the basilar membrane bows downward, transduction channels close in the outer hair cells, which undergo *hyperpolarization* and cell elongation, accentuating downward movement of the basilar membrane which recalls endolymph back under the tectorial membrane; in this manner transduction channels close in inner hair cells, causing cell hyperpolarization and reduced neurotransmitter release.

3. ROLE OF NERVOUS SYSTEM

3.1. Auditory Nerve

The cochlea receives innervation from the auditory (or cochlear) nerve, a branch of cranial nerve VIII (Ruggero, 1982). Sensory cells somata (about 30,000) are found in the spiral ganglion and their dendrites contact nearby hair cells: 95% of neurons, termed type I cells, contact inner hair cells; the remainder afferent neurons, named type II, innervate the outer hair cells, which represent over three-quarters of the receptor cell population. The axons of afferent neurons project to the brainstem cochlear nucleus. A type I neuron generally contacts a single hair cell through a myelinated large and fast conducting fiber, thus their information reaches the brain within a few tenths of a millisecond; type II neurons, instead, sends processes to contact 5 to 100 outer hair cell by thin, unmyelinated and slow conducting fibers. Both afferent fiber types project centrally into the cochlear nucleus in the brain stem: inner hair cells and type I neurons are the main channel for sound-evoked information to reach the hierarchically upper structures in the brainstem, whereas outer hair cells contribute very little direct information about sound.

The stimulation with a continuous pure tone originates a wave which, travelling along the basilar membrane, has different amplitudes at different points along the base-apex axis. Hair cells are tuned to a certain frequency: their frequency sensitivity (or characteristic frequency) depends on their position along the basilar membrane of the cochlea, due either to the above-described features of the basilar membrane, or to position-related structural differences between inner hair cells, enhancing the tuning. In fact, the ones near the base have shorter, stiffer stereovilli, which let them resonate to higher frequencies; on the contrary, the cells near the apex display longer and floppier stereovilli which make them resonate to lower frequencies; this position-based frequency selectivity of inner cells clearly describe a place coding of frequency. Aside, increases in sound *amplitude* cause an increase in the *rate* of action potentials in auditory nerve axons: then, sound intensity undergoes a rate coding at neuronal level, cooperation between neurons being required in order to code the full SPL range (0 to 120 dB SPL). The characteristic frequency of an acoustic nerve fiber is the frequency that evokes a response at the lowest sound pressure level, as low as 0 dB in the most sensitive range of hearing. The tuning curve, plotting the response area for a nerve fiber a graph of threshold sound pressure level vs. frequency, is extremely narrow at low sound levels, since the fiber responds only to a narrow band of frequencies near characteristic frequency, property likely linked to the active motility of the outer hair cells. The tuning curve is wider at high sound levels, in particular for frequencies below the characteristic frequency, likely reflecting most the passive mechanical characteristics of basilar membrane motion than outer hair cells electromotility. Fibers with the lowest characteristic frequencies innervate hair cells positioned at the cochlear apex, whereas fibers with higher characteristic frequencies contact hair cells located in progressively more basal regions, paralleling the pattern of basilar membrane vibration. This tonotopic mapping is preserved in the cochlear nucleus and along the central auditory pathway. Therefore, type I fibers respond to sound generating action potentials, often locked to particular phases within the cycle of the sound waveform following the phasic release of neurotransmitter depending by the AC receptor potential; both phase locking and AC receptor potential decrease for frequencies above 1 kHz.

Action potentials are then conducted toward the brain via discrete pathways which form a percept of the stimulus by extracting information about which nerve fibers are responding (place code, about frequency of sound, whereby neurons at different places code for different frequencies) and the rate and time pattern of the spikes in each fiber (information about sound intensity). Auditory nerve fibers with the same characteristic frequency show different sensitivity to sound intensity, and the difference between lower and higher thresholds can be as large as 70 dB. The sensitivity of response (SR) is correlated with the spontaneous firing rate of neurons, varying from one fiber to another over the range of 0 to 100 spikes/s. Three main groups of fibers have been classified on the basis of spontaneous firing: low SR (0.5 spikes/s), medium SR (0.5 to 17.5 spikes/s), high SR (17.5 spikes/s), the latter exhibiting higher sensitivities than the others. Low SR fibers play important roles in detecting changes in sounds at high intensities, because of both their low sensitivity, which causes them to respond mostly at high sound levels, and their lesser tendency to saturate. Information carried by the different SR groups may be kept somewhat separate in the brain stem: for example, low and medium SR fibers represent the largest afferents to the cochlear nucleus, preferentially innervating certain regions.

The response of a single auditory nerve fiber increases with sound level until it is saturated, that is to say the fiber no longer increases its firing rate. This mostly occurs within a dynamic range generally between 20 and 30 dB, sometimes greater. Such a narrow individual dynamic range does not match the large range in level of audible sound, from 0 to 100 dB. The auditory nerve can accurately signal within this large intensity range because fibers with the same characteristic frequency but lower sensitivity are recruited at higher sound levels, when fibers tuned to other characteristic frequencies also begin to respond, since tuning curves become broader.

3.2. Descending Control on Inner Ear

The superior olivary complex of the brainstem projects fibers to the inner ear; in particular, lateral olivo-cochlear neurons, the function of which is not well known, contact dendrites of type I auditory nerve fibers through small diameter axons, whereas medial olivo-cochlear neurons project to outer hair cells through cholinergic fibers (Guinan, 1996; Warr, 1992).

Acetylcholine activates a nicotinic receptor on the membrane of the outer hair cell, allowing Ca^2 influx and K^+ efflux through Ca^{2-} activated K^+ channels: in this manner the membrane results hyperpolarized, reducing the electromotility of the outer hair cell and the motion of basilar membrane; the responsiveness of inner hair cells and auditory nerve fibers is reduced and results shifted to higher sound levels. Consequently, this mechanism may control the gain of the cochlear amplifier to prevent saturation of responses, inducing suppression of responsiveness to unwanted sounds, protecting hair cells in the cochlea from damage due to intense sounds, and letting the fiber signal changes in sound intensity even at higher sound levels, being also able to underlie auditory focus in noisy environments.

3.3. Central Auditory Pathways

Starting from the cochlear nucleus, the auditory information travels toward the cerebral cortex via the thalamus, relaying in several brainstem nuclei with relevant functions (Rhode and Greenberg 1992). The cochlear nucleus is the best understood among auditory centers, being the region where parallel pathways in the auditory system begin. Cochlear nucleus neurons, excited by auditory nerve inputs, are classified following both morphological and functional criteria (tone burst-evoked firing pattern, map of response, laterality of response). On the basis of the *cellular firing patterns* in response to sound stimulation, cellular units in the cochlear nucleus are classified as "pauser" (pyramidal cells), "onset" ("octopus" cells), "primary-like with notch" (globular bushy cells), "chopper" (multipolar cells) and "primary-like" (spherical bushy cells). Like tuning curves, *response maps* plotted on graphs of sound level versus frequency show areas of excitation; however, they can also show areas of inhibition in the dorsal subdivision of the cochlear nucleus, the inferior colliculus, and at higher stages of the auditory system, since at these levels inhibitory influences are present, shaping responses. Five response types have been defined (types I-V) on this basis: type I responses have no inhibitory areas, the other types have progressively larger inhibitory areas. Type IV neurons correspond to pyramidal cells, the main projection neurons of the dorsal cochlear neuron. *Laterality of response* is defined as whether the neuron responds to the contralateral or ipsilateral ear and whether the response is excitatory or inhibitory. Many neurons in central auditory nuclei above the cochlear nucleus are binaural and can be influenced by sound presented to either ear. A predominant pattern, however, is for the neuron to be excited by sound in the contralateral ear, resulting from the fact that many central auditory pathways cross to the opposite side of the brain. The influence of the ipsilateral ear can be excitatory, inhibitory, or mixed. There are also uncrossed pathways; these pathways generate the response to the ipsilateral ear. Despite an influence of the ipsilateral ear, lesion studies indicate the functional importance of excitation from the contralateral ear. For instance, damage to the inferior colliculus or auditory cortex on one side decreases the ability to localize sounds on the opposite side. Thus, as in other sensory and in motor systems, one side of the brain is concerned primarily with function on the opposite side of the body. An important characteristic of most central auditory nuclei is tonotopic organization, the mapping of neural characteristic frequencies onto position. This feature is determined by basilar membrane features and is relayed into the central nervous system by CN VIII, resulting in regions in which neurons share the same characteristic frequency, called isofrequency laminae.

The cochlear nucleus projects in turn to the other auditory nuclei of the brain stem: superior olivary complex, nuclei of the lateral lemniscus, and inferior colliculus, important for determination of the location of a sound source. In fact, whereas sound frequency is mapped along the cochlea, in contrast to other sensory systems the external location of a sound source is not directly represented in the auditory receptor organ. In the auditory system, directional information is centrally determined, mainly in the brain, by comparing interaural differences in responses.

The location of azimuthal position of sound sources in space is predominantly determined by the auditory system at the brain stem level, by using two main binaural cues, respectively interaural time differences and interaural level differences, differently useful depending on the frequency of the sound (Brand et al, 2002; Wightman and Kistler 1993; Yin and Chan 1990). Regarding the former, sound reaches the ear nearest to the source earlier than the farther one, markedly depending on the azimuth of the source: interaural time differences can be then translated into phase differences in the sound waveforms at the two ears, particularly useful at low frequencies; however, they become less affordable for frequencies >1.5 kHz because the time interval needed for the sound to reach the farther ear could be sufficient for the waveform to repeat by a cycle or multiples. A second reason for differences are less important for localizing sounds at high frequencies is linked to the decline in phase locking for frequencies above 1 to 3 kHz.

Interaural level differences are dependent on the *sound shadow* action exerted by the head, which reduces the level of sound at the ear away from the source. These differences are significantly large only at high frequencies, being much smaller at low frequencies. Thus, interaural time differences are the major cues for sound localization at low frequencies (1 kHz), whereas interaural level differences for localization at high frequencies (3 kHz). The accuracy of azimuthal localization is good at both low and high frequencies, being less accurate at middle frequencies because the cues are more ambiguous in this range. The minimum discriminable angle for localization of a sound source approaches one degree of azimuth, corresponding to about 10 ms in interaural time and 1 dB interaural level differences.

Two neural circuits that provide sensitivity to interaural time or level differences are within the superior olivary complex, respectively found in the medial (MSO) and in lateral superior olive (LSO), and their inputs.

Originated from both left and right cochlear nuclei, the afferents for the MSO of each side are from primary-like units (spherical bushy cells), the activity of which preserves the timing and phase-locking features of the auditory nerve fibers. For low frequency sounds joining from a lateral source, a time difference will exist between phase-locked spikes from one side relative to the ones of the other side. During a continuous sound, this time difference between phase-locked spikes will repeat for each of the many waveforms.

An impulse takes time to travel along a fiber, that is the way an axon can be considered a *delay line*. In the model proposed by Jeffress, within the MSO neurons respond best when they receive coincident input from the two sides, if the delays were about equal. If we consider a series of neurons in the MSO, each receiving converging inputs from both cochlear nuclei in such a way that the afferents from each cochlear nucleus enter the series from opposite sides, we observe that, because of the same conduction speed in afferent fibers, neurons in the middle of the series can receive temporally coincident activation only when both cochlear nuclei are activated simultaneously, that is to say when sound simultaneously reach both ears because its source is located along the midline, equidistant from each ear. For sound sources located laterally to the midline, coincident activation will be received by neurons more laterally placed in the series: the topography of neurons receiving coincident activation is hypothesized to be the key mechanism allowing to exactly perceive the source location of a sound.

Neurons and circuits in the lateral superior olive (LSO) are sensitive to interaural level differences. LSO also receive bilateral inputs, excitatory from the ipsilateral side (joining from spherical bushy cells of the cochlear nucleus), whereas inhibitory from the contralateral side, in particular from globular bushy cells of the cochlear nucleus, and synapses on inhibitory neurons in the medial nucleus of the trapezoid body, which use the neurotransmitter glycine. LSO neurons compare the difference between sound levels at the two ears, being then excited when sound in the ipsilateral ear is of higher level, whereas inhibited when sound is of higher level in the contralateral ear. If sound is of equal level in the two ears, little neuronal response is observed because of a prevalent contralateral inhibition. These neurons are thus excited by sound sources located on the ipsilateral side of the head. The lateral superior olive projects centrally either excitatory fibers to the inferior colliculus on the opposite side, transforming this ipsilateral response to a contralateral one, or inhibitory fibers to the inferior colliculus of the same side. LSO is predominantly composed of neurons with high characteristic frequencies and has a tonotopic organization.

Almost all ascending inputs from lower brain stem centers converges at the inferior colliculus, a structure displaying several subdivisions. The *central nucleus is* organized tonotopically and receives direct input from the cochlear nucleus and binaural input from the MSO and LSO: the dorsolateral part of the nucleus receives low characteristic frequency input, included the one from MSO, whereas the ventromedial part is targeted by LSO and generally by high characteristic frequency fibers. In the colliculus, terminals from the MSO and LSO may have limited spatial overlap: due to the nature of the afferents, neurons in the dorsolateral part of the colliculus are mainly sensitive to interaural time differences, whereas cells in the ventromedial region of the nucleus are sensitive to interaural level differences. Since additional circuits for the generation of ITD sensitivity have not been identified, the colliculus appears to be sensitive to interaural time differences mainly by action of its inputs from the MSO. On the contrary, damaging the superior olivary complex does not abolish sensitivity to interaural level differences in the colliculus, which can be then created anew at levels above the LSO, either by the dorsal nucleus of the lateral lemniscus, that sends a large inhibitory projection to the colliculus, or by inhibitory mechanisms within the colliculus. Differently from other specialized mammals, in the human auditory system there is no evidence of a mapping of sound source location to position within the inferior colliculus.

The inferior colliculus transmits auditory information to both the superior colliculus, where a spatial map of sound is found, and the auditory cerebral cortex: in particular, neurons of the inferior colliculus project to the medial geniculate body (de Ribaupierre, 1997), where principal cells in turn project to the auditory cortex. The pathways from the inferior colliculus include a lemniscal (*core*) pathway and extralemniscal (*belt*) pathways.

3.4. Auditory Cortex

The auditory cortex includes several areas of the dorsal temporal lobe (Clarey et al, 1992). The ventral region of the medial geniculate nucleus sends the main projection to the primary auditory cortex (A1, or Brodmann area 41), which in humans lies on Heschl's gyrus of the temporal lobe, medial to the sylvian fissure, and contains a tonotopic representation of characteristic frequencies, that is to say an organized map reflecting the pattern of peripheral sensors, based on the frequencies that best stimulate the neurons. In particular, neurons with low characteristic frequencies are located rostrally, whereas those tuned to high frequencies are found at the caudal end of A1. Then, a smooth frequency gradient is evident in one direction, whereas iso-frequency contours are observed along the orthogonal direction. Due to larger inputs, representations of relevant frequencies are wider in comparison with representations of other frequencies. Other characteristics of auditory stimuli are also represented in A1, with less clear mapping rules: for example, at right angles to the axis of tonotopic mapping, a map of binaural interactions is evident.

Like other cortical areas, the auditory cortex is organized in cortical columns running across all of the cortical layers and oriented normally to the cortical surface. All neurons within a column have similar response characteristics (e.g., similar characteristic frequencies and types of responses to binaural sounds): regarding the latter, generally a cortical neuron is excited by the main ear (most often the contralateral one), whereas the opposite ear can be excitatory (EE neurons) or inhibitory (EI neurons), respectively displaying a summation or a suppressive interaction; depending on sound level, some neurons can show both summation and suppression interactions. Summation columns alternate with suppression columns, mainly in the A1 high frequency region. Neurons within a summation column tend to have large projections to the opposite hemisphere, whereas fewer contralateral projections are generally sent by suppression columns, unless for columns with neurons inhibited by contralateral ear and excited by ipsilateral ear. Thus, the auditory cortex can be subdivided into cortical columns responsive to every audible frequency and each type of binaural interaction.

Others parameters mapped onto the surface of primary auditory cortex are bandwidth (responsiveness to a narrow or broad range of frequencies), neuronal response latency, loudness, etc. The intersection between different maps is not still understood. In every case, in A1 neurons and subregions many independent variables of sound are represented, which permit selective sound discrimination on the basis of several independent and/or combined analyses.

Multiple regions surround A1, many of which show a tonotopic representation. These areas receive direct input from the ventral division of the medial geniculate nucleus, primarily in cortical layers IIIb and IV. Adjacent tonotopic fields have mirror-image tonotopy, since the direction of tonotopy reverses at the boundary between fields.

Actually, it is suggested by different Authors that primary or primary-like areas (*core*, 3 or 4 areas) are surrounded by 7 to 10 secondary areas (*belt*), the latter receiving input from the core areas of auditory cortex, as well as from thalamic nuclei, in some cases (Rauschecker et al, 1995). As revealed by recent functional MRI studies, in humans and monkeys core regions are primarily activated by pure tones, whereas complex sounds and narrow-band noise bursts activate the neurons of belt areas.

In the auditory cortex, many neurons with large receptive fields and broad tuning are sensitive to interaural time and level differences and therefore to spatial localization of sounds; however, no organized spatial map of sound is evident in any of the sound location sensitive cortical areas, differently from what observed in the midbrain (Buonomano and Merzenich, 1998; Cohen and Knudsen1999). These cortical neurons sensitive to sound spatial location are found along a sound-localization pathway starting from the central nucleus of the inferior colliculus and reaching (through the auditory thalamus) the A1 area, cortical association areas and the frontal eye fields, involved in gaze control, which are directly connected to brain stem tegmentum premotor nuclei mediating gaze changes, as well as to the superior colliculus.

Cortical pathways are required for more complex sound-localization tasks (forming an image of the sound source, remembering it, moving toward it, etc.), being less active if the task is only to indicate the side of the sound source.

As for the output from the primary visual and somatosensory cortex, the circuits originating from the auditory cortex are segregated into separate processing streams. In facts, the more rostral and ventral areas connect primarily to the more rostral and ventral areas of the temporal lobe, generally implicated in nonspatial functions, whereas the more caudal area projects to the dorsal and caudal temporal lobe, implicated in spatial processing. In addition, these belt areas and their temporal lobe targets both project to largely different areas of the frontal lobes. Caudal and parietal areas are more active when a sound must be located or moves, and ventral areas are more active during identification of the same stimulus or analysis of its pitch. Therefore, an oversimplified schema suggest that identification of auditory objects could be made by anterior-ventral pathways by analyzing spectral and temporal characteristics of sounds, whereas dorsal-posterior pathways could analyze sound source location and detection of source motion.

As for both visual and somatosensory systems, the auditory cortex massively projects back to lower areas: the ratio between descending fibers entering the sensory thalamus and axons projecting from the thalamus to the cortex is almost 10:1. Fibers from the auditory cortex contact the inferior colliculus, olivo-cochlear neurons and the dorsal cochlear nucleus. Through these projections, the auditory cortex can actively increase and adjust the responses of neurons in subcortical structures, in this way modulating and sharpening signal processing. On the contrary, a decreased cortical activity reduces thalamic and collicular responses. Therefore, the cortex exercises a top-down control of perception.

REFERENCES

Brownell, W. E., Bader, C. R., Bertrand, D., and de Ribaupierre, Y. (1985). Evoked mechanical response of isolated hair cells. *Science,* **227**: 194–196.

Brand, A., Behrend, O., Marquardt, T., McAlpine, D., and Grothe, B. (2002). Precise inhibition is essential for microsecond interaural time difference coding. *Nature,* **417**: 543–547.

Buonomano, D. V. and Merzenich, M. M. (1998). Cortical plasticity: From synapses to maps. *Annu. Rev. Neurosci.,* **21**: 149–186.

Clarey, J. C., Barone, P., and Imig, T. J. (1992). Physiology of thalamus and cortex. In *"The Mammalian Auditory Pathway: Neurophysiology"* (A. N. Popper and R. R. Fay, eds.), pp. 232–334. Springer-Verlag, New York.

Cohen, Y. E. and Knudsen, E. I. (1999). Maps versus clusters: Different representations of auditory space in the midbrain and forebrain. *Trends Neurosci.,* **12**: 128–135.

de Ribaupierre, F. (1997). Acoustical information processing in the auditory thalamus and cerebral cortex. In *"The Central Auditory System"* (G. Ehret and R. Romand, eds.), pp. 317–397. Oxford Univ. Press, New York.

Guinan, J. J., Jr. (1996). The physiology of olivocochlear efferents. In *"The Cochlea"* (P. Dallos, A. N. Popper, and R. R. Fay, eds.), pp. 435–502. Springer-Verlag, New York.

Hudspeth, A. J. and Corey, D. P. (1977). Sensitivity, polarity, and conductance change in the response of vertebrate hair cells to controlled mechanical stimuli. *Proc. Natl. Acad. Sci. USA,* **74**: 2407–2411.

Liberman, M. C., Gao, J., He, D. Z. Z., Wu, X., Jia, S., and Zuo, J. (2002). Prestin is required for electromotility of the outer hair cell and for the cochlear amplifi er. *Nature,* **419**: 300–304.

Pickles, J. O., Comis, S. D., and Osborne, M. P. (1984). Cross-links between stereocilia in the guinea-pig organ of Corti, and their possible relation to sensory transduction. *Hearing Res.,* **15**: 103–112.

Rauschecker, J. P., Tian, B., and Hauser, M. (1995). Processing of complex sounds in the macaque nonprimary auditory cortex. *Science,* **268**: 111–114.

Rhode, W. S. and Greenberg, S. (1992). Physiology of the cochlear nuclei. In *The Mammalian Auditory Pathway, Neurophysiology* (A. N. Popper and R. R. Fay, eds.), pp. 94–152. Springer-Verlag, New York.

Ruggero, M. A. (1992). Physiology and coding of sound in the auditory nerve. In *The Mammalian Auditory Pathway, Neurophysiology* (A. N. Popper and R. R. Fay, eds.), pp. 34–93. Springer-Verlag, New York.

Rybalchenko, V. and Santos-Sacchi, J. (2003). Cl-flux through a nonselective, stretch sensitive conductance influences the outer hair cell motor of the guinea pig. *J. Physiol.,* **547.3**: 873–891.

Warr, W. B. (1992). Organization of olivocochlear efferent systems in mammals. In *The Mammalian Auditory Pathway, Neuroanatomy* (D. B. Webster, A. N. Popper, and R. R. Fay, eds.), pp. 410–448. Springer-Verlag, New York.

Wightman, F. L. and Kistler, D. J. (1993). Sound localization. In *Human Psychophysics* (W. A. Yost, A. N. Popper, and R. R. Fay, eds.), pp. 155–192. Springer-Verlag, New York.

Yin, T. C. T. and Chan, J. C. K. (1990). Interaural time sensitivity in medial superior olive of cat. *J. Neurophysiol.,* **64**, 465–488.

Zheng, J., Shen, W., He, D. Z., Long, K. B., Madison, L. D., and Dallos, P. (2000). Prestin is the motor protein of cochlear outer hair cells. *Nature,* **405**: 149–155.

Chapter 2

GENETICS IN SENSORINEURAL HEARING LOSS

Alessandro Castiglione[*], *MD, PhD*
Department of Neurosciences and Complex Operative Unit
of Otorhinolaryngology, University Hospital of Padua, Italy

ABSTRACT

In the field of genetics, this decade will be characterized by the widespread use of so-called next-generation sequencers, first described in 2003, based on the human genome project publication essentially conducted through Sanger sequencing using the first generation of DNA-sequencers. Actually, before long, there was a rapidly growing demand for a new system, thus a new generation of non-Sanger-based sequencing technologies have been developed to sequence DNA at an unprecedented speed, thereby enabling impressive scientific achievements and novel biological applications. The premises and promises of similar events open a window on a next generation diagnosis of hearing losses. However, this new technology has to overcome the inertia of a field that has previously relied on Sanger-sequencing for 30 years. These new methods of DNA analysis are promising and could considerably reduce the time and cost of sequencing studies, up to the famous spot "the genome for $1,000". However, the use of technology does not necessarily suggest an infallible diagnosis and optimal treatment. There is a need to "manage" a substantial amount of information (that at best will be different and complementary) to extrapolate meaningful or rather more valuable conclusions than previously obtained, as well as interpretations and the resolution of ethical and legal aspects paradoxically require increasing amounts of time and money to manage such situations. In addition, recent increasing scientific evidences are revaluating the Lamarckian approach to hereditary conditions beside to the classical most famous Mendelian or Darwinian models. Even more surprising and is the advent of genetic therapy for an increasing number of diseases. In conclusion, all events seem to announce a revolutionary decade for future diagnosis and treatments of genetic hearing loss. In such

---

[*] Corresponding Author's Email: alessandro.castiglione@unipd.it. (Address: Via Giustiniani, 2 – Padova, 35128 – PD, Italy, tel. +39 049 8212051, fax. +39 049 8211994).

exciting, but also complex, context, the clinical approach needs to focus on the best and simplest solution.

In this chapter, a brief review and update about genetics of hearing loss will be reported in the light of those revolutionary events, in order to help and accompanied the reader in reflecting on the new role of clinician in a high rapidly changing context.

Keywords: genetics, hearing loss, syndromic hearing loss

INTRODUCTION

In the field of genetics, this decade will be characterized by the widespread use of so-called next-generation sequencers (Schuster 2008, Shaffer 2007), first described in 2003, based on the human genome project publication (2003) essentially conducted through Sanger sequencing using the first generation of DNA-sequencers. However, before long, there was a rapidly growing demand for a new system. Thus, a new generation of non-Sanger-based sequencing technologies have been developed to sequence DNA at an unprecedented speed, thereby enabling impressive scientific achievements and novel biological applications. However, this new technology has to overcome the inertia of a field that has previously relied on Sanger-sequencing for 30 years (Schuster 2008). To characterize the new "tools" available to geneticists, we should consider the following example: previously published literature has been passed from pen and inkwell to scanner and digital copier in less than ten years. With minor inconvenience, in the terms of the previous example, scanners were initially used to acquire only parts of a line at a time, and subsequently the need to recreate complete sentences, pages, chapters, books and libraries increased as a reference to allow this process. In addition, the "writers", "readers", "book-shops" and the original sources have not been completely adapted and remain based on older technology. However, these new methods of DNA analysis are promising and could considerably reduce the time and cost of sequencing studies, up to the famous spot sentence "the genome for $1,000" (Dondorp and de Wert 2013). Unfortunately, possessing a fantastic scanner does equate with being an excellent photographer or writer, and similarly the use of technology do not necessarily suggest an infallible diagnosis and optimal treatment. Thus, there is a need to "manage" a substantial amount of information (that at best will be different and complementary) to extrapolate meaningful or rather more valuable conclusions than previously obtained, for example interpretations and the resolution of ethical and legal aspects paradoxically require increasing amounts of time and money. Ironically, bioinformatics replies to the "genome for $1,000" spot with the "consequentially cost of $1 million for data analysis" (Mardis 2010). How could this paradox be avoided? How does this paradox affect clinical practice in general or specific cases? Although the aim of this chapter is not to resolve controversial scientific (or philosophical) debates, it can be argued that physicians, patients and readers benefit from the knowledge that there are too many questions about privacy and too many doubts concerning the accuracy and in other words, the interpretation of this information.

Even when the clinical management and professionals involved are perfect, occasionally the genetics of hearing loss can generate confusion in patients, physicians and geneticists (also), likely reflecting the complexity and knowledge of the field (Salvago et al. 2014, De Stefano, Kulamarva, and Dispenza 2012). Indeed, a syndrome can be well known and well described (i.e., hearing loss, goiter, suggestive tonal and speech audiometries, CT/MRI scans with enlarged vestibular aqueducts and/or Mondini deformity, and positive perchlorate tests), although it might be difficult to identify a mutation in the gene responsible for that condition (*SLC26A4*, and/or *FOXI1* and/or *KCNJ10*, etc.).

HEARING LOSS AND ITS GENETICS

Hearing impairment is one of the commonest clinical conditions, in particular at birth. It has been estimated that approximately 1-2 in 100 person has hearing concerns in the first decade of life (Martines et al. 2015, Dispenza, De Stefano, et al. 2013). The prevalence of childhood and adolescent hearing loss is around 3%. The causes of hearing loss differ and they can vary in severity and physiopathology: the etiology of hearing loss in children remains unknown in 30-40% of cases, non-genetic in 30-35%, genetic non-syndromic in 30%, and genetic syndromic in 3-5% (Bartolotta et al. 2014, Dispenza, Cappello, et al. 2013). Most of genetic conditions responsible for hearing loss appear in a non-syndromic form (60-75% of all genetic cases). The two most common genes involved in hearing loss are *GJB2* for the non-syndromic forms and *SLC26A4* the syndromic ones.

The main objective of correctly identifying a syndrome should only be the usefulness for the patients. If you have doubts or improper diagnostic instruments it would be more helpful to describe, more objectively as possible, all available clinical data. Giving a "name" should help patients in manage and communicate their conditions, promoting a multidisciplinary approach. It should be also remembered that there are not specialists or specialties that can singularly approach all syndromes, as well as there is no a syndrome that cannot keep advantage from all available specialties. Therefore, the main target should be investigating and exploring clinical and genetic conditions trying to bring benefits to whom that are suffering from. The correct diagnosis comes next.

Even if recent advances provide improvement in diagnosis, the most effective procedures to suspect a genetic cause of hearing loss still remains history and objective clinical examination essentially based on: 1) family history; 2) symmetry of clinical findings (bilateral hearing loss); 3) dysmorphic features 4) symptoms onset and/or progression.

Non-Syndromic Hearing Loss (Approximately 65% of All Genetic Causes of Hearing Loss): Audioprofiles of Dominant and Recessive Patterns

More than 60 genes have been so far associated with non-syndromic hearing loss. Mutations in the *GJB2* gene still remain the leading cause of non-syndromic sensorineural hearing loss on a genetic basis; however today the new NGS panels modify the number of mutations identified in a more varied and wide gene range, including *TMC1* and *TECTA* for example. A new useful approach especially for the non-geneticist specialist may be to consider audioprofiles in different transmission patterns: non-syndromic dominant (sexual or autosomal chromosomes), non-syndromic recessive (sexual or autosomal chromosomes) and mitochondrial. The definition of a specific audioprofile for genes and mutations provides a good genetic knowledge without neglecting the clinical contribution and consists practically in collecting clinical data (in essence they are condensed in the audiometric data being non-syndromic forms, or in any case of a single organ, ear in this case) of all patients with similar mutations matched by age and when possible also by sex. Obviously for these case history is essential and collecting data revealed interesting considerations: in most cases non-syndromic with recessive patterns show worse entity of hearing loss without o slow progression, with early symptoms onset; in contrast dominant pattern has less severe loss of hearing, but high rate of progression with late onset. A deepening of these topics concerns the residual function of the proteins that has been widely found in the truncating and non-truncating forms of connexin 26 with important correlations and responses on the clinical clinic. However, as desirable, it would be quite challenging to evaluate and estimate the residual function of mutated proteins for each gene potentially involved in hearing loss, in addition to the difficulty in collecting an adequate number of identical mutations for each gene.

Syndromic Hearing Loss, without Congenital Craniofacial Findings and Recessive Inheritance Pattern

Even if initial screening examinations indicate normal hearing, the child remains at risk. During infancy and early childhood, parents should be aware of, and questioned about, the child's hearing and language milestones. Some syndromes, such as Pendred, Alport, Refsum, neurofibromatosis type II, Usher, and osteopetrosis, may place the patient at risk for progressive hearing loss.

Pendred Syndrome (Prevalence 7,5:100000, approximately 5% of Cases of Congenital Hearing Loss), otherwise the FOXI1-SLC26A4/ KCNJ10 Genetic Variants Responsible for Ions Disorders in the Inner Ear)

Two clinical pictures come from mutations in the *SLC26A4* gene: (1) the syndromic form, called Pendred Syndrome, characterized by hearing loss, goiter and eventually hypothyroidism, with/without EVA or other inner ear malformations as Mondini deformity; (2) the non-syndromic form, called DFNB4 or non-syndromic EVA (when EVA is present), characterized by hearing loss with/without EVA or other inner ear malformations. Mutations in the *FOXI1* (5q34) gene can be also responsible for these conditions. *FOXI1* encodes for a transcriptional activator that allow the transcription of *SLC26A4* and it is fundamental to develop normal sense of hearing and balance. Furthermore, mutations in the inwardly rectifying K (+) channel gene *KCNJ10* (1q23.2) can be also associated with hearing loss in carriers of *SLC26A4* mutations The inner ear malformations, when present, are generally bilateral (even if unilateral involvement is not exceptional), and they not seem to affect the auditory rehabilitation through cochlear implantation (Benatti et al. 2013, Busi et al. 2012, Busi et al. 2015, Castiglione, Busi, and Martini 2013, Castiglione et al. 2014).

The type of hearing loss is mixed and variable from moderate to profound; the hearing impairment can be progressive and affected patients can benefit from binaural or bimodal auditory training with hearing aids or cochlear implantation. Considering the progression of the disease required a planning in prescribing auditory device that takes into account this concrete possibility. Even if a conductive component can be present, generally patients do not take advantages from bone conduction devices (Benatti et al. 2013, Busi et al. 2012, Busi et al. 2015, Castiglione, Busi, and Martini 2013, Castiglione et al. 2014).

Usher Syndrome (Ciliopathies Reflecting the Potential Effects of Variations in the Genes Encoding Actin-Based Structures and Tip Links in Inner Ear Cells)

There are 3 types of Usher Syndrome and 10 subtypes, which altogether account for the diagnosis of 3.5 cases per 100,000 births. Thus, this syndrome is one of the most common illnesses after Pendred Syndrome, characterized by hearing loss without major dysmorphic aspects. The genetics of Usher Syndrome are complex, reflecting the high number of genes potentially involved in this condition: *MYO7A*, *USH1C*, *CDH23*, *PCDH15*, *SANS*, *USH2A*, *VLGR1*, *WHRN*, *USH3A*, and *PDZD7* (Reiners et al. 2006). The majority of these genes are involved in the formation and constitution of specific structures (called tip-link) and actin filaments in inner ear cells. Notably, the cilia outside of the inner ear typically composed of tubulin (not actin); therefore, these structures are preserved in Usher Syndrome. However, syndromes that show similar aspects, such as Alström Syndrome, could result from mutations in genes encoding proteins and elements common to actin and tubulin, suggesting a wide clinical spectrum (and more severe) in Alström Syndrome. The retinal pigment epithelium contains both actin and tubulin filaments essential for melanosome activity. Retinitis pigmentosa in Usher and Alström Syndromes results from defects in actin and/or tubulin in the retinal pigment epithelium or photoreceptors.

Patients with Usher Syndrome develop hearing loss and vestibular and visual impairments. This disorder is inherited in an autosomal recessive pattern and characterized by progressive blindness resulting from retinitis pigmentosa, and moderate to severe sensorineural hearing loss. Usher syndrome has been classified into three types: Type I, characterized by severe to profound bilateral congenital hearing loss and poor or absent vestibular function with retinitis pigmentosa diagnosed by 10 years of age; Type II, characterized by mild to moderate hearing loss at birth and normal vestibular function with the onset of retinitis pigmentosa during late adolescence; Type III, characterized by progressive hearing loss and vestibular dysfunction with a variable degree of retinitis pigmentosa (Castiglione, Busi, and Martini 2013). Due to the lacking of visual reinforcement in spatial orientation, these patients can benefit from mandatory binaural auditory rehabilitation, when not contraindicated, with hearing aids or cochlear implants.

Jervell and Lange-Nielsen Syndrome (Prevalence 0.3: 100,000), or Genetic Variants of KCN1/KCNE1 Genes Responsible for Ions Disorders in the Inner Ear

Prolongation of the QT interval can come out from genetic defects in channel proteins, the same proteins that can be responsible for sensorineural hearing loss when expressed in the inner ear. These channels are critical in the function of the inner ear and heart muscle. The prolonged QT has the higher prevalence among this patients, and then is called Jervell and Lange-Nielsen syndrome when (and only if) it is accompanied by hearing loss; thus, by definition, 100% of patients have hearing loss that tends to be severe to profound. Mutations in the *KCNQ1*, and less commonly, the *KCNE1* gene, coding proteins that form potassium transport channels, are considered responsible for the Jervell and Lange-Nielsen syndrome.

Syndromic Hearing Loss with Congenital Craniofacial Findings and Dominant Inheritance Pattern

Describing morphological and clinical aspects still remains the best clinical practice involving the precise, thorough and accurate collection of signs and symptoms, suggesting that the accurate diagnosis of a syndrome is not an intuitive reaction when examining a patient. Indeed, patients must be examined from different point of views: frontal, lateral and ventral. Examiners must not estimate abnormalities through sight, but rather anomalies should be measured using appropriate instruments. These analyses should proceed stepwise, combining until the obtained knowledge facilitates the consideration of clinical aspects other specialists have previously described or defined. Useless tests or exams and needless considerations of all available tests for patients should be avoided. Even when the diagnosis seems accurate, 2-3 alternative solutions should also be considered to avoid misdiagnosis. Notably, having a mutation does not prevent the occurrence of other diseases, conditions or genetic disorders. In most cases, it is possible to hypothesize fragility in DNA repair or function, even when difficult to prove, thus a collection of different mutations could affect the phenotype.

BOR Syndrome and EYA1 Related Disorders (or Branchial Defects Potentially Resulting from Genetic Variants in EYA1, SIX5, and SIX5, Genes on the Axis of the Tbx1-Six1/Eya1-Fgf8 Genetic Pathway)

Branchio-oto-renal (BOR) syndrome is an autosomal dominant disorder comprising external, middle and inner ear malformations, branchial cleft sinuses, cervical fistulae, mixed or conductive hearing loss and renal anomalies with an estimate prevalence of 2-3:100000 newborns, responsible for approximately 2% of deaf children. BOR syndrome is perhaps one of the most frequent syndromes responsible for hearing loss, with most difficulties in defining and performing auditory rehabilitation. With respect to syndromes in otolaryngology, the BOR disorder represents the first ones among congenital malformations (together with the Treacher Collins syndrome). Furthermore, BOR syndrome is perhaps one with the widest clinically variable diseases with uncertain auditory assessment and rehabilitation. The best advice in these cases is to exclusively to rely on audiometric profiling and patient impressions, as there is no clear correlation between the observed malformations and the severity of hearing loss. Notably, all associated congenital conditions, mild or moderate, represent the natural hearing for these patients. Therefore, external interventions (surgery or hearing aids) might be considered "artificial" and "unacceptable". Indeed, experts must perform reconstructive surgery on the middle and external ears, and the results in terms of auditory function can be extremely disappointing, if not pejorative.

BOR syndrome primarily reflects mutations in *EYA1* (on chromosome 8, BOR type 1) *SIX 5* (on chromosome 19, BOR type 2) and *SIX1* (on chromosome 14, BOR type 3) genes, although we cannot exclude the involvement of other genes that play a role in the *Tbx1-Six1/Eya1-Fgf8* genetic pathway, which controls mammalian cardiovascular and craniofacial morphogenesis, as demonstrated for other branchial defects, such as Di George syndrome (Guo et al. 2011).

CHARGE Association (or Overlapping Features with DiGeorge Syndrome and Other Branchial Defects Resulting from Genetic Variations in the SMAD1/CHD7-FGF8/BMP Family/WNT1-OTX2-FOXA2-TBX1 Genetic Pathways)

When considering genetic hearing loss, the possibility of sharing new pathways with other syndromes should be considered, suggesting that these defects can be surprisingly similar (or different) (Corsten-Janssen et al. 2013, Guo et al. 2011, Liu et al. 2014, Payne et al. 2015, Schulz et al. 2014).

CHARGE association or syndrome has a birth prevalence of approximately 0.14 per 100,000 newborns. The acronym recalls the primary clinical manifestations of this syndrome, although the corollary of signs and symptoms are much more vast and complex, including iris or retinal colobomas, heart disease, choanal atresia, growth defects and developmental delays, genitourinary hypoplasia, external ear abnormalities, brain abnormalities, sensorineural hearing loss (up to 90% of cases), respiratory problems and cranial nerve hypoplasia (including the seventh and the eighth ones) with important functional deficits. This association reflects mutations in the *CHD7* gene in approximately two thirds of cases. The CHARGE association alone it is not an absolute limit to the rehabilitation program; indeed, expectations must be consistent with the clinical conditions, and in cases of cochlear implant, the expert medical team will generate nerve stimulation, and carefully evaluate hypoplasia and malformations. Bilateral or binaural rehabilitation is desirable.

Mutations in the MITF Pathway (Responsible for Waardenburg Syndrome)

The *MITF* promoter is partially regulated through the transcription factors *PAX3*, *SOX10*, *LEF1/TCF* and *CREB* during melanocyte development. In humans, mutations affecting the MITF pathway lead to pigmentary and auditory defects, collectively known as Waardenburg Syndrome (WS) (Lin and Fisher 2007). The *MITF* gene encodes a transcription factor that regulates the differentiation and development of melanocytes and the retinal pigment epithelium and is also responsible for the pigment cell-specific transcription of melanogenesis genes. Hearing deficiency stems from a requirement for melanocytes within the stria vascularis of the cochlea (inner ear), a requirement involving the maintenance of endolymphatic potassium for auditory nerve action potential. Waardenburg-associated mutations represent a striking epistatic series in which essentially every culprit gene is mechanistically associated with the regulation of MITF expression or activity. These genes, including Pax3, Slug, Sox10, endothelin 1, and endothelin receptor B, are transcriptional regulators of *MITF* expression (Pax3 and Sox10), transcriptional targets of *MITF* (Slug), or *MAPK* activators that directly phosphorylate *MITF* (ET1 and EdnrB) (Steel 1995, Chin, Garraway, and Fisher 2006). Mutations in *MITF* gene are also responsible for melanomas, but these mutations typically differ in type and effect from those causing pigmentary defects and deafness, thus leading to different phenotypes (Grill et al. 2013).

CONCLUSION: PERFORM SIMPLE TASKS WITH THE HIGHEST ATTENTION

In 2013, Stamatiou GA and Stankovic KM (Stamatiou and Stankovic 2013) published a fine analysis on a new point of view during the present new era of NGS to identify "genetic nodes" of several genes. The genes associated with hearing loss and deafness were identified through PubMed literature searches and the Hereditary Hearing Loss Homepage. These genes were assembled into 3 groups: 63 genes associated with nonsyndromic deafness, 107 genes associated with nonsyndromic or syndromic sensorineural deafness, and 112 genes associated with otic capsule development and malformations. Each group of genes was analyzed to identify the most interconnected nodal molecules. The nodal molecules of these networks included transforming growth factor beta1 (*TGFB1*) for Group 1, *MAPK3/MAPK1* MAP kinase (*ERK 1/2*) and the G protein coupled receptors (*GPCR*) for Group 2, and *TGFB1* and hepatocyte nuclear factor 4 alpha (*HNF4A*) for Group 3. These results were confirmed in different analyses, suggesting new investigations and treatments involving glutathione, protein kinase B (Akt) and nuclear factor kappa B (NFkB) (Muller and Barr-Gillespie 2015).

A potential solution for more demanding genetic analyses could involve separating the multitude of genes in variously articulated pathways of different lengths, assigning priority when possible, and subsequently analyzing these pathways, moving on to the next series when a non-conclusive mutation is identified; these analyses must continue until the changes that greatly impact pathological pathways are identified.

Not only wide analyses but also targeted analyses should be performed, and impacted pathways should be developed and designed, considering the clinical and diagnostic possibilities. At this point the quality of a pathway is fundamental and should be well known and defined as the metabolic pathway. Obviously, a long period of study and analysis to identify genetic variations (pathological conditions) is needed, as the cause-effect relationship does not always exhibit a desirable time of onset, and frequently, only the initial effects associated with disease causes are observed.

However, a genetic pathway is not always as linear as a classical metabolic pathway, rather metabolic pathways can be "modified" in different ways, whereas a genetic pathway can be "far" from linear, with sequential events, also influenced through time and the environment. Thus, the clinical phenotype is markedly helpful in defining the depth of the associated analysis.

REFERENCES

2003. "International consortium completes human genome project." *Pharmacogenomics* 4 (3):241. doi: 10.1517/phgs.4.3.241.22688.

Bartolotta, C., P. Salvago, S. Cocuzza, C. Fabiano, P. Sammarco, and F. Martines. 2014. "Identification of D179H, a novel missense GJB2 mutation in a Western Sicily family." *European Archives of Oto-Rhino-Laryngology* 271 (6):1457-1461. doi: 10.1007/s00405-013-2613-y.

Benatti, A., A. Castiglione, P. Trevisi, R. Bovo, M. Rosignoli, R. Manara, and A. Martini. 2013. "Endocochlear inflammation in cochlear implant users: case report and literature review." *Int J Pediatr Otorhinolaryngol* 77 (6):885-93. doi: 10.1016/j.ijporl.2013.03.016.

Busi, M., A. Castiglione, M. Taddei Masieri, A. Ravani, V. Guaran, L. Astolfi, P. Trevisi, A. Ferlini, and A. Martini. 2012. "Novel mutations in the SLC26A4 gene." *Int J Pediatr Otorhinolaryngol* 76 (9):1249-54. doi: 10.1016/j.ijporl.2012.05.014.

Busi, Micol, Monica Rosignoli, Alessandro Castiglione, Federica Minazzi, Patrizia Trevisi, Claudia Aimoni, Ferdinando Calzolari, Enrico Granieri, and Alessandro Martini. 2015. "Cochlear Implant Outcomes and Genetic Mutations in Children with Ear and Brain Anomalies." *BioMed Research International*.

Castiglione, A., S. Melchionda, M. Carella, P. Trevisi, R. Bovo, R. Manara, and A. Martini. 2014. "EYA1-related disorders: Two clinical cases and a literature review." *Int J Pediatr Otorhinolaryngol*. doi: 10.1016/j.ijporl.2014.03.032.

Castiglione, Alessandro, Micol Busi, and Alessandro Martini. 2013. "Syndromic hearing loss: An update." *Hearing, Balance and Communication* 11 (3):146-159. doi: 10.3109/21695717.2013.820514.

Chin, L., L. A. Garraway, and D. E. Fisher. 2006. "Malignant melanoma: genetics and therapeutics in the genomic era." *Genes Dev* 20 (16):2149-82. doi: 10.1101/gad.1437206.

Corsten-Janssen, N., S. C. Saitta, L. H. Hoefsloot, D. M. McDonald-McGinn, D. A. Driscoll, R. Derks, K. A. Dickinson, W. S. Kerstjens-Frederikse, B. S. Emanuel, E. H. Zackai, and C. M. van Ravenswaaij-Arts. 2013. "More Clinical Overlap between 22q11.2 Deletion Syndrome and CHARGE Syndrome than Often Anticipated." *Mol Syndromol* 4 (5):235-45. doi: 10.1159/000351127.

De Stefano, A., G. Kulamarva, and F. Dispenza. 2012. "Malignant paroxysmal positional vertigo." *Auris Nasus Larynx* 39:378-382.

Dispenza, F, F Cappello, G Kulamarva, and A De Stefano. 2013. "The discovery of the stapes." *Acta Otolaryngol Ital* 33 (5):357-359.

Dispenza, F., A. De Stefano, C. Costantino, D. Marchese, and F. Riggio. 2013. "Sudden Sensorineural Hearing Loss: Results of intratympanic steroids as salvage treatment." *Am J Otolaryngol* 34 (4):296-300.

Dondorp, W. J., and G. M. de Wert. 2013. "The 'thousand-dollar genome': an ethical exploration." *Eur J Hum Genet* 21 Suppl 1:S6-26. doi: 10.1038/ejhg.2013.73.

Grill, C., K. Bergsteinsdottir, M. H. Ogmundsdottir, V. Pogenberg, A. Schepsky, M. Wilmanns, V. Pingault, and E. Steingrimsson. 2013. "MITF mutations associated with pigment deficiency syndromes and melanoma have different effects on protein function." *Hum Mol Genet* 22 (21):4357-67. doi: 10.1093/hmg/ddt285.

Guo, C., Y. Sun, B. Zhou, R. M. Adam, X. Li, W. T. Pu, B. E. Morrow, A. Moon, and X. Li. 2011. "A Tbx1-Six1/Eya1-Fgf8 genetic pathway controls mammalian cardiovascular and craniofacial morphogenesis." *J Clin Invest* 121 (4):1585-95. doi: 10.1172/JCI44630.

Lin, J. Y., and D. E. Fisher. 2007. "Melanocyte biology and skin pigmentation." *Nature* 445 (7130):843-50. doi: 10.1038/nature05660.

Liu, Y., C. Harmelink, Y. Peng, Y. Chen, Q. Wang, and K. Jiao. 2014. "CHD7 interacts with BMP R-SMADs to epigenetically regulate cardiogenesis in mice." *Hum Mol Genet* 23 (8):2145-56. doi: 10.1093/hmg/ddt610.

Mardis, E. R. 2010. "The $1,000 genome, the $100,000 analysis?" *Genome Med* 2 (11):84. doi: 10.1186/gm205.

Martines, F., P. Salvago, C. Bartolotta, S. Cocuzza, C. Fabiano, S. Ferrara, E. La Mattina, M. Mucia, P. Sammarco, F. Sireci, and E. Martines. 2015. "A genotype–phenotype correlation in Sicilian patients with GJB2 biallelic mutations." *European Archives of Oto-Rhino-Laryngology* 272 (8):1857-1865. doi: 10.1007/s00405-014-2970-1.

Muller, U., and P. G. Barr-Gillespie. 2015. "New treatment options for hearing loss." *Nat Rev Drug Discov* 14 (5):346-65. doi: 10.1038/nrd4533.

Payne, S., M. J. Burney, K. McCue, N. Popal, S. M. Davidson, R. H. Anderson, and P. J. Scambler. 2015. "A critical role for the chromatin remodeller CHD7 in anterior mesoderm during cardiovascular development." *Dev Biol* 405 (1):82-95. doi: 10.1016/j.ydbio.2015.06.017.

Reiners, J., K. Nagel-Wolfrum, K. Jurgens, T. Marker, and U. Wolfrum. 2006. "Molecular basis of human Usher syndrome: deciphering the meshes of the Usher protein network provides insights into the pathomechanisms of the Usher disease." *Exp Eye Res* 83 (1):97-119. doi: 10.1016/j.exer.2005.11.010.

Salvago, P., E. Martines, E. La Mattina, M. Mucia, P. Sammarco, F. Sireci, and F. Martines. 2014. "Distribution and phenotype of GJB2 mutations in 102 Sicilian patients with congenital non syndromic sensorineural hearing loss." *International Journal of Audiology* 53 (8):558-563. doi: 10.3109/14992027.2014.905717.

Schulz, Y., P. Wehner, L. Opitz, G. Salinas-Riester, E. M. Bongers, C. M. van Ravenswaaij-Arts, J. Wincent, J. Schoumans, J. Kohlhase, A. Borchers, and S. Pauli. 2014. "CHD7, the gene mutated in CHARGE syndrome, regulates genes involved in neural crest cell guidance." *Hum Genet* 133 (8):997-1009. doi: 10.1007/s00439-014-1444-2.

Schuster, S. C. 2008. "Next-generation sequencing transforms today's biology." *Nat Methods* 5 (1):16-8. doi: 10.1038/nmeth1156.

Shaffer, C. 2007. "Next-generation sequencing outpaces expectations." *Nat Biotechnol* 25 (2):149. doi: 10.1038/nbt0207-149.

Stamatiou, G. A., and K. M. Stankovic. 2013. "A comprehensive network and pathway analysis of human deafness genes." *Otol Neurotol* 34 (5):961-70. doi: 10.1097/MAO.0b013e3182898272.

Steel, K. P. 1995. "Inherited hearing defects in mice." *Annu Rev Genet* 29:675-701. doi: 10.1146/annurev.ge.29.120195.003331.

Chapter 3

CONGENITAL SENSORINEURAL HEARING LOSS

*Sara Ghiselli[1,2], MD, Bruno Galletti[1], MD,
Francesco Freni[1], MD, PhD, Rocco Bruno[1], MD
and Francesco Galletti[1], MD*

[1]University of Messina, Department of Human Pathology of the Adult
and of the Developmental Age "G. Barresi," ENT Section, Messina, Italy
[2]IRCCS "Burlo Garofalo," Trieste, Italy

ABSTRACT

Congenital hearing loss (CHL) is defined as the hearing loss present at birth and, consequently, before speech development. It is one of the prevalent chronic conditions in children and the main sensor neural disorder in developed countries. The estimated prevalence of permanent bilateral CHL is 1-3 per 1000 live births in developed countries.

CHL is caused by genetic factors in more than 50% of the cases. Genetic hearing loss may be the only clinical feature (non-syndromic or isolated forms) or may be associated with other symptoms (syndromic forms).

Non-syndromic hearing loss is extremely heterogeneous. About 80% of the cases are autosomal recessive, 15-24% are autosomal dominant and 1-2% are X-linked. Furthermore, less than 1% of CHL resulting from mitochondrial mutations and it presents with a characteristic matrilineal pattern of transmission. Typically, autosomal recessive hearing loss is congenital whereas autosomal dominant is often progressive. The most frequent isolated form of genetic hearing loss in white population of Europe and United States is the gap junction protein beta 2 gene (GJB2) mutation that is the gene encoding connexin-26.

Syndromic form represents about the 30% of the cases of CHL and literature reports more than 400 syndromes where hearing loss is accompanied with physical or laboratory findings. Responsible genes are known for many of these scenarios.

A genetic diagnosis is required for different reasons, in particular for choosing appropriate therapeutic options, for treating associated medical problem (syndromic forms) and for predicting the progression of the degree. New treatments and screening strategies are available for identifying the responsive gene, e.g., Next Generation DNA sequencing that allows the simultaneous analysis of a large number of genes causing CHL with a higher probability of gene identification.

This paragraph will describe the different genes and clinical features involved in CHL both in isolated and in syndromic form.

Keywords: congenital hearing loss, genetic hearing loss, deafness

INTRODUCTION

Congenital hearing loss (CHL) is defined as the hearing loss present at birth and, consequently, before speech development.

It is one of the prevalent chronic conditions in children and the main sensor neural disorder in developed countries.

The estimated prevalence of permanent bilateral CHL is 1-3 per 1000 live births in developed countries and it varies between 19-24 newborns in sub-Saharian Africa and South Asia respectively.

The prevalence of the hearing loss increase until 3-4 per live birth [1] during the first 5 years of life when considering the progressive hearing loss genetically programmed.

Late diagnosis or treatment has consequences on different child developmental area. CHL affect speech development, language acquisition and it has an impact in brain plasticity and cognitive development. The hearing impairment, if it is not properly treated, move to isolating themselves to society and may decrease work opportunity in adult life.

For these reasons, it is very important an early diagnosis and an early right treatment of the CHL. Universal newborn hearing screening program has allowed a reduction of the time of reimbursement of the child with different type and degree of deafness and a consequent reduction of the associated disabilities.

Moreover, different economic studies underline that untreated hearing loss has a high social cost during the life (e.g., in the USA amount to $1.1 milion for person) and this cost decrease by 75% in case of early intervention and treatment [2]. Schulze-Gattermann showed that pediatric cochlear implantation provides positive cost-benefit ratios compared with hearing aid users especially if the child is implanted before the age of 2 years [3].

The benefits are not only economic but also in quality of life and school cost (moreover in country where there are special school for deaf people) [4].

Psychological reaction to a cochlear implant (CI) may be influenced by the temperament of the implanted subject [5].

More than 50% of the CHL is caused by genetic factors but it is difficult found the specific etiologic diagnosis. In fact, may be only one mutation in a specific gene or different mutations in different genes. Moreover may be an association with environmental prenatal factors (e.g., infections, prematurity, neonatal intensive care unit recovery).

Genetic hearing loss may be the only clinical feature (non-syndromic or isolated forms) or may be associated with other symptoms (syndromic forms).

Approximately 30% of the CHL considered syndromic and the remaining 70% being non-syndromic.

Non-syndromic hearing loss is extremely heterogeneous. About 80% of the cases are autosomal recessive, 15-24% are autosomal dominant and 1-2% are X-linked.

Typically, autosomal recessive hearing loss is congenital whereas autosomal dominant is often progressive.

The loci linked to non-syndromic CHL are conventionally named using a prefix followed by a suffix integer: DNFA for autosomal dominant loci, DFNB for autosomal recessive loci and DFN for X-linked loci.

The syndromic form can be differentiated from nonsyndromic hearing loss by the presence of associated symptoms in other organ systems. Syndrome that involve hearing loss are currently more than 400 and in some cases deafness is not present at birth but it appears later.

Know the different gene implicated in hearing loss is very important because it allows to give information, at the proband and his family, with specific genetic counselling about prognosis and recurrence. A genetic diagnosis is required also for choosing appropriate therapeutic options, for treating associated medical problem (in syndromic forms) and for predicting the progression of the degree.

Researcher and clinicians can always be informed about gene implicate in CHL (number, mutation and loci) consulting the Hereditary Hearing loss Homepage (http://hereditaryhearingloss.org) or http://ghr.nlm.nih.gov.

New treatments and screening strategies are available for identifying the responsive gene, e.g., Next Generation DNA sequencing and genetic panels that allow the simultaneous analysis of a large number of genes causing CHL with a higher probability of gene identification.

This paragraph will describe the different genes and clinical features involved in CHL both in isolated and in syndromic form.

Non Syndromic CHL

Non Syndromic CHL_Autosomal Recessive Hearing Loss

The loci and genes for non-syndromic, autosomal-recessive deafness are presented in Tables 1.

Table 1. Genes related with autosomal recessive non-syndromic congenital hearing loss

Locus	Gene	Chromosomal Location	Protein	Function
DFNB1	GJB2 GJB6	13q11–q12	Connexin 26 Connexin 30	Gap junction (ion haemostasis)
DFNB2	MYO7A	11q13.5	Myosin VIIa	Transport
DFNB3	MYO15	17p11.2	Myosin Xva	Transport
DFNB4	SLC26A4	7q31	Pendrin	Acid-base balance of endolymph (ion haemostasis)
DFNB5		14q12		
DFNB6	TMIE	3p21		
DFNB7	TMC1	9q13–q21		
DFNB8	TMPRSS3	21q22.3		
DFNB9	OTOF	2p23.1	Otoferlin	Fusion of synaptic vescicle with Ca^{+2}
DFNB10	TMPRSS3	21q22.3		
DFNB11		9q13–q21		
DFNB12	CDH23	10q21–q22	Cadherin 23	Lateran and tip links (adhesion)
DFNB13		7q34–q36		
DFNB14		7q31		
DFNB15		3q21.3–q25.2/19p13.3–p13.1		
DFNB16	STRC	15q15	Stereocilin	TM attachment links (adhesion)
DFNB17		7q31		
DFNB18	USH1C	11p15.1	Harmonin	Scaffolding protein (adhesion)
DFNB20		11q25–qter		
DFNB21	TECTA	11q23–q25	α-tectorin	Stability and structure of TM
DFNB22	OTOA	16p12.2	Otoancorin	TM attachment to nonsensory cell (adhesion)
DFNB23	PCDH15	10q21.1	Protocadherin 15	Lateran and tip links (adhesion)
DFNB27		2q23–q31		
DFNB29	CLDN14	21q22.1	Claudin 14	Tight junction
DFNB30	MYO3A	10p11.1	Myosin IIIA	Transport
DFNB31	WHRN	9q32–q34	Whirlin	Scaffolding protein (adhesion)
DFNB32		1p22.1–p13.3		
DFNB33		9q34.3		
DFNB35		14q24.1–q24.3		
DFNB36	ESPN	1p36.3	Espin	Actin crosslinking and bundling
DFNB37	MYO6	6q13	Myosin VI	Regualtion of exocytosis, stereocilia anchoring
DFNB38		6q26–q27		
DFNB39		7q11.22–q21.12		
DFNB40		22q11.21–q12.1		
DFNB42		3q13.31–q22.3		
DFNB44		7p14.1–q11.22		
DFNB46		18p11.32–p11.31		
DFNB48		15q23–q25.1		
DFNB49	TRIC	5q12.3–q14.1	Tricellulin	Tight junction
DFNB53	COL11A2	6p21.3	Type XI collagene α2	Stability and structure of TM
DFNB55		4q12–q13.2		
DFNB91	GJB3	1p35–p33	Connexin 31	Gap Junction (ion haemostasis)

GJB2 (Connexin 26) – DFNB1A

The most frequent isolated form of genetic hearing loss in white population of Europe and United States is the gap junction protein beta 2 gene (GJB2) mutation that is the gene encoding connexin 26. Mutations in the GJB2 gene are responsible for as much as 50% of pre-lingual, recessive deafness.

GJB2 gene is located on chromosome 13q11 (DFNB1) and it was described for the first time in 1994 but the first mutation in the locus were observed in 1997 [6].

Connexins are a large family of protein with four transmembrane domains, which have been implicated in gap-junctional intercellular communication. Connexins are membrane proteins and core components of gap junctions (GJs), which are intercellular communication channels that are important for recycling potassium ions from the hair cells to the endolymph during auditory transduction.

These proteins are present in the cell membranes of the epithelial cells and connective tissue of the cochlea and are responsible for maintaining an electrical potential in the cochlea thanks to an exchange of neurotransmitters, metabolites and potassium ions [7].

Gene inheritance are autosomal recessive in most cases; however, there are been reported forms with a autosomal dominace pattern of inheritance [8].

More than 300 mutations in the GJB2 gene are reported in the literatures and some of these are observed in various population: 35delG mutation in the Caucasian population, 235delC in the Asian population, 167delT in the Jewish population and p.Trp24 in population of India, Bangladesh, Slovenia and Romania.

Incidence varies in the different European country: it is highest in the Mediterranean country and lowest in the north. In fact, c.35delG allele accounted for 65.5% of mutated chromosomes in the south of Italy [9-11].

The 35delG mutation consists of a deletion of a guanine (G) in a sequence of six Gs extending from position 30–35 leading to a frameshift and premature stop codon at nucleotide 38 [12, 13].

GJB2 mutations are correlated to a neurosensorineural hearing loss of different degree dependent on genotype. It has been show that patients with two truncating mutations have significantly more severe hearing impairment than truncating/missense compound heterozygotes and that patients with two missense mutations have even less hearing impairment [14, 15].

GJB6 (Connexin 30) – DFNB1B

In the same locus of the GJB2 mutation (DFNB1), another gene, related to congenital hearing loss, has been found: GJB6.

Also this gene encoding for a gap-junction protein, connexin 30 (Cx30), that is expressed in the same inner-ear structures as connexion 26. In fact, both connexins are functionally related and Cx30 is co-expressed with Cx26 in the fibrocytes of the spiral ligament, basal cells of stria vascularis, spiral limbus, and supporting cells in the organ of Corti [16-18].

Genetic transmission is autosomal recessive and can be connected to either two GJB6 deletions (rare) or one GJB6 deletion and one GJB2 variant on opposite chromosome [19].

Mutation in Connexin 30 is characterized by bilateral and stable prelingual, mild-to-profound sensorineural hearing impairment and affected individuals have no other associated medical findings.

MYO7A (Myosin VIIA) – DFNB2

Myosins are a family of actin-based molecular motors that use energy from hydrolysis of ATP to generate mechanical force.

The function of the unconventional myosins is to regulate intracellular membrane traffic.

The MYO7A gene is a typical unconventional myosin consisting of 48 coding exons that is express in cochlea and in the retina of the mammalian.

Phenotype presentation is characterized by both vestibular dysfunction and hearing loss because in the inner ear, only the cochlear and vestibular sensory hair cells expressed the myosin VIIA gene.

Deafness is non-syndromic, congenital, profound and it is transmitted in autosomal-recessive manner [20].

MYO15A (Myosin XV) – DFNB3

MYO15A is a part of myosin family. In the inner ear, it has the function of the transportation of different proteins.

Mutation in this gene leads to a profound congenital hearing loss [21].

SLC26A4 (Pendrin) – DFNB4

Mutations in the *SLC26A4* gene are reported to be the most frequent cause of hereditary hearing loss in East Asia, and the second most common cause worldwide, after Connexin 26 (*GJB2*) gene mutations.

Mutations in the SLC26A4 gene are associated with two clinical pathway: Pendred syndrome or autosomal recessive non-syndromic deafness (DFNB4). Because of the variable expressivity and overlap of the clinical features, the two conditions may be considered as subsets of the spectrum of clinical manifestations of one single genetic entity.

Both disorders have similar audiologic characteristics which may be associated with abnormalities of the inner ear. In Pendred syndrome besides congenital sensorineural deafness, goiter or thyroid dysfunctions are frequently present.

The temporal bone abnormalities ranging from enlarged vestibular aqueduct (EVA) to Mondini dysplasia. To explain these abnormalities, it has been hypothesized that SLC26A4 controls fluid homeostasis in the membranous labyrinth, which in turn affects development of the bony labyrinth.

Hearing loss is common bilateral, often severe to profound degree with prelingual onset but, in some case deafness can arise in late childhood to early adulthood.

SLC26A4 gene encodes a transmembrane protein, pendrin, which functions as a transporter of chloride and iodide.

The human pendrin is expressed in the inner ear, mainly in endolymphatic sac and hair cells, and in the follicular cells of the thyroid.

Impaired function of pendrin was associated with endolymph acidification, leading to auditory sensory transduction defects. It is believed that its function in normal inner ear is related to pH homeostasis whereas in the thyroid, have a function in electroneutral iodide/chloride exchanger [22, 23].

OTOF (Otoferlin) – DFNB9

Mutations in the OTOF gene cause two disorders: nonsyndromic prelingual deafness and less frequently, temperature-sensitive nonsyndromic auditory neuropathy/dyssynchrony.

In auditory neuropathy auditory brain stem responses (ABRs) are absent and otoacoustic emissions (OAEs) are present but, however, with time OAEs disappear.

Deafness is bilateral, prelingual onset and with severe to profound degree and without inner-ear anomalies.

Otoferlin gene encoding for a transmembrane domain at the C-terminus predicted to have a cytoplasmic location and three Ca2þ-binding C2 domains. A function in Ca2þ-triggered synaptic vesicle membrane fusion was hypothesized [24].

CDH23 (Otocadherin) – DFNB12

The CDH23 gene is a very large gene that encodes for an intercellular adhesion protein (Otocadherin).

The study of Astuto et al. has been show that the DFNB12 phenotype demonstrated a large intra- and interfamilial variation, with hearing loss ranging from moderate to profound deafness and age at diagnosis between 3 months and 6 years [25].

USH1C (Harmonin) – DFNB18

The USH1C gene encodes a PDZ domain-containing protein, harmonin detecting in the sensory areas of the inner ear, especially in the cytoplasm and stereocilia of hair cells.

Mutations in this gene were described to cause congenital profound, non-syndromic, sensorineural deafness and severe balance deficits.

Alteration in USH1C gene is related to Usher syndrome the most frequent cause of combined deaf-blindness in man [26].

TECTA (α-Tectorin) – DFNB21

TECTA encodes α-tectorin, one of the major non-collagenous extracellular matrix components of the tectorial membrane that bridges the stereocilia bundles of the sensory hair cells. For this reasons, mutations in this gene have a dominant-negative effect that disrupts the structure of the tectorial membrane.

Mutations in the TECTA gene have been shown to be responsible for both autosomal dominant nonsyndromic hearing impairment and autosomal recessive sensorineural pre-lingual non-syndromic deafness [27].

COL11A2 (Collagen 11α2) – DFNB53

COL11A2 protein encodes the collagen type XI alpha-2. Mutations in this gene cause a non syndromic profound hearing loss can it be non-syndromic autosomal-dominant or autosomal-recessive [28].

Non Syndromic CHL_Autosomal Dominant Hearing Loss

On the contrary that the autosomal-recessive forms of deafness, autosomal-dominant forms are usually post-lingual and progressive [29].

The loci and genes for non-syndromic, autosomal-dominant deafness are presented in Tables 2.

Table 2. Genes related with autosomal dominant non-syndromic congenital hearing loss

Locus	Gene	Chromosomal Location	Protein	Function
DFNA1	DIAPH1	5q31	Diaphanous 1	Actin polymerisation (cytoskeleton)
DFNA2	KCNQ4 GJB3	1p34	KCNQ4 Connexin 31	Voltage-gated K⁺ channel Gap Junction (ion haemostasis)
DFNA3	GJB2 GJB6	13q12	Connexin 26 Connexin 30	Gap Junction (ion haemostasis)
DFNA4	MYH14	19q13	Nonmuscle myosin heavy chian XIV	Transport
DFNA5	DFNA5	7p15		
DFNA6	WFS1	4p16.3	wolframin	
DFNA7		1q21-q23		
DFNA8/12	TECTA	11q22-q24	A-tectorin	Stability and structure of TM
DFNA9	COCH	14q12-q13	Cochlin	Structures of the spiral limbus
DFNA10	EYA4	6q22-q23	Eyes absent 4	Regulation of transcription
DFNA11	MYO7A	11q12.3-q21	Myosin VIIa	Transport
DFNA13	COL11A2	6p21	Type XI collagen α2	Stability and structures of TM
DFNA14	WFS1	4p16.3	wolframin	
DFNA15	POU4F3	5q31	Class 3 POU	Regulation of transcription
DFNA16		2q23-q24.3		
DFNA17	MYH9	22q12.2-q13.3	Non muscle myosin heavy chain IX	transport
DFNA18		3q22		
DFNA20/26	ACTG1	17q25	γ-actin	Building cytoskeleton
DFNA21		6p21-p22		
DFNA22	MYO6	6q13	Myosin VI	Regulation of exocytosis, anchoring stereocilia
DFNA23		14q21-q22		
DFNA24		4q35-qter		
DFNA25	SLC17A8	12q21-q24	VGLUT-3	Regulation of exocytosis and endocytosis of glutamate
DFNA28	TFCP2L3	8q22	Transcription factors CP2-like 3	Regulation of transcription
DFNA30		15q25-q26		
DFNA36	TMC1	9q13-q21		
DFNA38	WFS1	4p16	wolframin	

DIAPH1 (Diaphanous) – DFNA1

Expression of DIAPH1 gene was demonstrated in many tissues including cochlea and skeletal muscle.

The gene DIAPH1 is involved in cytokinesis and establishment of cell polarity and the regulation of polymerization of actin (major component of the cytoskeleton of the hair Cells) is related to the role in hearing impairment [30].

KCNQ4 – DFNA2

Mutation in this gene affect potassium channels also present in the cochlea of mammalian provoke an alteration of the ion recycling into the endolymph at the level of the basolateral membrane of the outer hair cells.

Consequently, KCNQ4 gene mutation causes a progressive hearing loss more prominent in high frequencies [31].

GJB2 (Connexin 26) – DFNA3

Whereas the GJB2 gene is the major gene responsible for non-syndromic, recessive deafnes, there is some controversy as to the role of GJB2 in dominant deafness (DFNA3).

Autosomal-dominant hearing loss shows a different phenotype, consisting of pre-lingual to late-childhood onset, mild to profound, progressive hearing loss [32].

Mutations in the GJB2 gene are also responsible for autosomal-dominant syndrome with keratoderma and sensorineural deafness (Vohwinkel syndrome) and other forms of autosomal-dominant palmoplantar keratoderma with deafness [33].

TECTA (a-Tectorin) – DFNA8/DFNA12

TECTA gene encoding a non-collagenous component of the tectorial membrane in the inner ear (a-tectorin). Mutations of this gene disrupt the structure of the tectorial membrane, leading to inefficient transmission of sound to the mechanosensitive stereociliary bundles of the hair cells [34].

The hearing loss was congenital, non-progresive, moderate to severe, involved mainly the middle frequencies.

EYA4 – DFNA10

EYA4 is part of family transcriptional activators protein (EYA1-4) that facilitate normal embryonic development. Mutation in EYA1 causes BOR (Brachio-Oto-Renal) syndrome whereas mutation in EYA4 causes isolated hearing loss.

Deafness is progressive, moderate to profound and bilateral [35].

WFS1 – DFNA 6/14/38

WFS1 encodes a transmembrane protein (wolframin) the function of which is currently unknown.

In the most part of the cases, mutation in WFS1 is responsible for Wolfram syndrome but can be, also, a cause of non-syndromic low-frequency sensorineural hearing loss.

In this non syndromic case deafness is characterized by slowly progressive, low-frequency (<2000 Hz) sensorineural hearing loss [36].

SYNDROMIC CHL

Syndromic CHL_Autosomal Recesive Hearing Loss

Usher Syndrome

Usher syndrome prevalence ranging from 1/6000 to 1/10000 and it represent the 3-5% of infant hearing loss.

It is characterised by bilateral hearing loss and visual deficiency (until the blindness).

There are three subtypes based on severity of the deafness, vestibular dysfunction and the onset of visual impairment: USH1, USH2 and USH3.

Visual deficiency is due to retinitis pigmentosa: a gradual retinal degeneration leading to decreased night vision, loss of peripheral vision, and blindness.

In USH1 subtype can be found severe to profound congenital hearing loss, congenital vestibular dysfunction and progressive to severe blindness (started with might blindness in childhood).

Table 3. Genes associated with Usher syndrome subtypes

Subtype	Genes	Protein	Protein Function
USH1B	MYO7A	Myosin VIIA	Actin-based motor protein
USH1C	USH1C	Harmonin	scaffold protein
USH1D	CDH23	Cadherin23	Cell adhesion
USH1F	PCDH15	Protocadherin 15	Cell adhesion
USH1G	USH1G	SANS	Scaffold protein
USH1J	CIB2	CIB2	Calcium and integrin binding protein 2
USH2A	USH2A	usherin	Cell adhesion
USH2C	GPR98	VLGR1	Adhesion G protein-couple receptor VI
USH2D	DFNB31	whirlin	scaffold protein
USH3A	CLRN1	Clarin1	Auxiliary subunit of ion channels

USH2 patients have moderate to severe CHL, no vestibular dysfunction and retinitis pigmentosa started between the ages 10 to 40.

In the USH3 subtype there are progressive hearing loss, variable vestibular dysfunction and retinitis pigmentosa started from the age of 20.

The gene and loci associated with Usher syndrome is show in Table 3 [37].

Pendred Syndrome

Prevalence of Pendred syndrome is 7.5/100.000 newborns.

Pendred syndrome comprises a phenotypic spectrum of sensorineural hearing loss (SNHL), vestibular dysfunction and abnormal iodine metabolism.

SNHL is usually bilateral, progressive, from mild to profound degree and can be congenital or with a later onset.

Frequently there are associated temporal bone abnormalities (enlarged vestibular aqueduct with or without cochlear hypoplasia).

Abnormal iodine metabolism develop euthyroid goiter sometimes detected at birth, but often not clinically evident until 8 years of age. Often this patient have thyroid dysfunction, ranging from euthyroid to hypothyroidism.

In at least 50% of patients with Pendred syndrome, the molecular diagnosis is established by identification of biallelic pathogenic variants in SLC26A4 or double heterozygosity for one pathogenic variant in SLC26A4 and one pathogenic variant in either FOXI1 or KCNJ10 [38, 39].

Jervell and Lange-Nielsen Syndrome

It is estimate that prevalence of Jervell and Lange-Nielsen syndrome is 1.6 to 6 per 1.000.000 people worldwide.

This syndrome is characterized by severe-profound hearing loss, prolongation of the QT interval at basal ECG and sometimes T-waves abnormalities, and by an increased susceptibility to life-threatening ventricular arrhythmias.

KCNQ1, KCNE1 are the gene associated with the syndrome and they encode potassium channels found in the stria vascularis of the cochlea and in the heart [40].

Wolfram Syndrome

This syndrome is characterized by diabetes mellitus, diabetes insipidus, optic atrophy and deafness.

Often there are progressive neurologic abnormalities (cerebellar ataxia, peripheral neuropathy, dementia, psychiatric illness, and urinary tract atony), and other endocrine abnormalities

Sensorineural hearing loss is slow progressive emerging in late childhood. Median age at death is 30 years [41].

Pompe Disease

Pompe disease is a rare multi-systemic metabolic myopathy associated at conductive or sensorineural hearing loss in almost 50% of the cases.

This syndrome is caused by autosomal recessive mutations in the acidic alpha glucosidase (GAA) gene [42].

Syndromic CHL_Autosomal Dominant Hearing Loss

Waardenburg Syndrome

Prevalence of the Waardenburg syndrome is 1/42.000 and it represents 2-5% of infant hearing loss.

This syndrome is characterized by sensorineural hearing loss, abnormal pigmentation of the skin and hair, dystopia canthorum, heterochromia iridis and pinched nose.

There are four subtypes based on the presence or absence of the additional symptoms: WS1, WS2, WS3 and WS4.

WS1 and WS2 are the most frequent and WS1 is characterized by dystopia canthorum, wide-set eyes. WS3 is characterized by dystopia canthorum and musculoskeletal abnormalities of the upper limbs whereas WS4 is associated with Hirschprung diseases.

Gene involved in WS1 is PAX3 and MITF in WS2, these genes are involved in the regulation of melanocyte [43].

Brachio-Oto-Renal Syndrome

Brachio-Oto-Renal (BOR) syndrome is characterized by sensorineural or conductive hearing loss, cup-shaped pinnae, preauricular pits, branchial cleft fistulae and bilateral renal anomalies.

Prevalence of this disease is 1/40.000 and it is 2% of infant hearing loss [44].

Stickler Syndrome

Stickler syndrome is characterized by progressive sensorineural hearing loss with cleft palate, abnormal development of the epiphysis, vertebral abnormalities and osteoarthritis; myopathy, retinal detachment and vitreoretinal degeneration (only in Types 1 and 3).

The prevalence is about 7/7.500 to 1/9.000 newborns.

There are five subtypes based on the collagene gene involved: in type I COL2A1 is involved, COL11A1 in Type II and COL11A2 in Type III. Types IV and V are transmitted in recessive autosomal manner [45].

Treacher Collins Syndrome

Treacher Collins syndrome is characterized by microtia and malformed ears, midface hypoplasia, downslanting palpebral fissures, coloboma of outer 1/3 of lower eyelids, and micrognathia.

TCOF1, POLR1C and POLR1D are the three genes associated to this syndrome [46].

Syndromic CHL_X-Linked Hearing Loss

Alport Syndrome

Alport syndrome is characterizeb by progressive sensorineural hearing loss, renal disorders (glomerulonephritis, haematuria (and renal failure) and ocular abnormalities.

COL4A3, COL4A4 and COL4A5 are the three genes associated with Alport syndrome. All encoding for a collagen protein [47].

CONCLUSION

A genetic diagnosis for congenital hearing loss is required for different reasons, in particular for choosing appropriate therapeutic options, for treating associated medical problem (syndromic forms) and for predicting the progression of the degree [48].

New treatments and screening strategies are available for identifying the responsive gene, e.g., Next Generation DNA sequencing that allows the simultaneous analysis of a large number of genes causing CHL with a higher probability of gene identification.

REFERENCES

[1] IJA 2012; 51:512-528.
[2] Keren, R., Helfand, M., Homer, C., McPhillips, H., and Lieu, T. A. (2002) Projected cost-effectiveness of statewide universal newborn hearing screening. *Pediatrics,* 110 (5): 855–864.
[3] Schulze-Gattermann, H., Illg, A., Schoenermark, M., Lenarz, T., Lesinski-Schiedat, A. (2002) Cost-benefit analysis of pediatric cochlear implantation: German experience. *Otol Neurotol.,* Sep; 23(5):674-81.
[4] Martini, A., Bovo, R., Trevisi, P., Forli, F., Berrettini, S. (2013) Cochlear implant in children: rational, indications and cost/efficacy. *Minerva Pediatr.,* Jun; 65(3):325-39.

[5] Mento, C., Galletti, F., Freni, F., Logo, P., Testini, G., Rizzo, A., Settineri, S. (2016) The role of temperament in traumatic hearing loss: a single case study of a cochlear-implanted patient. *International Journal of Adolescent Medicine and Health.* 28 (1): 107-13.

[6] Guilford, P., Ben Arab, S., Blanchard, S., Levilliers, J., Weissenbach, J., Belkahia, A., Petit, C. (1994) A non-syndrome form of neurosensory, recessive deafness maps to the pericentromeric region of chromosome 13q. *Nat Genet.,* Jan; 6 (1): 24-8.

[7] Mielczarek, M., Zakrzewska, A., Olszewski, J. (2016) GJB2 sequencing in deaf and profound sensorineural hearing loss children. *Otolaryngol Pol.,* Jun 30; 70(3): 21-5.

[8] Kelsell, D. P., Dunlop, J., Stevens, H. P., Lench, N. J., Liang, J. N., Parry, G., Mueller, R. F., Leigh, I. M. (1997) Connexin 26 mutations in hereditary non-syndromic sensorineural deafness. *Nature,* May 1; 387(6628): 80-3.

[9] Amorini, M., Romeo, P., Bruno, R., Galletti, F., Di Bella, C., Longo, P., Briuglia, S., Salpietro, C., Rigoli, L. (2015) Prevalence of Deafness-Associated Connexin-26 (GJB2) and Connexin-30 (GJB6) Pathogenic Alleles in a Large Patient Cohort from Eastern Sicily. *Ann Hum Genet.,* Sep; 79 (5): 341-349.

[10] Martines, F., Salvago, P., Bartolotta, C., Cocuzza, S., Fabiano, C., Ferrara, S., La Mattina, E., Mucia, M., Sammarco, P., Sireci, F., Martines, E. (2015) A genotype–phenotype correlation in Sicilian patients with GJB2 biallelic mutations. *European Archives of Oto-Rhino-Laryngology,* 272 (8), pp. 1857-1865.

[11] Bartolotta, C., Salvago, P., Cocuzza, S., Fabiano, C., Sammarco, P., Martines, F. (2014) Identification of D179H, a novel missense GJB2 mutation in a Western Sicily family. *European Archives of Oto-Rhino-Laryngology,* 271 (6), pp. 1457-1461.

[12] Zelante, L., Gasparini, P., Estivill, X., et al. (1997) Connexin26 mutations associated with the most common form of non-syndromic neurosensory autosomal recessive deafness (DFNB1) in Mediterraneans. *Hum Mol Genet;* 6: 1605–1609.

[13] Denoyelle, F., Weil, D., Maw, M. A. et al. (1997) Prelingual deafness: high prevalence of a 30delG mutation in the connexin 26 gene. *Hum Mol Genet*; 6: 2173–2177.

[14] Snoeckx, R. L., Huygen, P. L., Feldmann, D., Marlin, S., Denoyelle, F., Waligora, J., Mueller-Malesinska, M., Pollak, A., Ploski, R., Murgia, A., Orzan, E., Castorina, P., Ambrosetti, U., Nowakowska-Szyrwinska, E., Bal, J., Wiszniewski, W., Janecke, A. R., Nekahm-Heis, D., Seeman, P., Bendova, O., Kenna, M. A., Frangulov, A., Rehm, H. L., Tekin, M., Incesulu, A., Dahl, H. H., du Sart, D., Jenkins, L., Lucas, D., Bitner-Glindzicz, M., Avraham, K. B., Brownstein, Z., del Castillo, I., Moreno, F., Blin, N., Pfister, M., Sziklai, I., Toth, T., Kelley, P. M., Cohn, E. S., Van Maldergem, L., Hilbert, P., Roux, A. F., Mondain, M., Hoefsloot, L. H., Cremers, C. W., Löppönen, T., Löppönen, H., Parving, A., Gronskov, K.,

Schrijver, I., Roberson, J., Gualandi, F., Martini, A., Lina-Granade, G., Pallares-Ruiz, N., Correia, C., Fialho, G., Cryns, K., Hilgert, N., Van de Heyning, P., Nishimura, C. J., Smith, R. J., Van Camp, G. (2005) GJB2 mutations and degree of hearing loss: a multicenter study. *Am J Hum Genet.* Dec; 77(6): 945-57.

[15] Salvago, P., Martines, E., La Mattina, E., Mucia, M., Sammarco, P., Sireci, F., Martines, F. (2014) Distribution and phenotype of GJB2 mutations in 102 Sicilian patients with congenital non syndromic sensorineural hearing loss. *International Journal of Audiology,* 53 (8), pp. 558-563.

[16] Del Castillo, I., Villamar, M., Moreno-Pelayo, M. A., del Castillo, F. J., Alvarez, A., Tellería, D., Menéndez, I., Moreno, F. A. (2002) Deletion involving the connexin 30 gene in nonsyndromic hearing impairment. *N Engl J Med.* Jan 24; 346 (4): 243-9.

[17] J. Sun, S. Ahmad, S. Chen, W. Tang, Y. Zhang, P. Chen, X. Lin. (2005) Cochlear gap junctions coassembled from Cx26 and 30 show faster intercellular Ca_2+ signaling than homomeric counterparts, *Am. J. Physiol. Cell Physiol.*; 288: C613–C623.

[18] Oh, S. K., Choi, S. Y., Yu, S. H., Lee, K. Y., Hong, J. H., Hur, S. W., Kim, S. J., Jeon, C. J., Kim, U. K. (2013) Valuation of the pathogenicity of GJB3 and GJB6 variants associated with nonsyndromic hearing loss. *Biochim Biophys Acta.* Jan; 1832 (1): 285-91.

[19] Petersen, M. B., Willems, P. (2006) Non-syndromic, autosomal-recessive deafness. *J Clin Genet.* May; 69 (5): 371-92.

[20] Weil, D., Lévy, G., Sahly, I., Lévi-Acobas, F., Blanchard, S., El-Amraoui, A., Crozet, F., Philippe, H., Abitbol, M., Petit, C. (1996) Human myosin VIIA responsible for the Usher 1B syndrome: a predicted membrane-associated motor protein expressed in developing sensory epithelia. *Proc Natl Acad Sci USA*; 93: 3232–3237.

[21] Robertson, N. G., Lu, L., Heller, S., Merchant, S. N., Eavey, R. D., McKenna, M., Nadol, J. B. Jr, Miyamoto, R. T., Linthicum, F. H. Jr, Lubianca Neto, J. F., Hudspeth, A. J., Seidman, C. E., Morton, C. C., Seidman, J. G. (1998) Mutations in a novel cochlear gene cause DFNA9, a human nonsyndromic deafness with vestibular dysfunction. *Nat Genet.* Nov; 20 (3): 299-303.

[22] Everett, L. A., Morsli, H., Wu, D. K., Green, E. D. (1999) Expression pattern of the mouse ortholog of the Pendred's syndrome gene (Pds) suggests a key role for pendrin in the inner ear. *Proc Natl Acad Sci USA.* 96: 9727–9732.

[23] Wémeau, J. L., Kopp, P. (2017) Pendred syndrome. *Best Pract Res Clin Endocrinol Metab.* Mar; 31 (2): 213-224.

[24] Yasunaga, S., Grati, M., Cohen-Salmon, M., El-Amraoui, A., Mustapha, M., Salem, N., El-Zir, E., Loiselet, J., Petit, C. (1999) A mutation in OTOF, encoding otoferlin,

a FER-1-like protein, causes DFNB9, a nonsyndromic form of deafness. *Nat Genet;* 21: 363–369.

[25] Astuto, L. M., Bork, J. M., Weston, M. D., Askew, J. W., Fields, R. R., Orten, D. J., Ohliger, S. J., Riazuddin, S., Morell, R. J., Khan, S., Riazuddin, S., Kremer, H., Van Hauwe, P., Moller, C. G., Cremers, C. W. R. J., Ayuso, C., Heckenlively, J. R., Rohrschneider, K., Spandau, U., Greenberg, J., Ramesar, R., Reardon, W., Bitoun, P., Millan, J., Legge, R., Friedman, T. B., Kimberling, W. J. (2002) CDH23 mutation and phenotype heterogeneity: a profile of 107 diverse families with Usher syndrome and nonsyndromic deafness. *Am J Hum Genet;* 71: 262–275.

[26] Reiners, J., van Wijk, E., Märker, T., Zimmermann, U., Jürgens, K., te Brinke, H., Overlack, N., Roepman, R., Knipper, M., Kremer, H., Wolfrum, U. (2005) Scaffold protein harmonin (USH1C) provides molecular links between Usher syndrome type 1 and type 2. *Hum Mol Genet.* Dec 15; 14 (24): 3933-43.

[27] Legan, P. K., Lukashkina, V. A., Goodyear, R. J., Kössl, M., Russell, I. J., Richardson, G. P. (2000) A targeted deletion in alpha-tectorin reveals that the tectorial membrane is required for the gain and timing of cochlear feedback. *Neuron;* 28: 273–285.

[28] Chen, W., Kahrizi, K., Meyer, N. C., Riazalhosseini, Y., Van Camp, G., Najmabadi, H., Smith, R. J. (2005) Mutation of COL11A2 causes autosomal recessive non-syndromic hearing loss at the DFNB53 locus. *J Med Genet;* 42: e61.

[29] Petersen, M. B. (2002) Non-syndromic autosomal-dominant deafness. *Clin Genet;* 62: 1–13

[30] Lynch, E. D., Lee, M. K., Morrow, J. E., Welcsh, P. L., León, P. E., King, M. C. (1997) Nonsyndromic deafness DFNA1 associated with mutation of a human homolog of the drosophila gene diaphanous. *Science;* 278: 1315–1318.

[31] Kubisch, C., Schroeder, B. C., Friedrich, T., Lütjohann, B., El-Amraoui, A., Marlin, S., Petit, C., Jentsch, T .J. (1999) KCNQ4, a novel potassium channel expressed in sensory outer hair cells, is mutated in dominant deafness. *Cell*; 96: 437–446.

[32] Chaib, H., Lina-Granade, G., Guilford, P., Plauchu, H., Levilliers, J., Morgon, A., Petit, C. (1994) A gene responsible for a dominant form of neurosensory nonsyndromic deafness maps to the NSRD1 recessive deafness gene interval. *Hum Mol Genet.* 3: 2219–2222.

[33] Kelsell, DPW-L., Houseman, M. J. (2001) Connexin mutations in skin disease and hearing loss. *Am J Hum Genet;* 68: 559–568.

[34] Verhoeven, K., Van Laer, L., Kirschhofer, K., et al., (1998) Mutations in the human a-tectorin gene cause autosomal dominant non-syndromic hearing impairment. *Nat Genet;* 19: 60–62.

[35] Hildebrand, M. S., Coman, D., Yang, T., Gardner, R. J., Rose, E., Smith, R. J., Bahlo, M., Dahl, H. H. (2007) A novel splice site mutation in EYA4 causes DFNA10 hearing loss. *Am J Med Genet A.* Jul 15; 143A(14): 1599-604.

[36] Young, T. L., Ives, E., Lynch, E., Person, R., Snook, S., MacLaren, L., Cater, T., Griffin, A., Fernandez, B., Lee, M. K., King, M. C. (2001) Non-syndromic progressive hearing loss DFNA38 is caused by heterozygous missense mutation in the Wolfram syndrome gene WFS1. *Hum Mol Genet;* 10: 2509–2514.

[37] Mathur, P., Yang, J. (2015) Usher syndrome: Hearing loss, retinal degeneration and associated abnormalities. *Biochim Biophys Acta.* Mar; 1852 (3): 406-20.

[38] Reardon, W., Trembath, R. C. (1996) Pendred syndrome. *J Med Genet.* Dec; 33 (12):1037-40.

[39] Bruno, R., Aversa, T., Catena, M., Valenzise, M., Lombardo, F., De Luca, F., Wasniewska, M. (2015) Even in the era of congenital hypothyroidism screening mild and subclinical sensorineural hearing loss remains a relatively common complication of severe congenital hypothyroidism. *Hearing Research* September; 327: 43-47.

[40] Martini, A., Volo, T., Ghiselli, S. (2011) Heart problems and deafness: Are they more common than supposed? *Audiological Medicine;* 9 (1): 1-3.

[41] Karzon, R., Narayanan, A., Chen, L., Lieu, J. E. C., Hershey, T. (2018) Longitudinal hearing loss in Wolfram syndrome. *Orphanet J Rare Dis.* Jun;13(1):102.

[42] Musumeci, O., Catalano, N., Barca, E., Ravaglia, S., Fiumara, A., Gangemi, G., Rodolico, C., Sorge, G., Vita, G., Galletti, F., Toscano, A. (2012) Auditory system involvement in late onset Pompe disease: A study of 20 Italian patients. *Molecular Genetics and Metabolism;* 107 (3): 480-484.

[43] Read, A. P., Newton, V. E. (1997) Waardenburg syndrome. *J Med Gen*; 34: 656-655.

[44] Smith, R. J. H. (1993) Branchiootorenal Spectrum Disorders. In: Pagon, R. A.; Adam, M. P.; Ardinger, H. H., et al., editors. *Gene Reviews (R).* Seattle (WA).

[45] Rose, P. S., Levy, H. P., Liberfarb, R. M., Davis, J., Szymko-Bennett, Y., Rubin, B. I., Tsilou, E., Griffith, A. J., Francomano, C. A. (2005) Stickler syndrome: clinical characteristics and diagnostic criteria. *Am J Med Genet A.;* 138A:199–207.

[46] Kadakia, S., Helman, S. N., Badhey, A. K., Saman, M., Ducic, Y. (2014) Treacher Collins Syndrome: the genetics of a craniofacial disease. *Int J Pediatr Otorhinolaryngol.;* 78: 893–898.

[47] Koffler, T, Ushakov, K., Avraham, K. B. (2015) Genetics of Hearing Loss – Syndromic. *Otolaryngol Clin North Am.*; 48 (6): 1041–1061.

[48] Martines, F., Maira, E., Ferrara, S. (2011) Age-related hearing impairment (ARHI): A common sensory deficit in the elderly. *Acta Medica Mediterranea*, 27 (1), 47-52.

Chapter 4

NEUROPLASTICITY AND SENSORINEURAL HEARING LOSS

Francesco Dispenza[1,2,*]*, MD, PhD, Alessia Maria Battaglia*[2]*, MD, Gabriele Ebbreo*[2]*, MD, Alessia Ceraso*[2]*, MD, Vito Pontillo*[3]*, MD and Antonina Mistretta*[2]*, MD*

[1]Istituto Euromediterraneo di Scienza e Tecnologia – IEMEST, Palermo, Italy
[2]U. O. C. Otorinolaringoiatria Azienda Ospedaliera Universitaria Policlinico P. Giaccone, Palermo, Italy
[3]Otolayngology Unit, Department of Basic Medical Science, Neuroscience and Sensory Organs, University of Bari Aldo Moro, Bari, Italy

ABSTRACT

Neuroplasticity is the ability of central nervous system to modify his own functions based on changes of external or internal factors, and it's the basis for numerous physiologic and pathologic events in otology. Sensorineural hearing loss implies a cochlear deficit but also modifications from acoustic tract up to auditory cortex. It determines morphofunctional changes, through neuroplasticity, that may be influenced by cochlear implants and hearing aids. There are many trials that shown a remarkable hearing development in deaf infant after cochlear implant or usage of hearing aids. However, many questions remain around the right time to act, due to the greatest neuronal response in younger children. Animal experimentation has shown also tonotopic changes in cortical and subcortical areas after cochlear lesions, that depends upon age and damage extension, as neuronal reorganization differ from neonatal and adults. In this chapter we'll discuss about central neuronal network modifications, after sensorineural hearing loss, emphasizing clinical consequences, in particular the usefulness of early diagnosis and rapid treatment.

---

[*] Corresponding Author's Email: francesco.dispenza@gmail.com.

Keywords: neural plasticity, hearing loss, deafness, neuroplasticity, brain

INTRODUCTION TO NEUROPLASTICITY

Since Rita Levi Montalcini's studies on anatomic changes to auditory pathways after experimental lesions of chick embryo, neuroplasticity has been widely recognized, and with that neuronal capacity to change itself in reaction to stimuli and lesions (Levi-Montalcini 1949). Mechanisms of neural plasticity have been the focus of interest in research for many decades. Plasticity is based in part on changes in synaptic function (synaptic plasticity), on change in synchronization in the neuronal networks, and on change in inter-neuronal connection patterns within neuronal networks (Thomas et al., 2018, Martines et al., 2015).

This may be associated on synaptic strengthening as postulated by Hebb's studies. Exactly as he said "When an axon of cell A is near enough to excite a cell B and repeatedly or persistently takes part in firing it, some growth process or metabolic change takes place in one or both cells such that *A*'s efficiency, as one of the cells firing *B*, is increased. The synaptic strengthen works through changes in pre-synaptic and postsynaptic areas. It could work on augmented release probability of neurotransmitters, incremented number of release sites or vesicles n the pre-synaptic neuron, while on receptor sensitivity and quantity of elicitable receptors in the post-synaptic neuron (Wang, Ko, and Kelly 1997).

This phenomenon may also explain the way of *Central Nervous System (CNS)* development, through the repeated stimulation of genetically determined neural pathway that leads improvement and development of some functions. A neuron is linked to many different other neurons but is activated just by some.

Neuroplasticity may explain the phantom limb's etiology or in auditory area, tinnitus's etiology. Certain types of tinnitus could arise from auditory neurons that somehow develop self-perpetuating activity. With our understanding that the brain is full of networks it is easy to conceive of local circuits being reinforced to the point of reverberation that in the auditory cortex may determine tinnitus (Eggermont 2012). Also the vestibular compensation after an issue involving one of the vestibular organs should be related to the neural plasticity (Lorusso et al., 2017, Dispenza et al., 2015, Dispenza, Kulamarva, and De Stefano 2012, Dispenza and De Stefano 2012, Dispenza et al., 2011).

Neuroplasticity is heavily studied on its variability during lifespan. The capacity for reorganization of the brain is more extensive during development. Especially in neonatal age comes a gargantuan synaptogenesis that last until the five years of age, followed by a dendritic pruning. Therefore comes the children ability to learn and grow at wonderful speed. An explanation may be that, in developing animals, due to immaturity of neuronal membranes and ionic channels, cortical postsynaptic potentials are known to have a longer duration. This has the effect of naturally boosting synaptic plasticity, as individual postsynaptic potentials can more easily temporally overlap. Temporal summation can by that cause a strong depolarization of postsynaptic cells. The eventual consequence of this effect is higher plasticity during early development. This phenomenon has a clinical effect, since most aspects of learning and intellectual functions may be acquired only in earlier age.

NEUROPLASTICITY IN THE AUDITORY SYSTEM

The neuroplasticity of the auditory system was object of study of expert otologists all over the world, in order to understand the mechanism and the relationship with different area of *CNS* (Dispenza et al., 2011, De Stefano et al., 2011, De Stefano, Kulamarva, and Dispenza 2012).

It has been shown that a pre-lingual sensorineural hearing loss may cause cognitive and relational developmental deficits; while in adults the development of an auditory deficit is associated with dementia and decreased attention (Contrera et al., 2017, Salvago et al., 2017). Alterations of cerebral white and gray matter have been reported in patients with hearing loss (Yang et al., 2014). Focal deficits of the white matter of the superior temporal gyrus for deaf children in prelingual age and volumetric decreases in gray matter in areas adjacent to the auditory cortex in individuals with bilateral hearing loss were demonstrated (Husain et al., 2011). Yang compared T1 weighted sequences and task free fMRIs of 14 adult patients with hearing impairments of moderate severity and 19 controls: Voxel based morphometry *(VBM)* showed decreased gray matter volume in bilateral posterior cingulate, lingual and the amplitude of low frequency fluctuation, calculated to analyze brain activity, was decreased in bilateral precuneus, left inferior parietal lobule, right inferior frontal gyrus and insula, and increased in right inferior and middle temporal gyrus (Figure 1) (Yang et al., 2014).

Boyen also applied VBM analyses to MRIs of normal-hearing control subjects, hearing-impaired subjects without tinnitus and hearing-impaired subjects with tinnitus. The two hearing impaired groups had well matched audiograms for frequencies of 8 kHz. VBM analyses revealed that both hearing impaired groups, compared to healthy controls, had GM volume increased in the superior and middle temporal gyrus and limbic areas and decreased in the superior frontal gyrus, frontal areas, occipital lobe and hypothalamus (Boyen et al., 2013).

Increased amplitude of low frequency fluctuation may determine a neuroplastic change in response to hearing loss. Many reviews showed that hearing loss brain adapt through unimodal and cross-modal plasticity (Kral 2007).

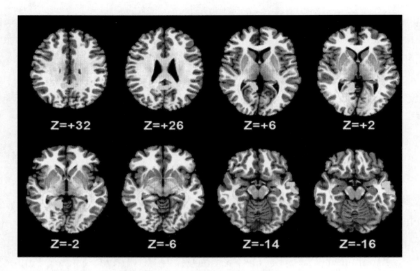

Figure 1. Brain areas with decreased gray matter. Modified from: Yang et al., Hearing Research 316 (2014) 37-43.

UNIMODAL PLASTICITY

Unimodal plasticity is the capacity of changing the neuronal pathway inside a single area; in the auditory area it mostly deal with tonotopic modifications and relations between primary auditory cortex and higher order cortex. It's a good idea to propose Merzenich studies on deaf cats.

An experiment studied cats treated shortly after birth with the ototoxic aminoglycoside amikacin, which resulted in a basal cochlear hair cells lesion. Though ABR evaluations it was assessed that the stimuli for low frequency sounds could still be transmitted, but it was gone for high frequency sound. Over time, auditory cortex showed normal representation of low frequencies, but the cortical region deprived of normal input by the partial cochlear deafferentation now contains neurons that are all tuned to 6 to 8 kHz. Thus there was an abnormally overrepresentation of the still captable frequency in the auditory cortex. Also, one of these subjects however showed an injury both on basal and apical cochlea. This kitten also developed a cortical frequency map in which there was a very large iso-frequency area where all neurons have a common 6.6-kHz frequency tuning (Kaas, Merzenich, and Killackey 1983).

Qualitatively, similar results are also found at the cortical level if the lesions are made in an adult animal, as showed by Robertson and Irvine studies and many others. At the level of the auditory cortex, after cochlear lesions were induced in the adult animal, the pattern of reorganization of tonotopic maps was similar to that of the developing neonate (Rajan and Irvine 1998). However, intuitively, considerable differences should be expected in the extent of the cortical tonotopic map reorganization in subjects with lesions made in early development compared with those made in adulthood since the importance of early sensory stimulation in driving the development of the mature brain has already been discussed. In fact, if we study the subcortical reorganization in adult and developmental animals many differences may be exposed.

It was showed that determining a cochlear lesion in a developmental animals lead to subcortical modifications along the auditory brain steam, with a tonotopic map reorganization, at inferiors colliculi and thalamo particularly, in large part reflecting what occurs at cortical level. Such subcortical reorganization apparently does not occur for similar lesions made in the adult. The age of induction of hearing loss, neonatal, childhood or adult does not appear to affect the outcome; increased spontaneous ring rates, increased neural synchrony and reorganization of the cortical tonotopic map (Harrison 2001).

Therefore neonatal induced hearing loss also results in reorganization of the tonotopic map in the inferior colliculus, which does not occur after adult acquired hearing loss (Eggermont 2017).

Dealing with neural pathway modifications between higher order auditory cortex and primary auditory cortex, we should remember that higher order auditory cortex maturity come necessarily from long term hearing experience, especially in developmental subject. We can expose Sharma's studies on prelingual deaf children. It showed in early implanted deaf childern an increasing amplitude and decreasing latency of wave P1 and an appearance of wave N1 with cochlear implant stimulation, whereas late-implanted children, especially those implanted in late teens, do not develop wave N1. Since N1 wave is generated in the higher order cortex we can assume that without auditory stimuli in early age, those areas doesn't develop and become significantly compromised (Sharma et al., 2002). Also, higher order cortex tends to reorganize cross-modally, leading to interaction with visual, and possibly others areas, in an attempt to compensate through visual and other stimuli to the auditory deficit.

CROSS-MODAL PLASTICITY

Cross modal plasticity works with connections between different areas. In Bertrand and Sharma studies, it was proved an higher order auditory cortex activation in response to a radial modulated visual grating stimulus giving the effect of apparent motion, in prelingual deaf children with cochlear implants, using CVEP. While normally hearing children show cortical activation of areas tipically associated with visual procession, while the CI children demonstrated additional activation of right lateral temporal cortex for the higher order N1 and P2 CVEP components (e.g., right inferior, middle, and superior temporal gyrus). Furthermore, speech perception performance in background noise using a clinical test (BKB SIN) was significantly negatively correlated with CVEP latency for CI children, such that poorer speech perception was associated with earlier CVEP N1 latency However, it appears that auditory reactivity is maintained despite cross-modal re-organization by vision (Bertrand et al., 2012).

Sandamn showed that even in adult crossmodal plasticity happens as well, since its studies showed an increased activation in the auditory cortex during CVEP, in both prelingually and postlingually deaf adults compared to the normal hearing group. Also increased CVEP amplitude over temporal cortex is associated with poor speech perception in quiet and noise environment (Chen et al., 2016).

Currently it is not well defined how long it takes to develop cross-modal plasticity in adults. A case report study showed a visual activaction of auditory cortex at least three months after sudden hearing loss, which increased over time, up to increasing its efficiency up to one year. Interestingly, there was a positive association between N1 amplitude at CVEP and speech perception. These findings are from a single case study and they should be interpreted cautiously (Glick and Sharma 2017).

Another area related to higher order cortex of deaf patients in cross modal plasticity it's the post-central gyrus of somatosensory cortex. As in, numerous studies showed a simultaneous activation of both somatosensory and auditory area cortical during cortical somatosensory evoked potentials (CSSEP) and, when treated with cochlear implants, even in cortical auditory evoked potentials (CAEP) In this case, findings of cross modal plasticity are related to poor speech perception performance as well (Cardon and Sharma 2018).

Even if visual cortex may be recruited by higher order auditory cortex, to evolve speech and communication by other mean than auditory input in hearing loss, many doubts remain over usefulness of somatosensory recruitment and many authors suggest this may happen, instead of a functional modification, due to close proximity of somatosensory and auditory cortices and the overlapping of somatosensory and auditory neurons subcortically, as a result of hearing impairment (Glick and Sharma 2017).

Cross modal plasticity take part also in relations to contralateral auditory cortex as in Khosla et al., study, especially in unilateral hearing loss (Khosla et al., 2003).

Normal-hearing subjects show significant latency and amplitude differences between ipsilateral and contralateral peaks for all components of the CAEP, with contralateral source activities that were typically larger and peaked earlier than the ipsilateral activities. However, in unilateral hearing loss, the patients showed a reduction of both amplitude and latency differences, when the best hearing ear was stimulated. Thus, unilateral hearing loss leads to a more synchronous and symmetrical activation of the auditory cortex (Eggermont 2017).

All this studies showed the higher order auditory cortex is the main protagonist of cross-modal plasticity as it's the one to get in relation both with visual and somatosensory auditory cortex, but also with frontal area and controlateral auditory area. It takes parts in language development and speech perception, it's heavely binded to the auditory input in normal people, even if it's relation with the visual and other area it's already proved by McGurk effect. However in absence of hearing experiece, the representation between higher order cortex and primary order cortex remain to a rudimentary level, and the higher order cortex due to their strong inputs also from nonauditory areas, take-over new functions and undergo crossmodal reorganization.

NEUROPLASTICITY AND COCHLEAR IMPLANTS

Cochlear implants are surgically implanted hearing aids used on patients with severe to profound sensorineural hearing loss in both ears to provides a sense of sound. In cochlear implants, cochlear transduction pass through a microphone then comes the spectral analysis through a bank of bandpass filters within a speech processor. At the very end, the output of each bandpass filter is directed to one for up 24 intra-cochlear electrodes positioned to stimulate auditory nerve fibers at tonotopically appropriate position along the cochlear spiral.

Electrical stimulation of the auditory nerve by cochlear implants evokes a pattern of activity, which differs from that evoked by acoustical stimulation in the normal ear. The spread of activation in the auditory nerve is much larger with electrical stimulation than with acoustical stimulation (Middlebrooks, Bierer, and Snyder 2005). Even the most focused stimulation strategies, as with the tripolar electrode configuration (Kral et al., 2002), do not come close to the acoustical stimulation and, in addition, are not favorable in cases of patchy degeneration of the auditory nerve. Moreover, randomness in the temporal firing pattern with electrical stimulation is much less than it is in the normally activated auditory nerve partially due to the loss of spontaneous activity in "deaf" auditory nerve fibers. Electrical stimulation at a high rate such as used in modern cochlear implants might induce a slight increase in randomness of the firing patterns because of refractory periods and sub-threshold electrical stimulation. Last but not last, simultaneous activation of several electrodes can lead to unwanted current flows between the active electrodes. Therefore, interleaved stimulation is used, which further biases the temporal excitation pattern when compared to natural acoustic-evoked activity.

Thus, after cochlear implantation, most of the representations of sounds in the nervous system have to be rebuilt to fit the characteristics of the new coding of auditory input.

Without auditory brainstem lesions, the outcome of cochlear implantation depends heavily on central factors, that is, its functional status and its plasticity (Kral and Tillein 2006).

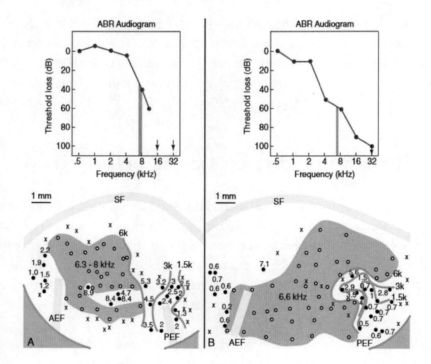

Figure 2. Cortical tonotopic maps that developed in two cats with neonatal basal cochlear lesions. Kittens were treated with the ototoxic aminoglycoside amikacin to produce basal lesions to the cochlea, the effects of which are reflected in the auditory brainstem response (ABR)–derived audiograms (upper panels). A, In this subject, the cochlear lesion was confined to the basal region. B, In this subject, hair cell damage was maximal at the cochlear base, but scattered hair cell loss extended up to apical regions. Shading indicates regions in which all neurons have similar tuning properties. AEF, anterior ectosylvian fissure; PEF, posterior ectosylvian fissure; SF, sylvian fissure (Modified from: Cumming's Otolaryngology, Head and Neck Surgery, sixth edition, chapter 132 "Neural Plasticity in Otology: 2042).

Many speculations were born about effects of cross modal plasticity in hearing recovery. Lee's studies have shown that delayed hearing-aided subjects presented the signs of cross-modal plasticity, and were less responsive to cochlear implant with greater difficulty in learning language and speech; the subjects who received an early prosthesis were often free of signs of cross-modal plasticity and respondent better.

These studies, however, had the defect of referring to the difference in timing of prosthesis, for which an ulterior study was performed on adult subjects suffering from post-lingual deafness and it was highlighted how the subjects with activation of the auditory cortex at CVER responded poorly to the hearing aids (Lee et al., 2001). Therefore it is possible to speculate that signs of cross modal plasticity can be exploited to evaluate the expectation of response to the cochlear implant. However, another study plasticity showed that cochlear implantation progressively regressed to a response only of the visual cortex in response to VCER.

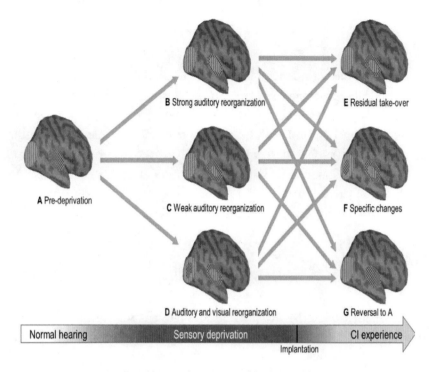

Figure 3. Schematic sketch illustrating cortical reorganization patterns resulting from sensory deprivation and hearing restorationwith a CI. "Cortical reorganization in postlingually deaf cochlear implant users: intra-modal and cross-modal considerations." Modified from: Stropahl et al., Hearing Research, Elsevier, 343(2017): 128-137.

Therefore, the concept remains that cross-modal plasticity is an adaptive response to deafness, which acts by potentiating the functioning sensory cortex areas and of the frontal cortex for TOP-BOTTOM response mechanisms to compensate for the auditory deficit. It is possible that in some subjects this phenomenon happens so well that even after prosthetics there is no recovery of the normal function of the auditory cortex, while, paradoxically, those who do not effectively highlight spoken language. The results discussed above have relevance for decisions regarding cochlear implants in congenitally deaf children (Kral and Tillein 2006). One question that has often been asked is whether the caretakers of children with cochlear implants should keep signing with these children, or if this would be counterproductive for learning and maintaining a language through spoken words using the cochlear implant? Arguments for both alternatives have been made. Signs accompanying spoken language might facilitate learning by appropriately activating the semantic auditory system with the associative language networks already established in the brain. On the other hand, signing might prevent the reassignment of high order auditory cortex to the auditory modality, and thus it may counterproductive in learning spoken language.

CONCLUSION

In this chapter we have evidenced how neuroplasticity plays a very important role in the regulation of cortical neuronal networks in response to inputs of various kinds, and in different age. In the case of deafness in the prelingual period, an early prosthetic implant allows the development of normal and physiological neuronal networks at the level of primary auditory cortex and higher order, as well as between areas, and promotes the stimulation that the central nervous system needs for development. Otherwise, in working between the different areas, in attempt to compensate for function, this can lead to a disadvantage in normal recovery after hearing aids.

REFERENCES

Bertrand, J. A., M. Lassonde, M. Robert, D. K. Nguyen, A. Bertone, M. E. Doucet, A. Bouthillier, and F. Lepore. 2012. "An intracranial event-related potential study on transformational apparent motion. Does its neural processing differ from real motion?" *Exp Brain Res* 216 (1):145-53. doi: 10.1007/s00221-011-2920-8.

Boyen, K., D. R. Langers, E. de Kleine, and P. van Dijk. 2013. "Gray matter in the brain: differences associated with tinnitus and hearing loss." *Hear Res* 295:67-78. doi: 10.1016/j.heares.2012.02.010.

Cardon, G., and A. Sharma. 2018. "Somatosensory Cross-Modal Reorganization in Adults With Age-Related, Early-Stage Hearing Loss." *Front Hum Neurosci* 12:172. doi: 10.3389/fnhum.2018.00172.

Chen, L. C., P. Sandmann, J. D. Thorne, M. G. Bleichner, and S. Debener. 2016. "Cross-Modal Functional Reorganization of Visual and Auditory Cortex in Adult Cochlear Implant Users Identified with fNIRS." *Neural Plast* 2016:4382656. doi: 10.1155/2016/4382656.

Contrera, K. J., J. Betz, J. Deal, J. S. Choi, H. N. Ayonayon, T. Harris, E. Helzner, K. R. Martin, K. Mehta, S. Pratt, S. M. Rubin, S. Satterfield, K. Yaffe, E. M. Simonsick, and F. R. Lin. 2017. "Association of Hearing Impairment and Anxiety in Older Adults." *J Aging Health* 29 (1):172-184. doi: 10.1177/0898264316634571.

De Stefano, A., F. Dispenza, L. Citraro, A. G. Petrucci, P. Di Giovanni, G. Kulamarva, N. Mathur, and A. Croce. 2011. "Are postural restrictions necessary for management of posterior canal benign paroxysmal positional vertigo?" *Ann Otol Rhinol Laryngol* 120 (7):460-4.

De Stefano, A., G. Kulamarva, and F. Dispenza. 2012. "Malignant paroxysmal positional vertigo." *Auris Nasus Larynx* 39:378-382.

Dispenza, F, and A De Stefano. 2012. "Vertigo in childhood: a methodological approach." *Bratisl Med J* 113:256-259.

Dispenza, F, A De Stefano, C Costantino, D Rando, M Giglione, R Stagno, and E Bennici. 2015. "Canal switch and re-entry phenomenon in benign paroxysmal positional vertigo: difference between immediate and delayed occurrence." *Acta Otolaryngol Ital* 35:116-120.

Dispenza, F, G Kulamarva, and A De Stefano. 2012. "Comparison of repositioning maneuvers for benign paroxysmal positional vertigo of posterior semicircular canal: advantages of hybrid maneuver." *Am J Otolaryngol* 33:528-532.

Dispenza, F., R. Gargano, N. Mathur, C. Saraniti, and S. Gallina. 2011. "Analysis of visually guided eye movements in subjects after whiplash injury." *Auris Nasus Larynx* 38:185-189.

Eggermont, J J. 2012. *The Neuroscience of Tinnitus*: Oxford University Press.

Eggermont, J. J. 2017. "Acquired hearing loss and brain plasticity." *Hear Res* 343:176-190. doi: 10.1016/j.heares.2016.05.008.

Glick, H., and A. Sharma. 2017. "Cross-modal plasticity in developmental and age-related hearing loss: Clinical implications." *Hear Res* 343:191-201. doi: 10.1016/j.heares.2016.08.012.

Harrison, R. V. 2001. "Age-related tonotopic map plasticity in the central auditory pathways." *Scand Audiol Suppl* (53):8-14.

Husain, F. T., R. E. Medina, C. W. Davis, Y. Szymko-Bennett, K. Simonyan, N. M. Pajor, and B. Horwitz. 2011. "Neuroanatomical changes due to hearing loss and chronic tinnitus: a combined VBM and DTI study." *Brain Res* 1369:74-88. doi: 10.1016/j.brainres.2010.10.095.

Kaas, J. H., M. M. Merzenich, and H. P. Killackey. 1983. "The reorganization of somatosensory cortex following peripheral nerve damage in adult and developing mammals." *Annu Rev Neurosci* 6:325-56. doi: 10.1146/annurev.ne.06.030183.001545.

Khosla, D., C. W. Ponton, J. J. Eggermont, B. Kwong, M. Don, and J. P. Vasama. 2003. "Differential ear effects of profound unilateral deafness on the adult human central auditory system." *J Assoc Res Otolaryngol* 4 (2):235-49. doi: 10.1007/s10162-002-3014-x.

Kral, A. 2007. "Unimodal and cross-modal plasticity in the 'deaf' auditory cortex." *Int J Audiol* 46 (9):479-93. doi: 10.1080/14992020701383027.

Kral, A., R. Hartmann, J. Tillein, S. Heid, and R. Klinke. 2002. "Hearing after congenital deafness: central auditory plasticity and sensory deprivation." *Cereb Cortex* 12 (8):797-807.

Kral, A., and J. Tillein. 2006. "Brain plasticity under cochlear implant stimulation." *Adv Otorhinolaryngol* 64:89-108. doi: 10.1159/000094647.

Lee, D. S., J. S. Lee, S. H. Oh, S. K. Kim, J. W. Kim, J. K. Chung, M. C. Lee, and C. S. Kim. 2001. "Cross-modal plasticity and cochlear implants." *Nature* 409 (6817):149-50. doi: 10.1038/35051653.

Levi-Montalcini, R. 1949. "Development of the acoustico-vestibular centers in the chick embryo in the absence of the afferent root fibers and of descending fiber tracts." *J Comp Neurol* 91:209-242.

Lorusso, F., F. Dispenza, G. Martinciglio, A. Messina, A. Battaglia, and S. Gallina. 2017. "Postural changes in patients undergoing hyoid surgery for OSAS." *EuroMediterranean Biomedical Journal* 12 (29):140-143. doi: 10.3269/1970-5492.2017.12.29.

Martines, F., P. Salvago, C. Bartolotta, S. Cocuzza, C. Fabiano, S. Ferrara, E. La Mattina, M. Mucia, P. Sammarco, F. Sireci, and E. Martines. 2015. "A genotype–phenotype correlation in Sicilian patients with GJB2 biallelic mutations." *European Archives of Oto-Rhino-Laryngology* 272 (8):1857-1865. doi: 10.1007/s00405-014-2970-1.

Middlebrooks, J. C., J. A. Bierer, and R. L. Snyder. 2005. "Cochlear implants: the view from the brain." *Curr Opin Neurobiol* 15 (4):488-93. doi: 10.1016/j.conb.2005.06.004.

Rajan, R., and D. R. Irvine. 1998. "Absence of plasticity of the frequency map in dorsal cochlear nucleus of adult cats after unilateral partial cochlear lesions." *J Comp Neurol* 399 (1):35-46.

Salvago, P, S Rizzo, A Bianco, and F Martines. 2017. "Sudden sensorineural hearing loss: is there a relationship between routine haematological parameters and audiogram shapes?" *Int J Audiol* 56:148-153.

Sharma, A., M. Dorman, A. Spahr, and N. W. Todd. 2002. "Early cochlear implantation in children allows normal development of central auditory pathways." *Ann Otol Rhinol Laryngol Suppl* 189:38-41.

Thomas, E, F Martines, A Bianco, G Messina, V Giustino, D Zangla, A Iovane, and A Palma. 2018. "Decreased postural control in people with moderate hearing loss." *Medicine (United States)* 97:e0244. doi: 10.1097/MD.0000000000010244.

Wang, J H, G Y Ko, and P T Kelly. 1997. "Cellular and molecular bases of memory: synaptic and neuronal plasticity." *J Clin Neurol Physiol* 14:264–293.

Yang, M., H. J. Chen, B. Liu, Z. C. Huang, Y. Feng, J. Li, J. Y. Chen, L. L. Zhang, H. Ji, X. Feng, X. Zhu, and G. J. Teng. 2014. "Brain structural and functional alterations in patients with unilateral hearing loss." *Hear Res* 316:37-43. doi: 10.1016/j.heares.2014.07.006.

In: Sensorineural Hearing Loss
Editors: F. Dispenza and F. Martines
ISBN: 978-1-53615-048-3
© 2019 Nova Science Publishers, Inc.

Chapter 5

NEURORADIOLOGY OF THE HEARING SYSTEM

Cesare Gagliardo[1,*], *MD, PhD, Silvia Piccinini*[2-3], *MD*
and Paola Feraco[4-5], *MD*

[1]Section of Radiological Sciences, Department of Biomedicine, Neuroscience and Advanced Diagnostic, University of Palermo, Palermo, Italy
[2]Department of Neuroradiology,
University Hospital of Modena, Modena, Italy
[3]Audiology and Pediatric Otolaryngology Unit,
University of Parma, Parma, Italy
[4]Department of Radiology, Ospedale S. Chiara,
Azienda Provinciale per i Servizi Sanitari, Trento, Italy
[5]Department of Experimental, Diagnostic and Specialty Medicine,
University of Bologna, Bologna, Italy

ABSTRACT

Hearing loss is one of the most frequent indications for CT and MR examinations of the auditory system. Such a symptomatology is becoming increasingly common in today's society and is extremely disturbing for patients. Causes may involve the auditory pathway at any level.

In most cases, neuroradiological examinations represents a mandatory step, within a multidisciplinary workup, towards final diagnosis, therapeutic plan and subsequent follow-ups. This chapter will introduce this critical topic starting from an imaging-based exposition of the anatomy and function of the auditory system. The chapter will include some hints on the choice of the best imaging examination to perform on each patient since the type of hearing loss determines which imaging study will yield the most diagnostic information. Practical coverage of the neuroradiological findings in conductive, sensorineural and mixed hearing loss forms will be presented. Ranging from

---

* Corresponding Author's Email: cesare.gagliardo@unipa.it; cesare.gagliardo@gmail.com.

congenital to acute and chronic causes, from children to adults, the role of imaging-based examinations will be illustrated for both common and uncommon diseases of the hearing system.

To increase reading and review experience, the authors will include concise descriptions (in a bullet outline format and/or in tables) of all the discussed key information related to anatomy, function and pathology. High-quality CT and MR images will support the reader in each paragraph for an optimal learning experience of the discussed topics.

1. INTRODUCTION TO THE ROLE OF IMAGING

Imaging techniques have historically supported the study of the auditory system which always required dedicated and optimized protocols to ensure a good visualization of its peculiar anatomy and related pathology.

Nowadays, Computerized Tomography (CT) and Magnetic Resonance Imaging (MRI) are the most used imaging modalities to investigate the auditory pathway at any level.

Conversely, the role of plain film radiographs has been significantly reduced and limited to specific applications over the past years (i.e., Stenvers' projection is still routinely used for intra- and/or postoperative evaluation of a cochlear implant lead).

Digital subtraction angiography (DSA) is still used in cases of hypervascular masses and vascular malformations involving the temporal bone or the auditory pathway.

Diagnostic ultrasounds found little use in this context if not for the evaluation of periauricular lesions or ultrasound-guided biopsies.

Nuclear medicine modalities, such as Positron Emission Tomography (PET) may be used for the assessment of temporal bone masses and/or nodal metastases.

Last but not least, dedicated devices such as cone beam CT (CBCT) that are more recently spreading worldwide, deserve mention since they have been successfully used for middle ear diseases [1], cochlear implants [2-4], cholesteatoma surgery [5-6], guidance of temporal bone surgery [7] and other specific pathologies such as otosclerosis [8-9].

CBCT equipment uses a rotating gantry on which an x-ray tube and a reciprocating solid state flat panel detector is attached [10]. This allows the operator to acquire a full dataset of the region of interest with a single 180-360° rotation of the gantry (scanning time varies from nearly 5 - using pulsed scans - to about 40 seconds). Because of their high spatial resolution (slice thickness could be in the order of some tens of microns), lower radiation dose, lower sensitivity to metallic and beam hardening artifacts and their reduced costs, these scanners have triggered a lively interest in the scientific community. Furthermore, the production of compact CBCT scanners enabled their usage in an office-based setting [10]. On the other hand, if compared to conventional CT, CBCT images are noisier because of the large volume being irradiated, are more sensitive to movement and distortion artifacts, partial volume averaging, undersampling and cone-beam effect. Last but not least, CBCT have a poor soft tissue contrast and their usage is substantially limited to oral and maxillofacial radiology [11].

1.1. Computerized Tomography (CT) Study Protocol

CT is the primary imaging modality for evaluating the osseous components of the temporal bone region [12-13]. The increasing number of multi-detector CT (MDCT) installations has been followed by the wide adoption of helical study protocols dedicated to high resolution temporal bone imaging. Nowadays, thanks to MDCT scanners, it is no longer necessary to ask patients to lay on the gantry in uncomfortable positions to obtain optimal study planes as we used to do in the past years with single-row-detector CT equipment using sequential study protocols. MDCT protocols (see Table 1) for temporal bone region are based on sub-millimetric (slice thickness should never exceed 1.0 mm), usually isotropic datasets and related multiplanar reconstructions (MPR). All temporal bone studies should be reconstructed using a bone algorithm and each side should be separately reconstructed using a magnified small field of view (FOV) for both axial and coronal planes. Reconstruction of the posterior fossa using soft-tissue algorithm with a wider FOV is recommended.

Table 1. Example of standard protocols for a 16 detector rows scanner (GE Brightspeed 16)

Acquisition parameters (helical scan type)	Protocol		
	<2y	>2y	*Adults*
Tube voltage (kV)	120	120	140
Tube current (mAs)	200	200	260
Axial thickness (mm)	0.625	0.625	0.625
Scan type	Helical full (0,7s)	Helical full (1s)	Helical full (1s)
Pitch	0.562:1	0.562:1	0.562:1
Speed (mm/rot)	5.62	5.62	5.62
Beam collimation (mm)	10	10	10
Interval (mm)	0.625	0.625	0.310
SFOV (cm)	10	10	24
DFOV (cm)	6	6	10
Scan durations (s)	11.44	16.33	9.3
N° of images	129	129	130
Matrix size	512 x 512	512 x 512	512 x 512
Maximum estimated $CTDI_{vol}$ (mGy)	52.04	74.34	143.70
DLP (mGy-cm)	478.21	682.93	750.09
Reconstruction kernel (window width/level)	Bone Plus - GE's hard/sharp kernel (4095/600)		

SFOV: Scan field of view; DFOV: Display field of view; CTDIvol: computed tomography dose index; DLP: dose-length product

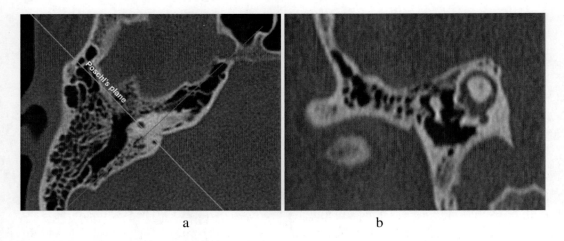

Figure 1. a) Axial CT passing through the superior semicircular canal (SSCC) with superimposed DICOM references lines for a MultiPlanar Reconstruction (MPR) among Poschl's plane obtained by tilting the MPR plane parallel to the SSCC; b) the whole SSCC is fully exposed on the obtained MPR.

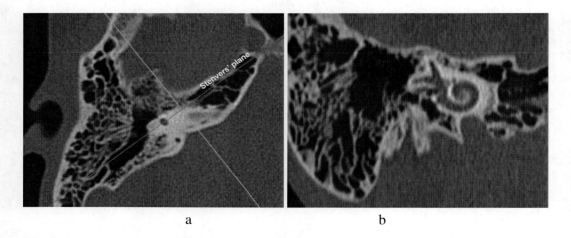

Figure 2. a) Axial CT passing through the superior semicircular canal (SSCC) with superimposed DICOM references lines for a MultiPlanar Reconstruction (MPR) among Stenvers' plane obtained by tilting the MPR plane perpendicular to the SSCC; b) the cochlea is exposed from basal turn to apex on the resulting MPR plane.

If a MDCT scanner is not available (or if reformatted coronals from the axial scans are not possible/adequate), direct coronal images should be considered. To ensure a direct coronal plane, the patient is asked to lay in the prone position with the head tilted back (for patients who cannot tolerate this position, supine positioning with a pillow under the shoulders and the head tilted posteriorly should be tried). For direct coronal plane imaging, the gantry should be perpendicular to the infraorbital-meatal line. The typical planning should be from the level of the posterior temporo-mandibular joint anteriorly, through the entire mastoid air cells posteriorly.

If a MDCT scanner is available, high resolution temporal bone imaging is obtained with the patient placed supine and the head in a neutral position. The gantry of the scanner should be angled parallel to the infraorbital-meatal line. Two topograms (one in the anterior-posterior projection and one lateral) are usually scanned to plan the study ensuring the full coverage of the region of interest. The typical axial planning should start from the arcuate eminence superiorly and the mastoid tip inferiorly. The excursion of the scan is planned to avoid including the eyes in the pathway of the x-ray beam to reduce the radiation dose to the lens. Coronal MPRs are usually obtained tilting the plane perpendicular to the infraorbital-meatal line. Considering the three-dimensional (3D) nature of the scanned dataset additional reformations, with no compromises in terms of image spatial resolution, are possible and could result in being very useful in specific cases. For example, if a superior semicircular canal dehiscence is suspected, Poschl plane (Figure 1) among the short temporal bone axis (obtained by tilting the MPR plane parallel to the superior semicircular canal) should be considered [14]. Similarly, Stenvers' plane (Figure 2) among the long temporal bone axis (obtained by tilting the MPR plane perpendicular to the superior semicircular canals) should be considered to evaluate a cochlear implant lead [15].

Intravenous (i.v.) administration of contrast medium is usually not indicated for temporal bone imaging but may be helpful when evaluating patients with acute mastoiditis in order to evaluate adjacent vascular structures such as the transverse sinus, to investigate the involvement of the mastoid and/or the perimastoid dissemination of a disease, or if a temporal bone tumor is suspected.

1.2. Magnetic Resonance Imaging (MRI) Study Protocol

MRI is the primary imaging modality for evaluating the non-osseous components of the temporal bone region [16-17]. A high field strength MRI scanner ($\geq$1.5T) is typically used together with a phased array head coil (8-, 16- or 32-channels). The use of dedicated surface coils can improve the signal/noise ratio at the cost of a lower depth and reduced FOV. MRI is the first imaging examination requested in case of suspected retrocochlear pathology and cranial nerve dysfunction. One of the most common indications for an MRI examination of the temporal bone is sensorineural hearing loss [18-19]. MRI is also useful in patients with CT-defined infections or neoplasms to determine if there is an involvement of the intracranial compartment.

Even if MDCT is still the preferred modality if a labyrinthine or cochlear lesion is suspected or in patients with subjective pulsatile tinnitus, there are specific lesions (such as cochlear schwannomas or labyrinthine hemorrhages) and cases (such as patients with objective pulsatile tinnitus - audible bruit) that could be better detected and studied by MRI.

During the MRI examination, the patient lays in the supine head-first position. A fast (low resolution) T2-weighted three plane localizer is scanned. Axial sequences are planned parallel to the line passing through both internal auditory channels (IACs) and perpendicular to the brain stem; the number of slices must be sufficient to cover the ROI from the hippocampus up to the line of the first cervical verbal body. Coronal sequences are planned parallel to the line passing through both internal auditory channels (IACs) on the coronal plane and parallel to the brain stem on the sagittal plane. The number of slices must be sufficient to cover the ROI from the posterior border of sphenoid sinus up to the fourth ventricle anterior wall. An example of an MRI protocol for the evaluation of the temporal bone is reported in Table 2; to ensure a good visualization of the peculiar anatomy and related pathology of this region a small FOV is used and slice thickness should not exceed 3 mm with no interslice gap. Axial and coronal T1-weighted pulse sequences acquired before and after administration of i.v. contrast agent should be included (at least one post-contrast T1-weighted sequence with fat saturation should be scanned as well). Nowadays, thin section 3D constructive interference in steady-state (3D-CISS) T2-weighted sequences are mandatory [20]. This technique has different names for each vendor: fast imaging, employing steady-state acquisition (FIESTA) by GE, true fast imaging with steady-state precession (FISP) by Siemens, balanced fast field echo (FFE) by Philips, and true steady-state free precession (SSFP) by Toshiba. 3D CISS sequences are very useful in the assessment of cranial nerves anatomical variations, pathologies and vascular conflicts and compressions. To evaluate the intracisternal tract of the 7th and 8th cranial nerves (CNs), oblique sagittal reformatted CISS images perpendicular the internal auditory channel are highly suggested (Figure 3). Thick slab MPRs using a maximum intensity projection (MIP) algorithm obtained from 3D CISS sequences are commonly used to visualize internal ear structures such as labyrinthine structures, the endolymphatic sac and to evaluate the extent of a cochlear dysplasia in cases of congenital or developmental hearing loss (Figure 4). Poschl like plane is commonly used in pediatric cases when a cranial nerve deficiency is suspected. If a cholesteatoma is suspected, non–echo planar (EP) diffusion weighted imaging (DWI) sequence has been demonstrated useful in differentiating typical findings of middle ear and/or mastoid infections from cholesteatomas larger than 2 mm [21]. Non-EP DWI is also useful in post-surgical evaluations. Conventional EP-DWI are more sensitive to susceptibility artifacts which typically affect this region with little to no practical applications. Additional dedicated sequences should be considered in case of intracranial or nasopharyngeal extensions of a disease.

Table 2. Example of standard protocols for 1.5T scanners using a dedicated 8-channel phased-array head coil

Parameters	MRI scanner: 1.5T Philips Achieva / 1.5T GE HDxT				
Pulse sequence	2D Ax T1w TSE / FSE	2D Ax and Cor T2w TSE SPIR / FSE FAT SAT	3D Ax B-FFE / FIESTA	2D Cor DWI / Ax DWI PROPELLER (b=0/1000m/s^2)	2D Ax T1w (Gd) SE	3D AX (Gd) FFE SPIR / SPGR FAT SAT
FOV (mm)	150x150 / 180x180	180x180 / 180x180	180x180 / 180x180	220x186 / 240x240	150x150 / 180x180	150x150 / 180x180
Matrix	224x178 / 256x224	256x202 / 256x256	308x307 / 352x320	124x87 / 384x384	208x166 / 256x224	208x208 / 256x256
N° of slices	12 /14	13 /14	75 / 64	18 /22	11 /14	50 / 64
Slice thickness (gap) mm	3 (0.3) / 3 (0.5)	3 (0.3) / 3 (0.5)	1 (-0.5) / 0.8	3 (0.3) / 3 (0.5)	3 (0.3) / 3 (0.5)	1.4 (-0.7) / 0.8
TE (ms)	10 / 20	90 / 85	3.5 / 2.2	77 / 93	15 / 20	4.6 / 3.4
TR (ms)	550 / 580	3000 / 4733	7.1 / 6.1	3713 / 6109	550 / 580	25 / 10.1
Number of excitations	3 / 2	3 / 4	2 / 3	4 / 3	3	1 / 1
Echo train length	3 / 18	17 / 22	n.a.	44 / 28	n.a.	n.a.
Acquisition time (m:s)	3:20 / 4:28	3:39 / 3:52	4:25 / 5:40	4:57 / 2:33	4:37 / 6:33	4:20 / 2:22

Ax: axial plane; Cor: coronal plane; T1w: T1 weighted; T2w: T2 weighted; TSE: Turbo Spin Echo; FSE: Fast Spin Echo; SPIR: Spectral Presaturation with Inversion Recovery; FAT SAT: Fat Saturation; B-FFE: Balanced gradient waveform Fast Field Echo; FIESTA: Fast Imaging Employing STeady-state Acquisition; DWI: Diffusion Weighted Imaging; PROPELLER: Periodically Rotated Overlapping ParallEL Lines with Enhanced Reconstruction (GE's radial k-space filling pattern used to reduce the effect of patient voluntary and physiologic motion and reduce magnetic susceptibility artifacts); SE: Spin Echo; Gd: sequence acquired after i.v. administration of gadolinium based contrast medium; FFE: Fast Field Echo; SPGR: SPoiled Gradient echo; m: minutes; s: seconds.

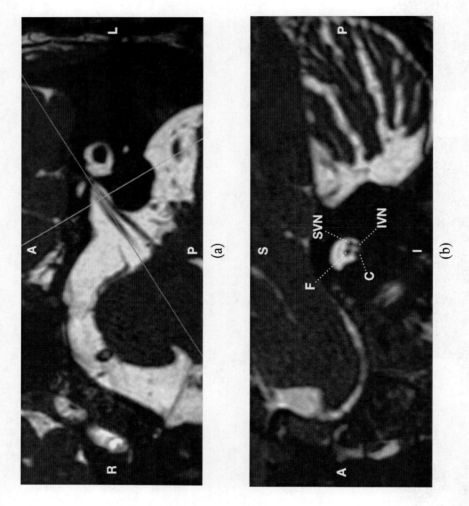

Figure 3. a) Axial 3D FIESTA passing through the left internal auditory channel (IAC) showing the intracisternal tract of the 7th (anterior) and 8th (posterior) cranial nerves; superimposed DICOM references lines shows the correct oblique orientation of a MultiPlanar Reconstruction (MPR) to evaluate the internal auditory channel tracts; b) the resulting MPR plane shows the typical four black dots into the IAC: the facial nerve (F) is in an anterior-superior location, the cochlear nerve (C) is in an anterior-inferior location, the superior and the inferior vestibular nerves (SVN and IVN respectively) are located posteriorly. A: anterior; P: posterior; S: superior; I: inferior.

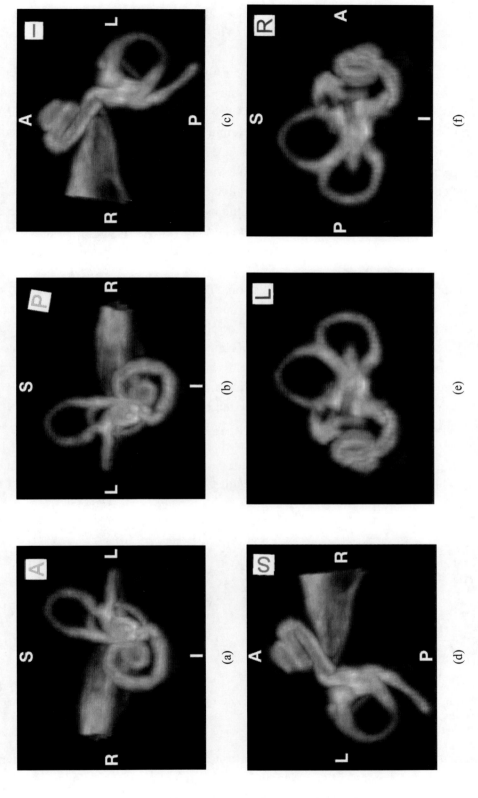

Figure 4. 3D Maximum Intensity Projection (MIP) reconstructions of the internal ear structures: anterior (a), posterior (b), inferior (c), superior (d), left (e) and right (f) orientations.

2. EXTERNAL EAR

Imaging plays a minor role in external ear pathology because it is usually evident at clinical evaluation. However, it becomes necessary if the EAC is obstructed or stenotic.

Aural dysplasia derives from a failure of the first branchial cleft to canalise EAC, implicating atresia or dysplasia. Clinical examination reveals a small and abnormal auricle (microtia) in association. In such cases, a CT scan is indicated before any surgical intervention to delineate the facial nerve canal. Aural dysplasia could be associated with congenital cholesteatoma or inner ear abnormalities which are usually minor [22, 23].

External otitis do not require imaging studies. If a necrotizing variant is present, imaging is recommended to evaluate periauricular involvement of the disease, because it spreads rapidly through bone and soft tissues. MRI is preferred if intracranial involvement is suspected [24].

In conductive deafness, stenotic EAC is sometimes difficult to evaluate, so a CT scan is required to exclude bone abnormalities such as fibrous dysplasia [25]. Fibrous dysplasia is a disease of young patients, conversely to esostosis that is usually in older people. Esostosis is a nodular elevation of bone involving tympanic bone, due to prolonged irritation of EAC secondary to cold water (Figure 5). Differential diagnosis includes osteoma that is usually seen as a unilateral, pedunculated bony lesion [26].

EAC cholesteatoma is rare; it is characterized by bony destruction and it usually has an iatrogenic origin after surgery. Trauma, focal osteitis, and cerumen retention are less frequent causes [27]. Keratosis obturans is an epidermal keratin plug in the EAC, often bilateral (Figure 6). On CT scan, it is a soft tissue mass associated with the widening of EAC, possibly with mild erosion of bony margins [28].

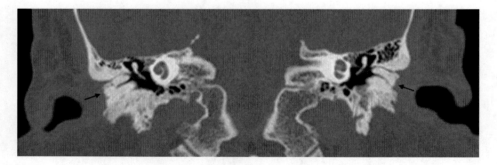

Figure 5. Bilateral EAC exostosis in a scuba diver with chronic exposure to cold water; coronal MPR of a MDCT scan show broad-based circumferential bony overgrowth of the osseous EAC (arrows) that severely reduces the width of the EAC (courtesy of Dr Giuseppe Tagliavia, "Centro di Radiologia Diagnostica srl" – Sciacca, Agrigento – Italy).

External ear cancers are rare; they demonstrate clinical symptoms similar to external otitis at the onset. They usually are squamous cell carcinoma or basocellular carcinoma. CT are required to evaluate surgical intervention; bone involvement is critical to surgical planning, especially when extending to temporomandibular joints or the middle ear. MRI is frequently associated in order to exclude perineural, perivascular or intracranial spread of the disease (Figure 7) [29, 30].

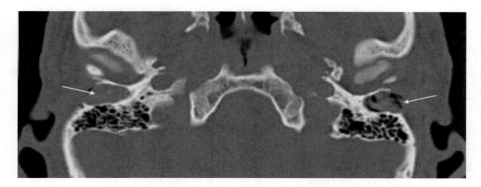

Figure 6. Bilateral EAC keratosis obturans; axial MDCT scan show bilateral soft tissue mass (arrows) within the bony EAC which enlarges the canal with no signs of bony erosion.

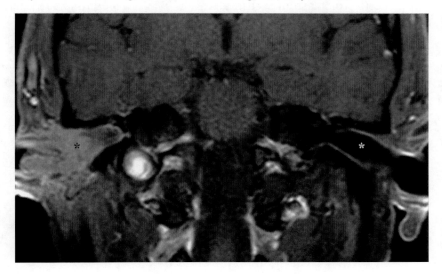

Figure 7. External ear cancer; coronal T1-weighted sequence with fat saturation acquired after i.v. administration of contrast medium. Contrast enhancing soft tissue mass (black asterisk) with undefined edges causing stenosis of right EAC and reaches the bony part of the EAC. Normal appearing contralateral EAC shows typical low signal due to its air content (white asterisk).

3. MIDDLE EAR AND MASTOID

The most frequent request for oto-neuroradiological examinations concern the middle ear.

The middle ear (or tympanic cavity), is the small, air-filled cavity, within the temporal bone located between the eardrum (tympanic membrane, TM) and the lateral bony wall of the internal ear. The tympanic cavity posteriorly communicates, through the *aditus ad antrum*, with the mastoid *antrum* and cells; anteriorly it communicates with the nasopharynx through the auditory tube (also known as Eustachian or pharyngotympanic tube) that allows it to equalize the air pressure inside the drum with atmospheric pressure lateral to the drum.

The tympanic cavity contains the three auditory *ossicles* (hammer or *malleus*, anvil or *incus* and stirrup or *stapes*) which transmit sound vibration from the tympanic membrane to the inner ear enabling the primary function of the middle ear itself (sound-conducting apparatus). Other components of the tympanic cavity are tendons of the *tensor tympani* and the *stapedius* muscles, the *chorda tympani* (branch of the facial nerve) and tympanic plexus (branches from facial and glossopharyngeal nerves).

The tympanic cavity is bounded by six walls which must be carefully evaluated during the assessment of oto-neuroradiological examinations: superior (or *tegmen tympani* or *paries tegmentalis*), inferior (or jugular wall or *paries jugularis*), anterior (or carotid wall), posterior (or mastoid wall), lateral (or *paries membranaceus*) and medial (or *paries labyrinthica*). The tympanic cavity is also divided into three levels: *epitympanum* (level above the TM; it houses the body of the malleus and the incus), *mesotympanum* (TM level; is the central and the biggest compartment of the middle ear cavity, it houses the long processes of malleus and incus, the stapes, oval and round windows, facial nerve and parts of the middle ear muscles and tendons) and *hypotympanum* (level below the TM, it houses no functional elements) [31]. In adults the tympanic cavity measures approximately $15 \times 15 \times 6$ mm but the width in the center part of the cavity is only 2 mm [32].

High resolution CT/MDCT imaging of the temporal bone represent the first line imaging modality for middle ear evaluation, surgical treatment planning and post-therapy follow-ups. MRI is usually performed as a second level investigation for specific clinical suspects.

3.1. Congenital Anomalies of the Middle Ear

Middle ear anomalies can be unilateral or bilateral but they are predominantly unilateral (70-90%). The incidence of middle ear malformations is approximately 1 in 3800 newborns. The etiopathogenesis of most malformations of the middle ear is still poorly defined. In all genetically determined malformations (syndromal and non-syndromal) one can assume a high frequency of spontaneous genetic mutations. The acquired ear malformations originate from exogenic injury during pregnancy. The noxae could comprise infections, chemical agents, malnutrition, radiation exposure, Rh incompatibility, hypoxia, atmospheric pressure changes and noise exposure. Deficiency or malfunction of the thyroid hormone can be also associated with ear malformations. However, in many cases, the actual cause is unknown [33].

Middle ear malformations are a rare cause of conductive hearing loss in children, especially when these conditions are not associated with malformations of the external ear. These anomalies are usually confused with serous otitis [34]. The clinical and surgical relevance of these disorders are strictly related to the associated anatomical development anomalies and malfunctions [31].

If a congenital conductive hearing loss (CCHL) is suspected, a high-resolution CT examination in order to evaluate the bony structures of the middle ear should be considered.

Congenital anomalies of the middle ear can be classified into major (associated with an involvement of the tympanic membrane and external ear) and minor (exclusive involvement of the middle ear) [34].

Minor middle ear anomalies include a change in the anatomy or size of the tympanic cavity or a reduced distance between anatomical structures of the middle ear and fixated ossicles (stapes ankylosis). In major anomalies, the ossicles are often involved. The most common isolated ossicle deformity involves the *stapes* suprastructure in terms of aplasia or hypoplasia, thickening, thinning or fusion of the stapes crura [33]. The *malleus* tends to be rarely involved in isolated middle ear malformations. The most frequent findings are deformities and hypoplasia of the head and of the manubrium of the malleus, fixations in the epitympanic recess and malleolo-incudal joint abnormality. The malleus can also be absent [31]. *Incus* malformations are dominated by absence or hypoplasia of the long process coexisting with incudo-stapedial joint separation. Less frequently, the long process may vary in position (horizontal rotation and fixation in the direction of the horizontally running tympanic segment of the facial nerve) or complete incus aplasia may be found. In addition, synostotic or synchondrotic incudo-malleolar joint abnormalities and epitympanic recess fixation have often been found [33].

The inner ear windows may be involved in middle ear anomalies in terms of a mobile stapes footplate or dysplasia/aplasia of the round or oval window. There may be anomalies of the oval window and, rarely, of the round window. Congenital agenesis of the oval window involves complete osseous obliteration of the oval window either by a concentric narrowing that produces a dimple-like depression along the medial tympanic wall or by a thick bony plate [33]. Almost 76% of the patients with congenital absence of the oval window presents with associated malformation of the facial nerve canal. The nerve can either limit the exposure of the oval window or it can cover the footplate completely. This condition may also be associated with conductive hearing loss [35].

Malformation and aberrant course of the facial nerve are frequently encountered; the common abnormalities include complete dehiscence of the tympanic segment, inferior displacement of the tympanic segment, and anterior and lateral displacement of the mastoid segment. The latter frequently obscures the round window.

Other malformations of the middle ear include a missing antrum, a pneumatized mastoid, cerebral spinal fluid (CSF) fistulas (indirect translabyrinthine or direct paralabyrinthine), congenital cholesteatoma (as known as congenital epidermoid), congenital dermoids, aberrant courses of arteries and veins, and malformations of the middle ear muscles.

The primary (congenital) cholesteatoma (Figure 8) counts as a congenital middle ear anomaly; a four-stage classification is used:

- *Stage I*: only one quadrant of tympanic membrane is affected with no ossicular involvement or mastoid extension;
- *Stage II*: multiple quadrants are affected but no ossicular involvement or mastoid extension;
- *Stage III*: ossicular involvement (includes erosion of ossicles and surgical removal for eradication of disease); no mastoid extension;
- *Stage IV*: mastoid extension (regardless of findings elsewhere).

Numerous classifications for middle ear malformations have been proposed. The classification of the minor malformations, proposed by Teunissen and Cremers [36], is based on the surgical aspects of the malformations, and subdivides them into four main groups:

1) Ankylosis or isolated congenital fixation of the stapes (footplate fixation and superstructure fixation);
2) Stapes ankylosis associated with other malformations of the ossicular chain (deformities of the incus and/or malleus, or aplasia of the long apophysis of the incus and bone fixation of malleus and/or incus);
3) Congenital anomalies of the ossicular chain with mobile stapes footplate (disruption of the ossicular chain, epytimpanic fixation or timpanic fixation);
4) Congenital aplasia or severe dysplasia of the oval and round windows (aplasia, dysplasia, prolapse of facial nerve or persistence of stapedial artery).

Kösling [37] described three degrees of severity of isolated middle ear malformations:

1) *Mild* malformations are those in which normal configuration of the tympanic cavity coexists with ossicular dysplasia;
2) *Moderate* malformations are characterized by hypoplasia of the tympanic cavity along with rudimentary or aplastic ossicles;
3) *Severe* malformations show aplastic or cleft-like tympanic cavity.

High-resolution CT is the best diagnostic imaging examination since it allows a correct visualization of bony structures. However, exploratory tympanotomy is the method that most reliably establishes the definitive diagnosis. All of these anomalies can be surgically corrected [31].

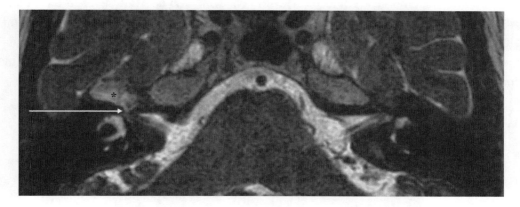

Figure 8. Primary (congenital) supralabytinthine cholesteatoma; axial CISS sequence passing through the IACs showing the cholesteatoma (black asterisk) with a inhomogeneous low- to high- signal with geniculate ganglion impairment (white arrow).

3.2. Acute Infections of Middle Ear

Infection of the middle ear cavity is termed otitis media; it is called otomastoiditis (OM) when inflammation process spreads to the mastoid. Otitis media could occur suddenly (acute otitis media, AOM) or, if it does not go away or happens repeatedly, could remain over months to years (chronic otitis media, COM).

A mixture of factors predisposes to otitis media, but Eustachian tube dysfunction is thought to be one of the most important factors. Congenital palate defects, host immunity, and viral or bacterial infection may all be contributing factors.

AOM is commonly seen in children and it is the most common bacterial infection among children.

Although AOM is generally considered a bacterial infection, there is ample evidence that respiratory viruses have a crucial role in the etiology and pathogenesis of this disease.

The presence of viruses in the middle ear fluid is important not only in regard to the aetiology and pathogenesis of acute otitis media, but also in regard to the outcome of the disease [38].

Symptoms include earache, fever, pain, otorrhea, conductive hearing loss (CHL) with a bulging and red tympanic membrane at otoscopy [39].

Although this infection can be well estimated on otoscopic examination, further questions concerning the extent of the disease, exact location, structures involved and possible bone erosion, will be addressed in detail only with neuroradiological examinations. CT is the imaging modality of choice for the assessment of CHL [40].

In AOM, high resolution temporal bone CT is routinely performed and may reveal soft tissue in the middle ear cavity (Figure 9), thickened tympanic membrane with bulging. Other features that could be seen in AOM include air-fluid level in the middle ear (effusion) and bony erosion [39]. MR is indicated when complicated inflammatory lesions are suspected to extend into the inner ear or towards the sigmoid sinus or jugular vein. MR is very sensible in identifying typical high signals from fluid collections in the middle ear cavity and mastoid antrum on T2-weighted pulse sequences.

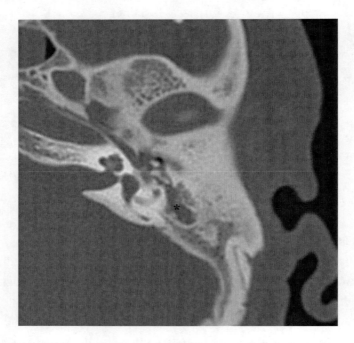

Figure 9. Acute otitis media; axial MDCT scan at the level of the IAC / middle ear showing soft tissue density in the middle ear cavity which extends to incorporate the ossicular chain and mastoid antrum (asterisk). Patient with a noticeable hypopneumatization of the temporal pyramid.

The clinical course of AOM is generally short: in the vast majority of patients the response of the immune system and the sensitivity of the germ to the administered antibiotic will be enough. However, acute otitis media can progress to severe complications, including acute mastoiditis, meningitis, and intracranial abscess [41]. In these cases contrast enhanced CT is useful to evaluate adjacent vascular structures such as the transverse sinus. MRI is mandatory if the intra-cranial dissemination of the inflammation process is suspected for a prompt diagnosis of cerebritis foci or to better characterize brain abscesses (late cerebritis).

Acute mastoiditis (AM), even if it could occur as an isolated process, is usually a complication of otitis media (Oto-Mastoiditis, OM) in which infection in the middle ear cleft involves the muco-periosteum and bony septa of the mastoid air cells. CT is usually the initial technique of choice for imaging patients with OM. Typical imaging findings are opacification of the tympanic cavity, mastoid antrum and air cells with bone erosion and/or destruction of the intramastoid bony septa (Figure 10) [42]. Contrast agent administration is recommended for better evaluation of perimastoid soft tissues and to exclude fearsome complications like dural venous sinus thrombosis [43]. MRI is mainly reserved for the detection, or detailed evaluation, of intracranial complications of OM. Typical MRI findings in patients with complicated OM are:

- opacification of the tympanic cavity and the mastoid with fluid-like signal intensity of intramastoid contents on T1- and T2-weighted imaging;
- diffusion weighted imaging (DWI) may show variable degrees of signal increase within the mastoid effusions; however, DWI is a mandatory sequence to detect purulent secretions and brain abscesses that are characterized by a bright signal intensity and a low signal on apparent diffusion coefficient (ADC) maps due to a restricted diffusion of water molecules movements within purulent collections;
- after administration of i.v. contrast, an intense intramastoid enhancement is commonly seen among the outer periosteum or the perimastoid dura.

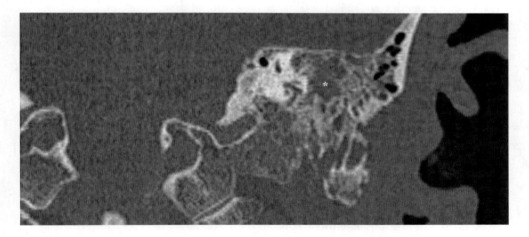

Figure 10. Patient with acute otomastoiditis; coronal MPR from a MDCT scan show typical soft tissue density into the middle ear cavity (asterisk) and mastoid cells with sign of erosion towards the infratemporal fossa (Bezold abscess).

According to Platzek [44], the diagnosis of AM is possible with a sensitivity of 100%, a specificity of 66% and an accuracy of 86%, with two of the following intramastoid findings on CT/MRI examinations: fluid accumulation, enhancement, or diffusion restriction.

In clinical practice, contrast-enhanced CT is still the preferable, first-line imaging technique due to higher accessibility, especially for urgent cases. Thus, MRI is:

- an alternative diagnostic tool for patients with contraindications to contrast-enhanced CT;
- a mandatory second level investigation to detect intracranial complications;
- recommended for paediatric patients due to its lack of ionizing radiation.

3.3. Chronic Otitis Media

The definition of chronic otitis media (COM) is based on clinical and pathological features.

When the inflammation of the middle ear persists at least 6 weeks and is associated with otorrhea through a perforated tympanic membrane, the diagnosis of chronic otitis media is placed.

Principal etiopathological factors of COM are infections of the upper respiratory tract, insufficiency of ciliary clearance and drainage of the Eustachian tube (Eustachian tube dysfunction), allergic history and familial predisposition. Symptoms include conductive hearing loss, vertigo, otorrhea and sometimes pain.

Chronic otitis media are classified in chronic suppurative otitis media (CSOM) and chronic otitis media with effusion (COME) [45].

CSOM is characterized by recurrent or persistent ear discharge (otorrhea) over 2 to 6 weeks through a perforation of the tympanic membrane.

COME is defined as the presence of fluid in the middle ear without symptoms or signs of infection and is the most common cause of acquired hearing loss in childhood.

Enabling an optimal visualization of bony structures and pneumatized spaces, CT is therefore the best diagnostic method to evaluate the involvement of temporal bone structures in patients with chronic inflammation of the middle ear [46].

On CT examination typical radiological signs of chronic otitis media are [39]:

- opacification or mucosal thickening in the tympanic cavity;
- obliteration of the epitympanum or Prussak's space by fibrous-inflammatory tissue (for tubal dysfunction, reduced transmucosal gas exchange, and development of otitis media);
- bone erosions and/or ossicular disorders;
- sclerosis and loss of aeration of the mastoid air cells;
- osteolysis of the bony septa and, in severe cases, osteomyelitis of the petrous temporal bone.

Since some ears with chronic inflammation develop cholesteatoma, chronic otitis media may be also classified into two groups: with or without cholesteatoma.

Cholesteatoma is a well-demarcated non-neoplastic lesion resulting from an abnormal accumulation of squamous epithelium usually found in the middle ear cavity and mastoid process of the temporal bone [45].

3.3.1. Chronic Otitis Media without Cholesteatoma

Post-inflammatory ossicular chain fixation is a common finding in patients with chronic otitis media and conductive hearing loss (Figure 11). On CT images, three distinctive forms of ossicular chain fixation can be evaluated:

- presence of fibrous tissue, usually in the niche of oval window, forming a so-called "peristapedial tent" (fibrous tissue may also be present anywhere in mesotympanum and epitympanum).
- tympanosclerosis, which reflects deposits of hyalinised collagen in the tympanic cavity. If it occurs in the tympanic membrane, it is called myringosclerosis. In the tympanic cavity, it may be present in any location, visible as focal calcified densities in the middle ear cavity, along tendons, also in direct apposition to the ossicular chain.
- formation of new bone, rarely seen in the tympanic cavity, usually in epitympanum. Visible as high density lamellar structures.

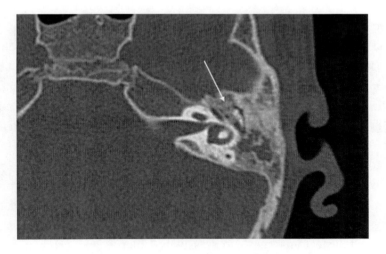

Figure 11. Chronic otomastoiditis with tympanosclerosis; axial MDCT scan showing non cholesteatomatous soft tissue density within the middle ear cavity and mastoid opacification. In this case calcific middle ear foci (arrow) is causing ossicular fixation resulting in conductive hearing loss; non cholesteatomatous ossicular chain erosion findings are present too.

Post-inflammatory ossicular chain erosion is rather rare in the case of a non cholesteatomatous disease but may seldom occur and will affect first the incus long process and lenticular process, followed by stapes head [47].

For best diagnostic accuracy on CT, images should be viewed using a correct bone window setting (large window width, e.g., 4000 HU; low window level, e.g., 0–200 HU).

Three distinctive signs should be carefully evaluated on axial CT images in order to exclude an ossicular erosion [39]:

- "ice cream cone" visible in the epitympanum, where the anterior ice cream cone consists of the malleus head and the posterior cone is made of the incus body and short process;
- "two parallel lines" visible in the mesotympanum, where the anterior line represents the malleus handle and the posterior line represents the incus long process;
- "two dots" visible in the mesotympanum where the lateral dot refers to the lenticular process and the medial dot to the stapes head; between the two dots the incudo-stapedial joint is well visible.

Post-inflammatory erosion sometimes involves walls of tympanic cavity. Based on CT multiplanar images, the following structures should always be carefully evaluated: bony walls of the lateral semicircular canal, bony walls of the tympanic segment of the facial nerve channel and the roof of the middle ear cavity (*tegmen tympani*) [39].

3.3.2. Chronic Otitis Media with Cholesteatoma

Occasionally, chronic suppurative otitis media is associated with a cholesteatoma within the middle ear. Cholesteatoma consists of squamous epithelium that is trapped within the middle ear cavity and mastoid process of the temporal bone. Granulation tissue and ear discharge are often associated with secondary infection of the desquamating epithelium [48]. In the setting of chronic middle ear inflammation, cholesteatomas arise as the result of tympanic membrane retraction or perforation [39].

Cholesteatoma can be either congenital (behind an intact tympanic membrane) or acquired, though the origins are indistinguishable with histology or imaging. Only the location of the lesion on CT/MRI, the clinical history of the patient, and the otologic status of the tympanic membrane could give some hints for a differential diagnosis [21]. If untreated, a cholesteatoma may progressively enlarge and erode the surrounding structures [45].

Since congenital cholesteatomas develop from embryonic epithelial rests, they can be located everywhere in the temporal bone from the external auditory channel to the middle ear, from the mastoid to the petrous apex or even in the squama of the temporal bone or within the tympanic membrane.

Acquired cholesteatomas are classified in primary and secondary but are uniquely localized in the middle ear (see Table 3):

- **"Primary acquired cholesteatomas"** (80% of all middle ear cholesteatomas) usually develop in the region of the pars flaccida behind an apparently intact tympanic membrane;
- **"Secondary acquired cholesteatomas"** (18% of all middle ear cholesteatomas) usually develop into the middle ear through a perforated tympanic membrane in the pars tensa region (rarely the pars flaccida); these cholesteatomas arising from the posterior tympanic membrane are likely to produce facial nerve exposure eroding the bony wall of the facial nerve canal and to destroy the stapedial suprastructure.

Table 3. Pars flaccida and pars tensa cholesteatomas main features

Pars flaccida cholesteatoma (attic or posterior epitympanic cholesteatoma)	Pars tensa cholesteatomas (sinus or posterior mesotympanic cholesteatoma)
Develop from the upper one-third portion of the tympanic membrane (pars flaccida or Shrapnell membrane).	Most often origins through a defect of the lower two-thirds portion of the tympanic membrane (pars tensa)
Soft tissue mass fills the Prussak's space, medial to attic wall and lateral to the ossicles (head of malleus and body of incus).	Soft tissue mass localized in the facial recess and sinus tympani of the tympanic cavity and in the mastoid region.
Erosion of the anterior portion of the lateral epitympanic wall is very common.	Extension of the soft tissue mass starts in the epitympanum medial to the ossicles
Initially ossicles are very often displaced medially.	Initially ossicles are displaced laterally (head of malleus and body of incus).
Ossicles erosion is frequent (most commonly long process of incus).	Ossicle erosion occurs to incus long process, stapedial superstructure and manubrium of malleus.

In elderly patients, a third special kind of cholesteatomas could be diagnosed: external auditory channel cholesteatomas. These lesions are subdivided into idiopathic and secondary [50]. The first are typically bilateral and located in the floor of the external auditory channel. The location and occurrence of the latter depends on the site of the inducing factor.

One last special group of cholesteatomas are the so called "mural cholesteatoma." These could mimic a mastoidectomy cave since they are the result of extensive lesions of the middle ear or of the mastoid which drain their fluid contents into the external auditory channel through the tympanic cavity leaving a wide empty cave often referred to as "automastoidectomy" [21].

When evaluating CT images for the presence of cholesteatoma (Figure 12), the following features should be addressed: ossicle erosion and displacement, bony walls of tegmen tympani and lateral semicircular canal, bony walls of tympanic segment and anterior genu of the facial nerve, possible extension of cholesteatoma towards sinus tympani and possible involvement of oval window niche [21].

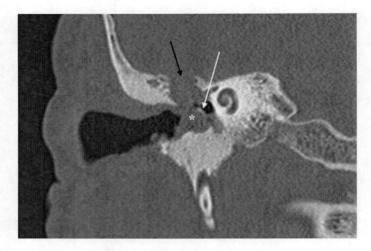

Figure 12. Chronic otomastoiditis with cholesteatoma; coronal MPR from a MDCT scan showing soft tissue density within the middle ear cavity (asterisk) with severe thinning of the tegmen tympani (black arrow), ossicular chain dislocation and severe erosion (white arrow).

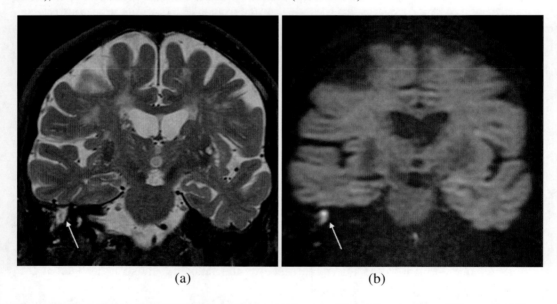

(a)   (b)

Figure 13. Chronic otomastoiditis with cholesteatoma (same patient shown in figure 12); coronal T2-weighted fast spin echo sequence with fast saturation (a) showing unspecific high signal intensity inflammatory tissue in the middle ear cavity (white arrow). A coronal non-echo planar DWI sequence (b) well demonstrate the cholesteatoma within the unspecific fluid collection as a bright comma shaped lesion (white arrow).

On MR images (Figure 13), typical cholesteatoma features include bright, hyperintense signal on diffusion-weighted MRI images (low signal on apparent diffusion coefficient maps), moderate signal intensity on T2-weighted images (lower than the signal that characterize the inflammatory tissue) and lack of enhancement on post-gadolinium T1-weighted sequences [21,49-50].

Chronic otitis media can cause both intracranial and extracranial complications [51, 52].

The most frequent complications of COM with cholesteatoma are [21]:

- erosion of the tegmen or sinus plate that could be thinned or completely eroded;
- erosion of the labyrinth with fistula formation appreciable as a loss of the endochondral bone overlying the labyrinth (labyrinthine fistula occurrence is one of the most common complications in chronic otitis media with cholesteatoma);
- extension of the cholesteatoma into the petrous pyramid;
- erosion of the facial nerve canal commonly resulting in a peripheral facial nerve paralysis.

Table 4. Most common pathologic entities to consider for cholesteatomas differential diagnosis

Pathologic entities	Cholesterol granulomas	Paragangliomas	Schwannomas (facial nerve and geniculate ganglion)	Facial nerve hemangiomas
MRI findings	- High signal on T1-w and T2w. - No contrast-enhancement.	Nodular contrast-enhancing mass on the cochlear promontory.	Characteristic tubular/oval enhancing mass along the tympanic segment of the facial nerve or of the geniculate ganglion.	-Mass with irregular poorly defined margins -Slightly hypointense/isointense on T1WI and hyperintense on T2WI -Bright contrast-enhancing oval lesions on postcontrast images.
CT findings	Bony erosion.	No bony erosion.	Enlarged facial nerve canal and/or geniculate fossa.	-Enlarged facial nerve canal and geniculate fossa. -The ossifying subtype causes a characteristic "honeycomb" morphology.
Others	-Blue tympanic membrane at otoscopic examination. - History of surgery or recurrent otitis media. - Usually DWI does not show diffusion restriction.	- Pulsatile mass at otoscopic examination. Common clinical symptom is rhythmic thumping in the ear.	Large tumors involving the tympanic segment of the facial nerve may be visible on otoscopic examination.	Primary symptoms are facial nerve palsy and hearing loss.

Sigmoid sinus thrombosis is a severe complication of chronic middle ear infectious diseases. In these cases, a contrast enhanced CT scan is mandatory to demonstrate the typical "empty triangle" or "delta" sign: the sigmoid sinus will appear surrounded by the normally enhancing dura that delimitate the un-enhancing thrombus inside the dural venous sinus [53]. MRI is more sensitive to detect thrombosis and assess intraluminal blood flow, and it may even show the involvement of adjacent structures.

In case of suspected infection/inflammation and/or complications (such as lateral semicircular canal fistula), an MRI examination including non-echo planar diffusion-weighted (non-EP DWI) and post-gadolinium T1-weighted sequences is mandatory. These will help differentiating the infection/inflammation from the cholesteatoma and it will show the status of the membranous labyrinth.

Since chronic otitis media with cholesteatoma (including precholesteatomatous states) is an aggressive form of otitis, surgical treatment is mandatory because of the higher risk for labyrinthine or intracranial complications.

The differential diagnosis checklist in case of suspected cholesteatomas includes: cholesterol granulomas, paragangliomas, schwannomas and facial nerve hemangioma (see Table 4).

3.4. Post-Operative Imaging

Surgery is widely used to treat various middle ear disorders such as chronic otitis media, cholesteatoma, otosclerosis, congenital malformations, traumas and tumours. The most common cause of failure in middle ear surgery include persistent suppurative process in middle ear / mastoid and recurrent and/or residual cholesteatoma [54]. Imaging needs to be able to differentiate residual or recurrent disease from granulation tissue, inflammatory tissue or fluid within the middle ear cavity and mastoid cavity. The examination of choice for a post-surgical follow-up is usually a non-contrast high-resolution temporal bone CT which provides information on the exact surgical procedure done and related findings [55-56]. The main role of CT is to allow a correct analysis of dense structures (bony tympano-mastoid walls, ossicular chain, prosthesis) [42]. Furthermore, CT easily detects an intra-tympanic soft tissue and its extension and margins within the postoperative middle ear. However, CT is not specific and so differentiation of granulation tissue in the middle ear cavity from other commonly encountered soft tissue masses such as cholesteatomas usually requires an MRI scan [56]. Despite this, CT is of great help for the assessment of the bony labyrinth and the facial nerve canal.

Conventional MRI scans have low specificity when it comes to differentiating granulation tissue from relapsing cholesteatoma [57]. As a matter of fact both the granulation tissue and the cholesteatoma show hypointense signal on T1 and hyperintense signal on T2 making the differentiation rather difficult. Many studies reported improved specificity of delayed (30-45 minutes) post-contrast T1-weighted sequences since the granulation tissue is poorly vascularized and contrast uptake may occur belatedly [55]. Cholesteatomas are not vascularized and so do not enhance: they typically appear bordered by a ring enhancement attached to the enhancing mucosa [55]. Diffusion-weighted imaging (DWI) is a helpful and effective method for distinguishing cholesteatomas from other soft tissues in post-surgical follow-ups; in particular, non-echo planar DWI has been shown to have a higher sensitivity and specificity in the diagnosis of postoperative chronic otitis media complications differentiating recurrent cholesteatoma from granulation tissue [55, 58].

However, De Foer [41] reported that MR imaging for detection of middle ear cholesteatoma can be performed by using non-EP DW imaging sequences alone since the combined use of DWI and delayed gadolinium-enhanced T1-weighted sequence yielded no significant increases in terms of sensitivity, specificity, negative and positive predictive values.

Some non-cholesteatoma lesions that show restricted diffusion have been reported in English literature and must be taken into account in the differential diagnosis checklist: residual haemorrhage after recent surgery, in ear patches containing silastic sheets or bone pate, cerumen located in the external ear canal, cholesterol granuloma and middle ear or mastoid abscess [55].

Pre-contrast T1-weighted sequences are mandatory to detect lesions with spontaneous high T1 signal intensity (cholesterol granuloma, fluid with high protein concentration, bleeding and fatty tissue) and to get information about the vascularity of the lesion. Fat suppression techniques may result useful too if the lesion is close to a fat containing structure. A careful analysis of the T1-weighted pre- and delayed post-contrast, T2-weighted images and DWI provide a sensitive and accurate method for differentiating soft tissue lesions. The most informative approach to imaging of post-surgical middle ear patients is the use of both CT and MR imaging examinations [55].

3.5. Otosclerosis

Otosclerosis is an autosomal dominant genetic disease with incomplete clinical penetrance and variable expression which involves the human otic capsule [59]. The typical clinical onset is in the third decade and is characterized with symptoms of conductive hearing loss (CHL) due to the impaired movement of the stapes; the disease is bilateral in a majority of cases with a female predilection (F:M ratio of ~2:1) [60]. Patients could also present sensorineural hearing loss (SNHL) or mixed hearing loss (MHL) and/or tinnitus [61]. Pathogenesis of otosclerosis is likely multifactorial and still incompletely understood: even if the genetic component is probably the most significant in determining the slowly progressive CHL, both viral (measles virus) and autoimmune (collagen auto-immunity) etiopathogenetic hypothesis have been investigated and accredited. Whatever the etiopathogenesis, otosclerosis is one of the leading causes of nonsyndromic deafness in adults [62-64].

Otosclerosis is an otodystrophy characterized by the replacement of the normal ivory-like enchondral bone of the otic capsule by immature and spongy vascular new bone; this process of remodeling occurs continuously and accounts for the progressive nature of the disease [65].

It is categorised into two types, fenestral and retrofenestral (or cochlear) otosclerosis. Retrofenestral otosclerosis rarely occurs without fenestral involvement and is considered a continuum of the fenestral otosclerotic process rather than a separate one. Imaging plays an important role in the diagnosis and management of otosclerosis.

In fenestral otosclerosis, demineralized foci of spongy bone typically occur in the region located anterior to the oval window (*fissula ante fenestram*) where a cleft of fibrocartilagenous tissue between the inner and middle ear is found (Figure 14). These typical demineralised foci location should not be confused with the so called "cochlear cleft" [66] that is particularly seen in up to 40% of children as a hypodense cleft in the cochlear otic capsule in the region anterior to the oval window; this finding has no pathological implication in the absence of a clinical evidence for otosclerosis or osteogenesis imperfecta and represent a potential imaging pitfall in children.

In patients with fenestral oteosclerosis, fixation of the stapes by foci located anterior to the oval window is found in 96% of cases. In slightly less than half the cases, demineralised foci are also present in other locations (oval window niche 30%, cochlear apex 12%, posterior to the oval window 12%); in 7% of cases a round window obliteration is found. Other even rarer sites of involvement are the promontory, round window niche and tympanic segment of the facial nerve [61]. CT is the tool of choice to investigate the eventual presence of otosclerotic lesions and its sensitivity to make the diagnosis was recently estimated as high as 90–95% [66]. Stapedectomy is used to treat fenestral otosclerosis and is commonly combined with the insertion of a stapes prosthesis to restore ossicular chain functionality. CT is useful to evaluate the position of radiodense prosthesis (dislocation is a common possible complication) and the typical findings of other post-surgical common complications. MRI will be useful to identify fibrotic changes in cases of labyrinthitis ossificans (Figure 15) [61].

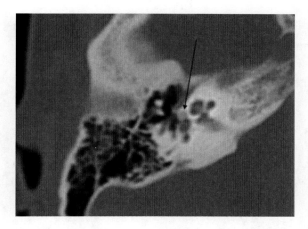

Figure 14. Fenestral otosclerosis; axial MPR from a MDCT scan showing an otospongiosis focus (arrow) close to the round window (not shown).

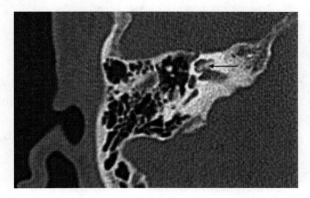

Figure 15. Labyrinthitis ossificans (arrow) could involve any part of the inner ear, in different grade (mild, moderate as shown in the figure, and severe). It is a sequela of an inflammatory process spreading into the membranous labyrinth through three ways: hematogenic, meningogenic (as shown in the figure), and tympanogenic disseminations. Unusual cause of labyrinth ossification are temporal trauma, long standing otosclerosis or tumors. It is a relative contraindication for cochlear implant.

Retrofenestral (or cochlear) otosclerosis, is much less common but nearly always associated with fenestral otosclerosis. Primary cochlear otosclerosis is relatively rare. The typical clinical presentation is a bilateral symmetrical SNHL or MHL or a pulsatile tinnitus. Demineralized foci of spongy bone are typically seen in the cochlear capsule, which may extend around the vestibule, semicircular canals and internal auditory canal (Figure 16). The classical imaging appearance of cochlear otosclerosis on CT is a distinctive pericochlear hypodense double ring sign (which is also known as the "4th ring of Valvassori") [61].

MRI is rarely used in the case of otosclerosis but is useful to demonstrate the osteolytic inflammatory process (during the "acute phase" of the disease) that occurs in the otic capsule as a consequence of the otospongiotic process. During this phase, the otospongiotic foci will show a T1 shortening on MRI pulse sequences acquired after i.v.

injection of gadolinium. MRI is also useful to investigate post-surgery complications (intravestibular granuloma, intralabyrinthine hemorrhage and bacterial labyrinthitis) [68].

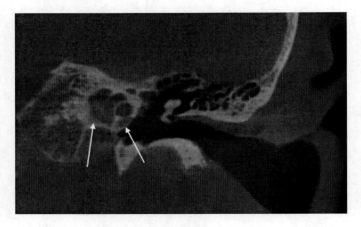

Figure 16. Cochlear otosclerosis; coronal MPR from CBCT scan showing the demineralized foci (arrows) around the basal turn of the cochlea in the otic capsule.

Fluorides and cochlear implantation (CI) are used to treat retrofenestral otosclerosis. Fluoride therapy may limit the growth of active otosclerotic foci and thereby prevent progression of SNHL. CI surgery in patients with otosclerosis may be challenging because of the high risk of partial insertion and misplacement of electrode arrays due to the ossification of the scala tympani in the basal turn of the cochlea [61].

4. INNER EAR

The inner ear is composed of a membranous labyrinth surrounded by a bony labyrinth.

The membranous labyrinth consists of utricle, saccule, semicircular canals, endolymphatic sac and duct, and cochlear duct [69]. CT and MRI may well demonstrate the inner ear structures and their abnormalities. CT has always been the preferred imaging modality to delineate the intricate osseous anatomy and malformations of the inner ear, but high-resolution MR imaging is used with increasing frequency to study the membranous labyrinth and eighth cranial nerve (vestibulocochlear nerve) [70–71].

4.1. Malformations

Congenital abnormalities of the inner ear are the most common cause of sensorineural hearing loss (SNHL). Inner ear malformations (IEMs) occur as a result of an interruption of the development of the ear itself during the first trimester of fetal development. The causes may be idiopathic, associated with an inborn genetic error or due to a teratogenic agent exposure [72]. The findings may be isolated or related to a specific syndrome (Table 5). Patients with congenital inner ear malformations often present with a variable degree of SNHL. Roughly 50% of cases of congenital SNHL can be linked to a genetic cause, with approximately 30% of these considered syndromic and the remaining 70% being nonsyndromic [73]. The abnormalities are usually bilateral and symmetric; these patients are commonly affected by a profound SNHL that could benefit from the use of hearing aids or may have an indication for a cochlear implant (CI).

Table 5. Hereditary syndromes commonly associated with SNHL and characteristic imaging findings

Hereditary syndrome associated with SNHL	Related imaging findings
Alagille syndrome	Absence of the PSCC with normal appearing LSCC
Branchio-oto-renal syndrome	Cochlear hypoplasia (apical turn); abnormal course of the facial nerve canal; funnel-shaped IAC with large porus acousticus; vestibular dysplasia; SCC hypoplasia; enlargement of the vestibular aqueduct; cochlear nerve deficiency; stenosis or atresia of the external auditory canal; middle ear and ossicular chain abnormalities; Eustachian tube dilation; absence of the stapedius muscle.
CHARGE syndrome	Small misshaped pinnae; small middle ear cavities; absence of the stapedius muscle; absence of the round and oval windows; hypoplasia of the incus and stapes; ossicular chain fixation; abnormal course of the tympanic facial nerve; SCC aplasia with associated vestibular dysplasia; cochlear nerve deficiency with atresia of the cochlear aperture; abnormalities of cochlear partitioning.
Klippel-Feil syndrome	Small pinnae with stenotic and downward sloping EEC; deformed caput mallei; rudimental incus head; shortness or absence of long process and absence of the whole incus; missing stapes head; fixed footplate; absence of footplate or of the the whole stapes.
Pendred syndrome	Modiolar deficiency; vestibular enlargement; absence of the interscalar septum between the upper and middle cochlear turn; endolymphatic sac enlargement.
Waardenburg syndrome	Vestibular aqueduct enlargement; widening of the upper vestibule; IAC hypoplasia; decreased modiolus size; aplasia or hypoplasia of the PSCC.
X-linked hearing loss with stapes gusher	Enlarged bulbous IACs; widened cochlear aperture (appearing as wide as communication between the basal turn of the cochlea and the IAC) with absence of the lamina cribrosa; cochlear hypoplasia with modiolar deficiency; widening of the bony canal for the labyrinthine segment of the facial nerve; dilation of the vestibular aqueducts.

Congenital malformations of the inner ear may be considered in two broad categories [74]: (a) malformations with pathologic changes that involve only the membranous labyrinth and (b) malformations that involve both the osseous and the membranous labyrinth (malformed otic capsules).

The majority of the causes of congenital hearing loss (80%) belong to the first group. There is no gross bony abnormality and, therefore, in these cases HRCT and MR imaging of the temporal bone reveal normal findings. The remaining 20% have various malformations involving the bony labyrinth and can be radiologically demonstrated by CT and MRI. In patients who are candidates for CI surgery, imaging provides preoperative information about the inner ear, the vestibulocochlear nerve, and the brain. CT and MRI together, can aid decision making about the best management strategy by facilitating the identification and characterization of inner ear malformations and any associated neurologic abnormalities.

Formerly, the Jackler et al. classification of IEMs was based on the time of developmental arrest during embryogenesis and anatomical development [75]. In 2002 Sennaroglu et al. [76] modified this classification and grouped the inner ear anomalies by their decreasing severity; Michel deformity (complete labyrinth aplasia), cochlear aplasia, common cavity, incomplete partition type 1 (IP-I or cystic cochleovestibular malformation), cochlear hypoplasia and incomplete partition type 2 (IP-II or classic Mondini deformity). There are a variety of IEMs and they all present in a different way: each group has different radiological findings that are very important in the management of deaf patients.

4.1.1. Complete Labyrinthine Aplasia (Michel Deformity)

Complete Labyrinthine Aplasia (CLA) is a rare malformation resulting in complete aplasia of the membranous labyrinth. It is caused by the developmental arrest of otic placode, early during the third week of fetal development [77]. It is the most severe among the deformities involving the osseous and membranous labyrinth.

According to radiological findings [78], three subgroups of CLA are present:

1) *CLA with hypoplastic or aplastic petrous bone* - In these cases CLA is accompanied by hypoplasia or aplasia of the petrous bone.
2) *CLA without otic capsule* - In this group of CLA, formation of the petrous bone is normal, but the otic capsule is hypoplastic or aplastic.
3) *CLA with otic capsule* - Formation of the petrous bone and the otic capsule is normal. Only in this group of CLA with otic capsule development, the labyrinthine segment of the facial canal is in its normal location.

On CT examinations there is a complete absence of inner ear structures (cochlea, vestibule and semicircular canals). The external auditory canal and middle ear cavity are usually normal because they do not arise from the otic capsule. Vestibulocochlear nerve is aplastic in patients with Michel deformity because they have no otic vesicle development. Patients present with a complete SNHL [77].

4.1.2. Cochlear Aplasia

Cochlear aplasia is the absence of the cochlea with formation of the utricle, saccule and semicircular canals. CT demonstrates an absent cochlea with a partially or completely formed vestibule and semicircular canals (SCCs) (Figure 17).

There are two subgroups [79]:

1) *Cochlear aplasia with normal labyrinth* - Vestibule and SCCs are normally developed;
2) *Cochlear aplasia with a dilated vestibule (CADV)* - Vestibule and SCCs show dilatation.

It is very important to differentiate CADV from a common cavity (CC) deformity.

Cochlear aplasia with a normal labyrinth is usually symmetric. In CADV, however, asymmetric development may be present; pathology may be due to genetic or environmental factors. Otic capsule development is always normal.

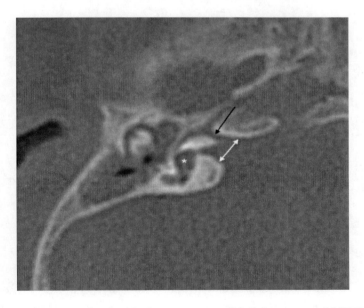

Figure 17. Cochlear aplasia associated with aberrant course of facial nerve; axial MDCT scan at the level of the IAC (double headed arrow). The cochlea is absent, a dilated vestibule can be identified (asterisk) and the intralabyrinthine segment of CN VII is antero-medially displaced (black arrow).

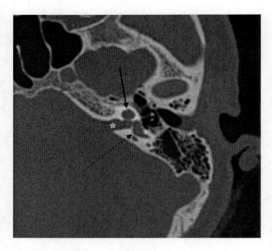

Figure 18. Incomplete partition type I (IP-1); axial MDCT scan showing typical cystic appearance of the cochlea and vestibule (severe case). The cochlea (black arrow) is featureless because of the absence of the modiolus and the interscalar septum; coexists vestibular dilatation (dotted arrow) and a wide IAC (asterisk).

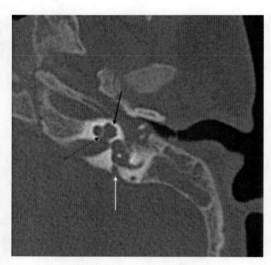

Figure 19. Incomplete partition type II (IP-II); axial MDCT scan. The apical part of the modiolus is defective giving the typical cystic appearance of the apex of the cochlea because of coalescent apical and middle turn (arrow). The defective modiolus is appreciable only in proximity of the medial side of the basal turn (dotted arrow). Coexists vestibule (asterisk) and vestibular aqueduct (white arrow) dilatation.

4.1.3. Common Cavity Deformity

A common cavity results from a developmental arrest in the 4th week of gestation and accounts for about 25% of all cochlear malformations [71]. CC deformity denotes a malformed inner ear in which the vestibule and cochlea are confluent with no internal architecture. Theoretically, this structure has cochlear and vestibular neural structures. There may be accompanying SCCs or their rudimentary parts.

It is important to differentiate CC from CAVD because CI in a CC may result in acoustic stimulation, whereas in CAVD no functional stimulation will occur with CI.

4.1.4. Cochlear Hypoplasia (CH)

In this deformity, there is a clear differentiation between cochlea and vestibule. In CH the dimensions are less than those of a normal cochlea with various internal architecture deformities. But the definition "cochlea with one and a half turns" should be used for hypoplasia (particularly type III), rather than for IP-II cochlea.

Patients have variable SNHL depending on the degree of development of the membranous labyrinth. CT shows a small cochlear bud, while the vestibule is usually enlarged. The SSCs are malformed in 50% of patients. Four different types of CH have been defined [80]: *(i) CH-I (Bud-like cochlea), (ii) CH-II (Cystic hypoplastic cochlea), (iii) CH-III (Cochlea with less than 2 turns), (iiii) CH-IV (Cochlea with hypoplastic middle and apical turns)* (Figure 20).

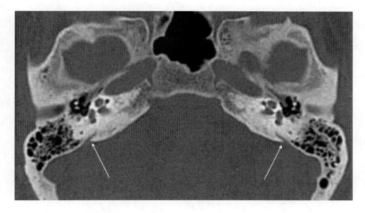

Figure 20. Patient with congenital sensorineural hearing loss with an enlarged vestibular aqueduct syndrome; axial MDCT scan showing bilateral slight enlargement of vestibular aqueduct and its operculum (arrows).

4.1.5. Incomplete Partitions

In incomplete partition (IP) anomalies there is a clear differentiation between cochlea and vestibule, with normal external dimensions and various internal architecture defects. Incomplete partitions constitute 41% of IEMs [79, 80] There are three different types of incomplete partition groups according to the defect in the modiolus and the interscalar septa:

1) **IP-I** (termed as "cystic cochleovestibular malformation" [79]). These represent approximately 20% of IEMs. In this anomaly, there is a clear differentiation between cochlea and vestibule. The fact that the vestibule is distinguishable from the cochlea makes it possible to differentiate an IP-I from a common cavity. Cochlea is accompanied by an enlarged, dilated vestibule (Figure 18). The

cribriform area between the cochlea and IAC is often defective, and all patients have a large IAC, predisposing them to increased risks for meningitis. All patients with IP-I and recurrent meningitis who have normal tympanic membranes but fluid filling the middle ear and mastoid, should have an exploration of the middle ear with special attention to the stapes footplate.
2) **IP-II** (classic Mondini deformity). In IP-II, the apical part of the modiolus is defective (Figure 19). It is the most common type of cochlear malformation, accounting for more than 50% of all cochlear deformities [74]. This anomaly was originally described by Carlo Mondini, and together with a minimally dilated vestibule and an enlarged vestibular aqueduct (EVA) constitute the triad of the Mondini deformity. The term "Mondini" should be used only if the above mentioned triad of malformations is present [76,81]. The apical part of the modiolus and the corresponding interscalar septa are defective, giving the apex of the cochlea a cystic appearance due to the confluence of middle and apical turns. The external dimensions of the cochlea are similar to that seen in normal cases. Therefore, it is not correct to define this anomaly as a cochlea with "one and a half turns" [80].
3) **IP-III**. In IP-III, cochlea has an interscalar septa but the modiolus is completely absent. IP-III cochlear malformation is the type of anomaly present in X-linked deafness [82]. It is the rarest form of incomplete partition cases, among 2% of all IEMs. The external dimensions of the cochlea (height and diameter) were found to be similar to the normal cochlea [83].

4.1.6. Enlarged Vestibular Aqueduct (EVA)

This describes the presence of an enlarged vestibular aqueduct in the presence of a normal cochlea, vestibule and SCCs (Figure 20). The difference between EVA and IP-II is that cochlea and vestibule are completely normal on HRCT and MRI [80]. Classically EVA is described when the midpoint between posterior labyrinth and operculum is larger than 1.5 mm on axial sections.

4.1.7. Malformations of the Vestibule and Semicircular Canals

The malformed canals are usually short and wide but may be narrow. In extensive malformations, the vestibule is dilated and forms a common lumen with the lateral canal. This type of abnormality, which has been described as "lateral semicircular canal–vestibule dysplasia," may be accompanied by a normal or malformed cochlea, depending on the stage of inner ear development at the time of embryologic arrest.

Aplasia of the semicircular canals is far less common than dysplasia. Absence of all semicircular ducts occurs frequently in patients with CHARGE syndrome (a combination of coloboma, heart anomalies, choanal atresia, retardation of growth and development, and genital and ear anomalies) [84, 85]. Isolated aplasia of the posterior semicircular duct has been described in patients with Waardenburg syndrome and Alagille syndrome [84].

It is essential to perform high-resolution CT to confirm the diagnosis of semicircular canal aplasia and to differentiate it from fibrous or calcified obliteration of the canals.

4.1.8. Abnormalities of the Vestibulo-Cochlear Nerve

With current MRI technique, it is possible to visualize the vestibulo-cochlear nerve. It may be normal to hypoplastic or absent (Figure 21). The absence of the cochlear nerve is definitely found in cochlear aplasia. While in the case of Michel deformity with absent IAC, the complete vestibulo-cochlear nerve is also absent and only facial nerve can be identified.

An hypoplastic vestibulo-cochlear nerve is particularly important in CC.

The amount of cochlear nerve fibers determines the hearing level and management strategy.

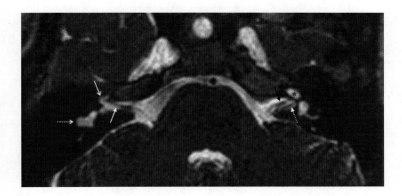

Figure 21. Cochlear nerve aplasia; axial 3D CISS sequence at the level of IACs showing right cochlear nerve aplasia with ipsilateral small bud cochlea (white arrow with empty head) and vestibular and lateral semicircular canal malformation (dotted line with empty head); the right facial nerve (white arrow) is antero-medially displaced. The left vestibulocochlear nerve (black arrow and white dotted arrow) is unremarkable as well as the visualised sections of the cochlea (basal turn, asterisk).

4.2. Infections

The inner ear infections usually refer to an inflammatory process of the membranous labyrinth, which typically manifests as an acute SNHL or vertigo. Labyrinthitis can be classified on the basis of the causative agent and can be considered infectious (bacterial, viral, or luetic) or non-infectious (trauma, autoimmune, or toxic).

A number of viruses, including measles, mumps, influenza, rubella, cytomegalovirus, and herpes are associated with acquired inner ear pathology [86]. CT and MRI are complementary in evaluating patients with labyrinthitis.

On the ot-neuroradiological point of view, three stages are described in labyrinthitis:

1) *Acute stage*: MR imaging demonstrates strong labyrinthine enhancement on gadolinium-enhanced T1-wheighted imaging; however, enhancement is not specific for an infectious aetiology because similar findings can be seen with non-infectious causes of labyrinthitis. On CT, the inner ear appears normal.
2) *Fibrous stage:* on CISS sequences is seen as loss of the normal fluid signal intensity in the membranous labyrinth [87]. Contrast-enhanced T1WI may demonstrate enhancement of the inner ear, not as strong as that in the acute phase. On CT, the inner ear will appear normal.
3) *Ossifying stage*: it appears on CT as calcification within the inner ear. MR imaging will demonstrate loss of normal hyperintense fluid signal intensity on CISS images, without enhancement on contrast-enhanced T1WI [88].

Fibrosing and ossifying labyrinthitis may be indistinguishable on MR imaging, and CT is necessary to determine the presence of inner ear ossification. This distinction is particularly important in candidates for cochlear implantation (CI) because significant ossification of the cochlea can make implantation more difficult, if not impossible, and often results in poor functional results [89].

When ossification of the labyrinth becomes very advanced, there may be no recognizable labyrinthine structures, in which case the chief differential consideration is labyrinthine aplasia.

4.3. Autoimmune Labyrinthitis

The diagnosis of autoimmune labyrinthitis is usually one of exclusion. Patients typically present with rapidly progressive fluctuating bilateral SNHL that responds to immunosuppressive agents. Usually these patients also have autoimmune disease such as Cogan syndrome, systemic lupus erythematosus, juvenile idiopathic arthritis, Wegener granulomatosis, Sjogren syndrome or antiphospholipid syndrome.

Autoimmune labyrinthitis appears similar to infectious forms of labyrinthitis on MR imaging and will demonstrate intense labyrinthine enhancement acutely on postcontrast T1WI [87, 88]. The imaging abnormalities often resolve with steroid treatment but may occasionally progress to fibrosing or ossifying labyrinthitis.

4.4. Imaging in Cochlear Implantation

Cochlear implantation (CI) is indicated for some patients with profound SNHL. Preoperative knowledge of the anatomic features of temporal bone may be critical for making the decision to perform CI. The majority of cases of SNHL result from degeneration of the hair cells in the organ of Corti. CI devices bypass the hair cells and directly stimulate the spiral ganglion cells. The electrode is inserted into the scala tympani via the round window or through an anteroinferior cochleostomy (Figure 22-23). Both MRI and high resolution CT in combination can provide surgically relevant information [90]. The goal of preoperative imaging is primarily to identify cochlear abnormalities, eighth-nerve deficiency, or anatomic variations that influence candidacy, ear selection, surgical approach, and prognosis. Special attention should be placed on the patency of the round window, size of the facial recess, course of the facial nerve, patency of the cochlea and presence of IAC [91].

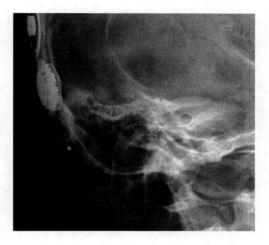

Figure 22. Cochlear implant visualization on plain film radiograph (Stenvers' view) performed for postoperative evaluation of a cochlear implant lead.

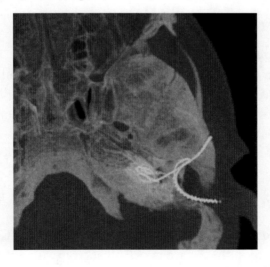

Figure 23. Cochlear implant in a patient with IP-II malformation; the image shows an axial thick-slab maximum intensity projection (MIP) reconstruction from a MDCT scan.

Cochlear anatomy, as well as the degree of residual hearing, may influence a surgeon's choice of electrode.

Once, evidence of an absent or severely dysplastic cochlear nerve, as in Michel deformity, was considered an absolute contraindication to cochlear implantation in any patient. More recently, implantation in children with an absent or deficient eighth nerve was performed with variable results. A potential alternative treatment for children with cochlear nerve deficiency is auditory brainstem implantation [92].

Other conditions that may preclude CI are active otosclerosis and bilateral acoustic schwannomas. Of course, active middle ear infections and fluid in the middle ear cavity should be noted to delay surgery.

5. Imaging of Cerebellopontine Angle and Internal Auditory Canal Lesions

Lesions of the cerebellopontine angle (CPA) and internal auditory canal (IAC) are frequent and represent 6%–10% of all intracranial tumors. Vestibular schwannomas and meningiomas are the two most frequent lesions and account for approximately 85%–90% of all CPA tumors [93, 94]. The other 10%–15% represents a group of lesions arising from the different structures found in these anatomical regions.

The detection of lesions at CPA and IAC is a diagnostic challenge for neuroradiologists. The diagnostic study with the greatest sensitivity and specificity in the evaluation of asymmetric sensorineural hearing loss (aSNHL) is MRI.

Currently, the MRI screening protocol for CPA lesions consists of high-resolution T2-weighted (T2w) sequences (see Paragraph 1.2 for CISS sequences) in combination with contrast-enhanced T1-weighted (GdT1w) sequences.

T2w has a very high diagnostic accuracy for the presence of CPA lesions in patients with aSNHL. However, GdT1w remains mandatory in the detection of smallest vestibular schwannomas as well as rare differential diagnoses [95].

Common lesions of the IAC/CPA include vestibular schwannomas, meningiomas, haemangiomas, lipomas, lymphomas, facial nerve tumours, and aneurysms.

5.1. Vestibular Schwannoma

Vestibular schwannoma (VS) is the most frequent tumour in the CPA (70-80% of all CPA masses). It arises from the Schwann cells that wrap the vestibulocochlear nerve at the glial-Schwann cell junction (Obersteiner-Redlich zone). VS are usually unilateral, not hereditary and occur sporadically; bilateral vestibular schwannomas are usually associated with a genetic disorder (neurofibromatosis type 2, NF2).

Most vestibular schwannomas develop from the inferior vestibular nerve in the IAC where they grow slowly (Figure 24). Then, eroding the posterior edge of the porus acusticus, it may give rise to a round component in the CPA cistern, giving the typical "ice cream on cone" pattern (Figure 25). Small, purely intracanalicular schwannomas exist, but may also present with a dumbbell extension in the cochlea or vestibule [96]. On the other hand, purely intracisternal vestibular schwannomas, without IAC involvement, have a large space to grow in before becoming symptomatic, and at imaging are always larger and heterogeneous due to cystic components or bleeding [97].

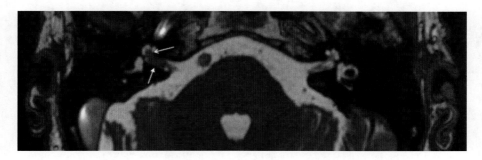

Figure 24. Intra-canalar vestibular schwannoma; axial CISS at the level of IACs showing a small mass which arise from the modiolus region (empty head arrow) and extends up to two/third of the IAC (arrow).

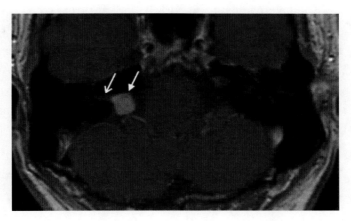

Figure 25. Vestibular schwannoma with typical "ice cream on cone" pattern; axial contrast enhanced T1-weighted sequence at the level of IACs showing an enhancing solid mass (arrow, the "ice cream") which arise from the IAC (empty head arrow, the "cone") and extends into the CPA cistern mass.

With CT, schwannomas are usually isodense and enhance after contrast administration. On MRI, they show T1 isointensity and T2 high signal intensity (Figure 26), but appear as a hypointense filling defect on T2- weighted high-resolution MR cisternography (CISS sequences), and enhance strongly on GdT1w. Enhancement of the adjacent meninges is possible in vestibular schwannoma and is not specific nor exclusive for meningiomas [98].

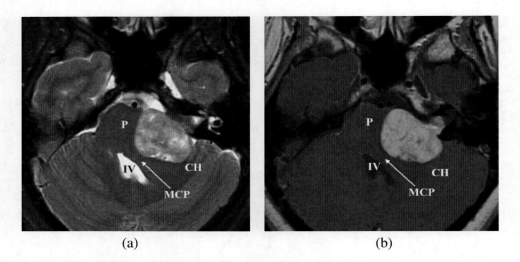

Figure 26. Giant solid vestibular schwannoma; axial T2-weighted turbo spin echo (a) and axial contrast enhanced T1-weighted spin echo (b) sequences at the level of left IACs showing a big solid mass extending from the IAC to the CPA cistern causing severe mass effect of the pons (P) and on the ipsilateral middle cerebellar peduncle (MCP) and cerebellar hemisphere (CH); the fourth ventricle (IV) is evidently compressed too.

There are three different MRI appearances of the tumor after Gd-administration: homogeneous (50–60%), heterogeneous (30–40%), and cystic (5–15%) [99].

MRI may also be used to optimize treatment planning with respect to several features of the lesion: (i) the size of the tumor; (ii) the distance between the lateral extremity of the intracanalicular portion of the tumor and the fundus because it affects the hearing prognosis and may modify the surgical approach; (iii) the intralabyrinthine signal intensity: poor hearing prognosis may be predicted by a low T2-signal intensity of labyrinth contents compared to the unaffected ear; (iv) the identification of the facial nerve and its position relative to the vestibular schwannoma [16].

5.2. Meningioma

Meningioma represents the second most frequent (10%– 15%) tumor of the CPA after VS [94]. Meningioma arises from arachnoid meningothelial cells and grows slowly in the CPA, independently from the internal auditory canal. It is usually located at the posterior aspect of the temporal bone or at the premeatal area, from where it can easily extend into the IAC, but without enlarging the porus [16]. At CT, meningiomas are hyperdense in 70% of the cases, calcified in about 20% and show a frequent adjacent bone reaction including hyperostosis and enostotic spur.

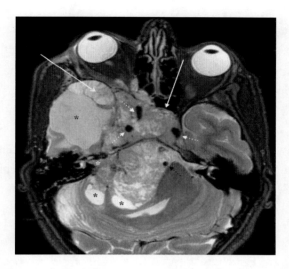

Figure 27. Skull base meningioma with multi-compartmental extension; axial T2-weighted turbo spin echo sequence with fat saturation. Heterogeneous mass with multiple intra-tumoral degenerative cysts and peritumoral arachnoid cysts (black asterisks). The tumour invades the pituitary fossa (white arrow) causing internal carotids arteries encasement (dotted arrows), the anterior cranial temporal fossa floor (white arrow with empty head) and orbital region, and the pontine and PCA cisterns extending into the right IAC (white asterisk) with basilar artery encasement (black dotted arrow) and mass effect on the pons and infratentorial brain structures with severe compression of the IV ventricle.

Meningiomas are isointense with the cortex on all sequences (Figure 27), and are strongly enhanced after i.v. contrast medium injection, usually homogeneously. The "dural tail sign," is particularly frequent in association with meningiomas, but not specific [98] and should suggest the diagnosis when observed.

5.3. Aneurysms

The vertebral and basilar arteries and some of their branches pass through the CPA cistern, where a tortuous segment or ectasia or even an aneurysm can develop. They account for a substantial part of non-tumoral lesions of the CPA that can lead to cranial nerves or brain stem compression [93]. In this location, intracranial aneurysms can arise from the postero-inferior cerebellar artery (PICA), the antero-inferior cerebellar artery (AICA), the vertebral artery (VA) or the basilar artery (BA) itself [100].

They may mimic vestibular schwannomas, especially on CT, because they appear as well defined round lesions that enhance after contrast administration. At MRI, aneurysms without internal thrombus have flow voids and pulsation artefacts on all spin echo sequences but demonstrate iso-to-high signal intensities and variable patterns of gadolinium uptake on T1-weighted images when intraluminal thrombus is present. MR angiography should then be performed to confirm the diagnosis, detect the parent artery and plan the possible therapeutic options.

5.4. Epidermoid Cyst

The epidermoid cyst is the third most frequent tumor of the CPA [93]. It is a congenital lesion arising from normal epithelial cells included during neural tube closure. It grows from the slow desquamation of the stratified keratinised epithelium that lines the cyst.

These tumors grow slowly, encasing nerves and arteries in the cisterns with a specific cauliflower-like outer surface [17]. On CT scans, epidermoid cysts appear hypoattenuating to CSF, and have characteristic irregular, lobulated margins. As opposed to an arachnoid cyst, epidermoid cysts produce no reaction to the adjacent bone structures.

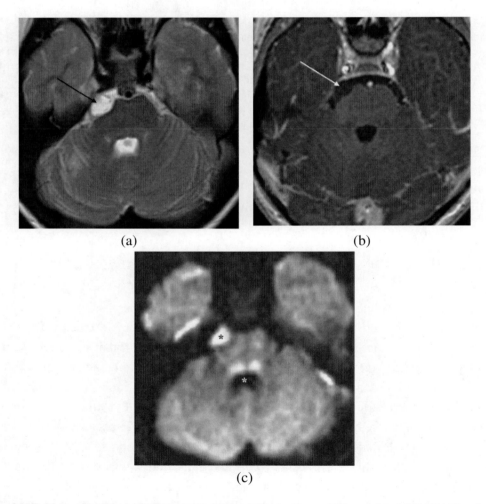

(a) (b)

(c)

Figure 28. Epidermoid cyst; axial T2-weighted (a), contrast-enhanced T1-weighted (b) and echo planar DWI (c) sequences at the level of the CPA / pontine cistern. A small lesion with CSF like signal on T2 and T1+Gd in the right CPA / pontine cistern is shown (arrows). DWI highlights the finding which show a typical bright signal (black asterisk) if compared to CSF (white asterisk within the IV ventricle).

With MRI, epidermoid cysts have slightly higher signal intensity than CSF on T1w and T2w images. However, based on signal intensity alone, it could be difficult to distinguish from arachnoid cysts on these sequences. T2-weighted FLuid Attenuated Inversion Recovery (FLAIR) and Diffusion Weighted Imaging (DWI) sequences are well known to allow differentiation between epidermoid and arachnoid cysts (Figure 28). DWI offers a finding specific for epidermoid cysts by showing a very bright signal [101]. DWI is also crucial in the postoperative follow-up as it allows confirmation of the presence of a possible residual tumour.

5.5. Arachnoid Cyst

An arachnoid cyst is a congenital, benign, intra-arachnoid pouch-like lesion filled with normal CSF. It is usually supratentorial, with about 70% being in the temporal fossa, mostly on the left side [17], anterior to the temporal poles. Only 10% of arachnoid cysts are located in the posterior fossa, where they most commonly develop in the CPA.

Spontaneous or traumatic intracystic haemorrhage can complicate arachnoid cysts, though this is uncommon in the posterior fossa [102].

At neuroimaging, attenuation and signal intensities of uncomplicated arachnoid cysts exactly match those of CSF on all sequences (Figure 29), and do not enhance after contrast media administration. The typical complete suppression of signal intensity on FLAIR sequence and the lack of diffusion restriction of these lesions on DWI easily help in the differential diagnosis with epidermoid cysts.

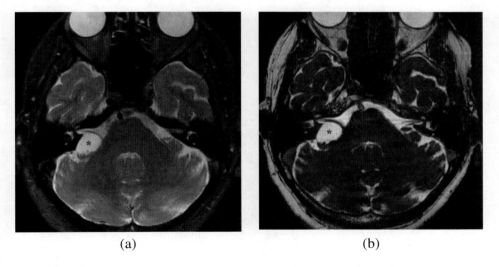

(a)   (b)

Figure 29. Arachnoid cyst; axial T2-weighted with fat-saturation (a) and high resolution CISS (b) sequences at the level of IACs. A lesion occupying the right CPA with CSF like signal on all pulse sequences is shown (asterisk); the cyst causes mild mass effect on the intracisternal tract of the vestibulocochlear nerve.

5.6. Lipochoristomas (Lipomatous Tumors)

Lipochoristomas are benign rare tumors (0.1% of all CPA tumours) that were thought to arise from cells of the meninx primitive and thus they were referred to as lipomas of the IAC/CPA. Nowadays they are more appropriately characterized as "lipomatous choristomas" since they arise from mesenchyme endogenous to the vestibulocochlear nerve [103]. They typically appear as homogeneous fatty lesions surrounding and encasing normal adjacent neurovascular structures with very dense adhesions, usually asymptomatic. Sometimes they may produce symptoms by compressing the adjacent cerebral structures, such as the cranial nerves [104]. Lipochoristomas typically show as hypoattenuating lesions on CT with a high signal on MRI T1-weighted images (promptly suppressed with fat saturations sequences) and no contrast enhancement on T1-weighted images acquired after i.v. administration of contrast medium (Figure 30). They usually show an indolent slow growth and conservative management with periodic imaging follow-ups is thus recommended. Those lesions which have a low fat content usually show an iso- or mildly hypo-intense signal on T1-weighted pulse sequences with appreciable signs of contrast enhancement after i.v. administration of gadolinium chelate [105].

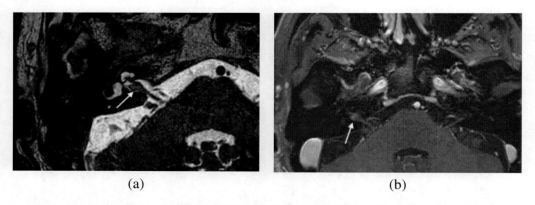

(a)   (b)

Figure 30. Lipochoristoma; axial CISS (a) and axial contrast-enhanced T1-weighted turbo spin echo sequence with fat saturation (b). A small lesion with fat-like signal on all pulse sequences is found (arrows) deep into the right IAC.

5.7. Dermoid Cyst

Dermoid cysts result from the congenital inclusion of cutaneous ectoderm. Intracranial dermoid cysts are usually supratentorial midline lesions containing a mix of fat, hair, calcifications and the products of sebaceous glands and desquamation of a keratinized epithelium. Dermoid cysts rarely arise in the CPA, and may be secondary to the caudal extension of a parasellar lesion [17].

At imaging, a dermoid cyst appears as a well-circumscribed fatty round mass with a thick peripheral capsule that may enhance. In case of rupture, the visualisation of fatty T1-hyperintense droplets in the sulci or a fat-fluid level in the ventricles is highly suggestive of the diagnosis.

5.8. Chordoma

Chordomas develop from remnants of the notochord and are located within the midline, near the clivus, from which they can expand into the CPA. Chondroid chordoma is a pathological subtype of chordoma that may arise more laterally in the petrous bone and grow directly in the CPA [106]. With CT, chordomas appear hypoattenuating soft-tissue mass associated with irregular bone erosion of the clivus. At MR imaging, chordomas usually appear as lobulated, large, hyperintense masses on T2w images with septa of low signal intensity. Slight enhancement is present.

5.9. Intra-Axial Tumors with CPA Involvement

Sometimes, an intra-axial or intraventricular tumor can be large enough to invade the CPA or to manifest as a CPA mass. In such a case, the intra-axial origin could almost be impossible to define (Figure 31). Diagnosis is difficult, but subtle signs like narrowing of the cisterns, irregularity of the tumor-brain interface, and edema are helpful.

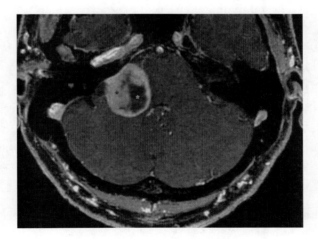

Figure 31. Glioblastoma; axial contrast-enhanced T1-weighted turbo spin echo sequence with fat saturation demonstrating a mostly solid and enhancing lesion (black asterisk) with some cystic / necrotic components (white asterisk) occupying the right CPA. In such a challenging case is not easy to understand the intra-axial exophytic nature of the tumor.

In this context, the most frequent diagnosis includes: pedunculated brainstem glioma, choroid plexus papilloma, lymphoma, hemangioblastoma, ependymoma, medulloblastoma, and dysembryoplastic neuroepithelial tumor (DNET) [17].

6. TRAUMATIC LESIONS OF THE TEMPORAL BONE

All the bones in our body are the result of an adaptation process [107]. The skull is no exception of what kind of trade-off the evolution process had to face: it must ensure maximum bone strength and resistance to protect its precious content from any external agent while maintaining a lightweight to ensure ease of head movements. A fracture, even considering the age-related physiological variations of our bones, will result when an external force hitting the skull will overcome its intrinsic elastic absorption capacity.

6.1. Temporal Bone Fractures

Nowadays, motor vehicle accidents are the most common cause of trauma. Almost two-thirds of road accidents are associated with head trauma even if the number of sports-, assault- and falls-related head trauma has increased in recent years [108, 109]. In severe head trauma cases, up to 8% of the patients will present a temporal bone fracture; if the patient has a skull fracture the probability that there is also a temporal bone fracture rises up to 22% [110]. Since many pathologic conditions could be associated with a temporal bone trauma a promptly imaging-based diagnosis is mandatory.

Temporal bone fractures can occur with or without brain injuries and are classified within the skull base traumatic lesions as laterobasal fractures.

Table 6. Features commonly associated with "otic capsule sparing" and "otic capsule violating" temporal bone fractures

Features	Kind of fracture	
	Otic capsule sparing	Otic capsule violating
Frequency	Common (70-90%)	relatively rare (10-30%)
Facial nerve injury	rare	frequent (2x)
Risk to develop CSF leak/fistula	low risk	high risk (4x)
Associated profound sensorineural and/or conductive hearing loss	low risk	high risk (7x)
Intracranial complications (subarachnoid hemorrhage, epidural hematoma)	rare	Frequent
Risk for meningitis	low	higher risk throughout life

Taking as reference the long axis of the temporal bone, they are historically classified as longitudinal, transverse (Figure 32) and mixed fractures (Figure 33) [111, 112]. However, this classification result was not always well correlated with the severity of clinical signs and symptoms. A new classification that distinguishes the temporal bone fractures in "otic capsule sparing" and "otic capsule violating" has been proposed (Table 6) [113]. While "otic capsule sparing" fractures are the most common (70-90%), the latter are rare (10-30%) and more frequently associated with complications such as cerebrospinal fluid leak or fistula, facial nerve injury, hearing loss and intracranial complication such as subarachnoid hemorrhage, epidural hematoma and meningitis [113-116]. A temporal bone fracture can also be classified as petrous or non-petrous [112].

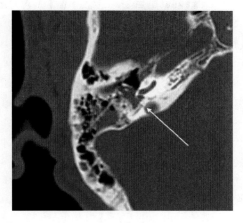

Figure 32. Transverse temporal bone fracture; axial MDCT scan (head trauma spiral CT protocol with 1mm thick slices) shows a transverse fracture line involving the right superior semicircular canal (arrow).

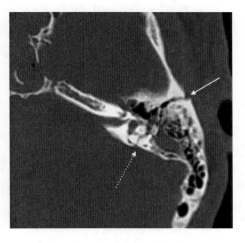

Figure 33. Mixed temporal bone fracture; axial MDCT scan (head trauma spiral CT protocol with 1mm thick slices) shows a longitudinal fracture line involving the left temporal bone pyramid base (arrow) and a transverse fracture line through the ipsilateral inner ear structures (dotted arrow).

The first, extending to the petrous apex or the otic capsule, is more frequently associated with cerebrospinal leak and facial nerve injury. The latter doesn't involve the petrous apex nor the otic capsule but may extend into the tympanic cavity or mastoid and is more frequently associated with conductive hearing loss [117].

Patients with severe head trauma are often unconscious and, after the emergency room evaluation, are commonly hospitalized in a neurosurgery unit. As soon as the patient's condition allows it, an otological assessment as well as facial nerve evaluation should be performed to facilitate the detection and treatment of potentially correctable middle ear and facial nerve injuries [116].

A high-resolution CT scan is the first-line imaging examination in patients with severe head trauma with or without suspected temporal bone injuries. On CT images, fracture lines must be differentiated from the so called "pseudofractures." The latter are normal linear structures very commonly seen on cross-sectional images and are related to the temporal bone anatomy (small canals) and its relationship with adjacent bones (fine sutures) that can mimic temporal bone fractures. If a pseudofracture is suspected, a comparison with the unaffected contralateral side may be helpful in the differential diagnosis. Identifying a small fracture line is not always easy since most polytrauma patients are studied with generic CT trauma protocols (thus slice thickness is rarely less than 1mm as for high resolution temporal bone imaging). If a patient arrives in the Radiology Department with a presumptive diagnosis of temporal bone fracture because of some typical physical findings (i.e., hemotympanum, postauricular ecchymosis and periorbital ecchymosis), an attendant sign of a temporal bone fracture could be the opacifications of mastoid cells, tympanic cavity and external auditory canal with or without blood-fluid levels. More rarely, pneumocephalus as a sign for an open skull base fracture or a brain injury or an extra-axial fluid collection or even small air bubbles in the glenoid fossa of the temporomandibular joint could be indirect signs of a temporal bone fracture [118].

6.2. Ossicular Injuries

Ossicular injuries are usually related to temporal, occipital or parietal region high energy trauma. The ossicular chain is more frequently damaged in longitudinal or mixed fractures of the temporal bone while it is rarely involved in patients with transverse fractures and other kinds of head trauma.

The most common CT finding is the dislocation of the ossicular chain. If an ossicular injury is suspected, multiplanar reconstructions will be helpful to detect the ossicular chain complex; the oval window region should always be carefully evaluated.

Incudo-malleolar and incudo-stapedial joint separation are the most common dislocation injuries; both are best seen on axial slices, the first as a gap between the body of incus and head of malleus and the latter as gap between the body of incus and head of malleus. The whole incudo-malleolar complex dislocation is usually due to an incudo-stapedial joint rupture.

Isolated dislocation of the incus is characterized by the "Y" sign on coronal slices [119] and is far more common than the isolated dislocation of the malleus because of the weaker ligamentary complex.

More rare are the dislocation of the stapes into the vestibulum (stapedio-vestibular dislocation); in these cases, a perilymphatic fistula is often seen and the identification of small air bubbles in the labyrinth could be an indirect sign of it.

Fractures of the single components of the ossicular chain are very rare and hard to identify if high-resolution CT protocols and multiplanar reconstructions are not used.

6.3. Contusio Labyrinthi (Labyrinthine Concussion)

In patients with a negative CT scan for temporal bone fractures but typical clinical signs of inner ear impairment after a head trauma, a traumatic lesion of the inner ear must be suspected. This could occasionally be associated with the opacifications of pneumatized areas of the middle ear in an otherwise negative CT examination. The only oto-neuroradiological examination that could provide a direct demonstration of such an impairment of the inner ear is MRI that could reveal an hyperintense intra-labyrinthine bleeding on T1-weighted sequences (Figure 34) with enhancement on involved inner ear structures on T1-weighted sequences performed after i.v. contrast administration (labyrinthine contusion or concussion). In such cases the risk of fibrosis and ossification of the labyrinth is possible but less frequent than in cases with transverse fractures of the temporal bone [120].

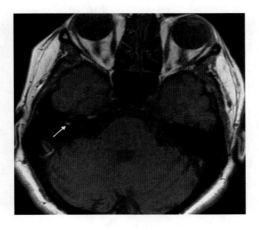

Figure 34. Labyrinthine concussion; axial T1-weighted spin echo sequence shows a small spot of T1 shortening (arrow) due to intra-labyrinthine haemorrhage in a patient with unremarkable CT examination after a head trauma.

6.4. Post Traumatic Hearing Loss

Sensorineural, conductive, or mixed hearing loss may all occur after a head trauma involving the temporal bone. After a trauma, use of a systematic approach to explore the main functional components of auditory pathways is highly suggested [121]. Since conductive hearing loss (CHL) is caused by the impairment of the ossicular chain, high-resolution CT will be the best imaging examination to investigate what part of it has been affected and how (dislocation or fracture). In cases of sensorineural hearing loss (SNHL), high resolution CT scan is still useful to identify indirect signs of inner ear impairment such as pneumolabyrinth and perilymphatic fistula, but it's not useful to detect a labyrinthine haemorrhage (see labyrinthine concussion paragraph) or brain axonal shearing injuries along the central auditory pathways. In these cases MRI is the more exhaustive neuroradiological examination to perform.

6.5. Facial Nerve Injury

Trauma (blunt, penetrating and iatrogenic) is the second most frequent cause of facial palsy; Bell's palsy is the most common and is still a diagnosis of exclusion [122, 123]. Most of the post-traumatic facial nerve injuries are caused by temporal bone fractures. Even if "otic capsule violating" fractures are relatively rare, they are those more commonly associated with facial nerve injury. Blunt trauma usually leads to nerve compression and subsequent edema and contusion. Post traumatic facial nerve transection is very rare. Even if most temporal bone injuries do not require an urgent surgical intervention, it has been demonstrated that in cases with a facial nerve injury, the earlier the facial nerve decompression is performed, the better the chances of a good recovery since bone fragments can prevent axonal regrowth [123]. Brodie and colleagues, analyzing 820 temporal bone fractures, identified the severity and the delay of onset as the two most important prognostic factors in recovery of post-traumatic facial paralysis [124].

To identify a facial nerve injury, the whole course of the nerve must be analyzed. On high resolution CT images, multiplanar reconstruction (MPR) will be extremely helpful for the identification of facial nerve canal post-traumatic lesions. Geniculate ganglion region, either in association with a transverse or an anterior longitudinal fracture, is the most common localization of traumatic facial nerve injury [124]; coronal is the one best plane to identify such a lesion. Lesions of the posterior genu or of the descending branch are commonly associated with a posterior longitudinal fracture; sagittal is the best imaging plane for a correct diagnosis. MRI is more sensible in investigating soft tissues and so is more useful in showing the damaged nerve at any level from the brainstem to the fundus of the internal auditory canal.

6.6. Vascular Injuries (Carotid Canal and Jugular Gulf Impairment)

The complex anatomy that characterizes the skull base and the temporal bone leads to the risk of injury also to vascular structures that pass through and which are in strict contact with nerby bony structures.

The internal carotid artery (ICA) enters the skull passing through the carotid canal and its petrous segment is located in the petrous part of the temporal bone. The carotid canal should be always carefully evaluated since patients with fractures that extend to it are at an increased risk for carotid artery injury. Complications associated with carotid artery injuries are associated with a worse prognosis and include vessel wall damage (Figure 35) such as dissection, transection or pseudoaneurysm but also complete occlusion and development of post-traumatic arteriovenous fistulas. CT angiography should be always performed when fractures involving the carotid canal are identified [118]. A brain MRI examination could be helpful to identify vascular brain injuries even in hyper acute phase by the use of Diffusion Weighted pulse sequences.

Veins could be injured after a blunt or penetrating head trauma as well. MDCT venography allowed the identification of traumatic dural venous sinus thrombosis in more than 40% of patients with skull fractures extending to a dural venous sinus or jugular bulb (Figure 36) [125]. Dural venous sinus thrombosis is also one of the unsuspected causes of delayed intracerebral hemorrhage following head trauma with fractures but delayed sinus thrombosis can occur even in the absence of skull fracture [126].

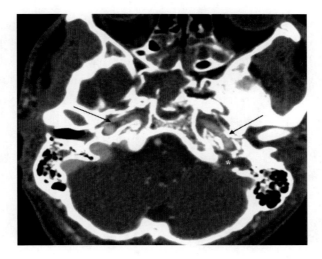

Figure 35. Post-traumatic internal carotid artery impairment; CT angiography (CTA) in a patient with multiple facial skeleton and skull base fractures following a severe head trauma. Both ICA canals are impaired with inhomogeneous intravascular enhancement and abnormal vessel contour of both ICAs (arrows). A brain MRI scan performed a few hours later revealed typical watershed territory stroke signs. Note the filling defect of the left jugular gulf (asterisk) as indirect sign of a post-traumatic traumatic dural venous sinus thrombosis (see Figure 36).

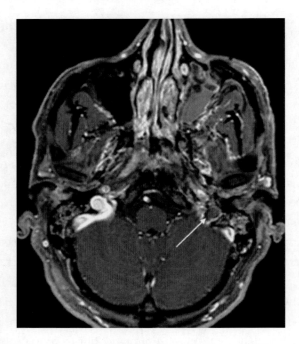

Figure 36. Post-traumatic dural venous sinus thrombosis; axial contrast enhanced T1-weighted turbo field echo sequence (same patient shown in Figure 35) further confirms the left jugular gulf thrombosis: normal enhancing vessel wall surrounding the nonenhancing thrombosed lumen ("delta sign").

7. Petrous Apex Lesions and Other Lesions of the Temporal Bone

Petrous apex lesions are usually an incidental finding while scanning the head with other indications [127]. However, it isn't uncommon that petrous apex lesions presented with nerve palsy, especially of the abducens nerve (6th cranial nerve) due to its proximity to the Dorello canal, next to petroclival fissure. Between the lateral and central skull base, petrous apex is located antero-medially to the inner ear with greater wing of the sphenoid and clivus as medial margins. It is in close relationship with Meckel cave, cavernous sinus, foramen lacerum, Eustachian tube and internal carotid artery (ICA) [128]. CT and MRI are complementary for differential diagnosis [129].

7.1. Leave-Me-Alone Lesions

Leave-me-alone lesions are the most frequent incidental findings and they include asymmetric pneumatization (Figure 37), asymmetric fatty marrow, trapped fluid effusion and variant of petrous apex ossification in the child population. The main imaging characteristic of this type of lesion is the preservation of bone margins and intra-lesion osseous septa. They usually do not require any imaging follow-ups [128, 130].

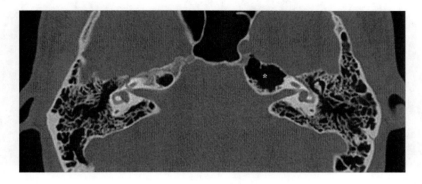

Figure 37. Asymmetric petrous apex pneumatization; axial MDCT scan showing a big air filled cell within the left petrous apex (asterisk).

7.2. Infections and Inflammatory Diseases

In adulthood, leave-me-alone lesions differential diagnosis is mainly represented by cholesterol granuloma (60%). Conversely to asymmetric fatty marrow, cholesterol granuloma is not suppressed with fat-saturation sequences, with a persisting hyperintense signal on T1 and T2 weighted images. Actually, cholesterol crystals are made by hemoglobin catabolism in a long course chronic inflammation process. Rarely does trapped fluid of the petrous apex effusion show slight hyperintensity on T1-weighted imaging due to proteinaceous material; in this case a 2-3 months follow-up imaging is recommended [131]. Mucocele should be also mentioned as T1-hyperintense petrous apex lesions in relation to its mucoid content, always considering the rarity of the lesions [132].

Trapped fluid effusion is a sterile retained fluid collection in a pneumatized petrous apex, whereas petrous apicitis is a suppurative infection usually extended from severe otomastoiditis or invasive sinusitis (Figure 38). On CT scan, opacification of the petrous air cells has blurred margins and could be combined with demineralization or erosion of the adjacent bone [128]. On MR imaging, fatty marrow has an inhomogeneous signal on T1 and on fat suppressed T2 images. Enhancement is usually intense after i.v. contrast administration, differently from trapped fluid effusion which has thin linear peripheral rim enhancement. Adjacent structures can be involved in uncontrolled infections leading to meningitis, thrombophlebitis or empyema. Nowadays, Gradenigo syndrome (characterized by the triad of suppurative otitis media, pain in the distribution of the trigeminal nerve, and abducens nerve palsy) or complicated petrous apicitis is extremely rare due to the wide use of antibiotics [133].

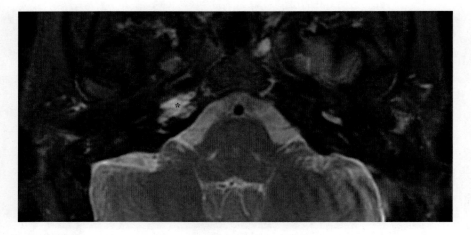

Figure 38. Petrous apicitis; axial T2-weighted turbo spin echo with fat saturation revealing an inhomogeneous fluid collection within the right petrous apex (asterisk).

Pseudotumor is a rare locally aggressive inflammatory disease of the soft tissues adjacent to petrous apex; differential diagnosis based on imaging characteristics is extremely difficult because of its intense enhancement after Gd administration that make it prone to be confused with tumors or invasive infections. Moreover, sometimes it presents bony erosion. A biopsy is necessary for the diagnosis [134].

7.3. Neoplasms

The most frequent neoplastic lesion located at the petrous apex is chondrosarcoma, representing 6% of all skull base tumors. It is a well-differentiated tumor arising from the cartilaginous remnants of the petro-occipital fissure. It can be associated with Ollier disease or Maffucci syndrome and occasionally with Paget disease. A CT scan is extremely useful to assess tumor characteristics because more than 50% of them presented calcifications of the matrix, usually rounded or curvilinear. The margins are lobulated and the adjacent bone is not sclerotic. On MRI, chondrosarcoma enhance avidly, whether homogeneously or not. In the differential diagnosis of a lytic enhancing soft-tissue mass centered on petrous apex, it should be considered chordoma that is usually more central located, and rhabdomyosarcoma in childhood population. Ewing sarcoma should also be included even if it is more rare [128, 130].

7.4. Non-Neoplastic Lesions

Fibrous-osseous lesions of the petrous apex are usually expressions of a widespread disease of the skull. Paget is a disease of the aged population, whereas fibrous dysplasia is typical of children and young adults. Fibrous dysplasia can be mono or polyostotic. Even if temporal bone is frequently affected, petrous apex involvement is uncommon. On MR imaging, monostotic disease can mimic malignancies due to avid enhancement after Gd contrast administration. Complications could be caused by foraminal narrowing [130]. Aneurysmal bone cyst involving temporal bone is extremely rare. Imaging appearance is similar to aneurysmal bone cyst involving any other osseous structures of the body and is characterized by bubble and multiloculated appearance, which demonstrates fluid-fluid levels and septal contrast enhancement on MR imaging. Histopathological confirmation is needed to exclude giant cell tumor of the bone [135].

Petrous apex is the election site of meningocele in intracranial idiopathic hypertension (IHH), due to chronic increased CSF pulsations. Meningocele area well-defined CSF-filled lesions laterally to the Meckel cave, sometimes containing Gassner ganglion. The treatment depends essentially on the presence of CSF leaks in relation to an extended scalloping of the bone [136]. In children, meningoceles located at the petrous apex combine usually with sphenoid wing aplasia in NF1 [137].

Petrous internal carotid artery aneurysms are mainly asymptomatic, so they are recognized as incidental expanding lesions of the petrous apex with smooth margins and no bony erosion. CTA or MRA is required for the diagnosis [128].

Cholesteatoma is the second most frequent petrous apex lesion after cholesterol granuloma; it can be congenital or acquired, respectively arising from epithelial remnants in petrous apex (congenital) or spreading from tympanomastoid region (acquired). Imaging characteristics of cholesteatoma are the same all over the temporal bone region (see Paragraph 3.3) [138].

7.5. Other Lesions of the Temporal Bone

There are multiple pathological conditions affecting temporal bone not only at the petrous apex but also the temporal squama, the mastoid or the otic capsule. The main differential diagnosis is between tumoral or non-tumoral lesions.

7.5.1. Tumor-Like Lesions

Epidermoid or dermoid cysts are typically located at CPA, as extra-axial intradural masses; rarely can they have an intradiploic location all over the skull (0.25% of all intracranial tumors), also affecting the temporal squama [139].

Acquired cholesteatoma usually affects the structures around the tympanic cavity; congenital origin of the lesion should be considered when an isolated mass is noted above the labyrinthine compartment or in the mastoid [140].

Cavitating otosclerosis could be mentioned as a tumor-like lesion when presenting as a focal well-circumscribed mass. Representing an inactive foci of cochlear otosclerosis, it has a fluid-filled cystic MR appearance, anteriorly located to the IAC or in the pericochlear region. If it is associated with enhancing areas after Gd administration, it should be a mixed active and inactive otosclerosis focus and differentiated from more aggressive lytic lesions (i.e., metastasis) [141].

7.5.2. Tumors

Temporal bone paragangliomas, Fisch's classification is based on tumor location and is strictly related to surgical management (Table 7) [142]. Paraganglioma is recognized as a locally aggressive highly vascular neuroendocrine tumor with bone, soft tissue and nerve involvement. They can be solitary or multicentric, sporadic or familial. On CT scan, it is usually noted as a lytic lesion near the jugular foramen, except for Class A and B paragangliomas that are limited to tympanic cavity [143]. Typical MR appearance is a salt-and-pepper lesion on T2w sequence, due to intratumoral flow-voids of vascular origin. An angiographic study should be always performed; CT angiography (CTA) or contrast enhanced - MR angiography (CE-MRA) demonstrate arterial vascularization of the lesion (Figure 39), because paragangliomas are also visualized in the early phase of the injection. Time of Flight (TOF) imaging is useful to recognize intralesional arterial vessels, if the dimension of the tumor are adequate to allow it. Digital Subtraction Angiography (DSA) should be necessary only in the presurgical stage. Nevertheless, the real extension of the disease is better delineated in the fat sat T1-w imaging acquired after Gd injection; volumetric acquisition is recommended in presurgical MR studies. PET/CT remains the gold-standard imaging for non invasive diagnosis [144, 145].

Table 7. Fish Classification of temporal bone paragangliomas

Class A (glomus tympanicum)	Limited to mesotympanum.
Class B (glomus hypotympanicum)	Limited to hypotympanum, mesotympanum, and mastoid without erosion of jugular bulb.
Class C	Involvement and destruction of infralabyrinthine and apical compartments. Sub- classification by degree of carotid canal erosion: • C1: no invasion of carotid; destruction of jugular bulb/foramen; • C2: invasion of vertical carotid canal between foramen and bend; • C3: invasion along horizontal carotid canal; • C4: invasion of foramen lacerum and along carotid into cavernous sinus.
Class D	Intracranial extension (D_e, extradural; D_i, intradural): • D_{e1}: up to 2cm dural displacement; • D_{e2}: more than 2cm dural displacement; • D_{i1}: up to 2cm intradural extension; • D_{i2}: more than 2cm intradural extension.

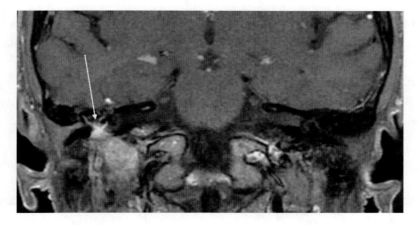

Figure 39. Paraganglioma; coronal MPR from a 3D contrast-enhanced T1-weighted turbo filed echo with fat saturation sequence revealing a lively enhancing lesion in the infralabyrinthine region of the right inner ear (arrow).

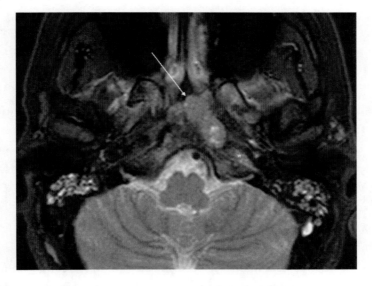

Figure 40. Nasopharyngeal squamous cell carcinoma; axial T2-weighted fast spin echo sequence with fat saturation showing a solid mass (arrow) extending through the pharyngotympanic tube (auditory tube) and infiltrating clivus bone structures with signs of petrous apex involvement (asterisk).

A differential diagnosis of temporal bone paraganglioma includes other lytic bone destructive lesions such as metastasis, plasmocytoma or endolymphatic sac tumor.

Metastasis can be located everywhere in the temporal bone. Bony destruction and multiple locations in the body are the best clues for diagnosis. If the abnormal growing cells composing the mass are plasma cells, it is called plasmacytoma. Plasmacytoma can be solitary, or as a part of myeloma with different treatment and prognosis. Metastasis and plasmacytoma have similar MRI features, showing an intense enhancing mass with irregular margins. Histopathological confirmation is needed [127].

Carcinoma arising from nasopharynx (Figure 40), pinna or EAC could extend into the temporal bone; in relation to the original location of the tumor, they could infiltrate the temporal bone anteriorly or laterally. Conversely, endolymphatic sac tumor is a rare low-grade papillary adenocarcinoma centered on the vestibular aqueduct, eroding through the posterior limit of the temporal bone; it is characterized by spiculae at the erosion margin on CT imaging and T1-shortening areas before Gd administration on MR imaging [145].

Intraosseous meningioma, schwannoma and hemangioma are extremely uncommon. Intraosseous meningioma has a mixed sclerotic and lytic appearance on CT scan and thick meningeal enhancement after Gd administration on MRI. Intraosseous schwannoma are a well-defined lytic lesion, homogeneously enhancing after Gd injection on MRI. Intraosseous hemangioma could have a trabeculated or honeycomb appearance on CT scan and a heterogeneous contrast enhancement, increasing during MRI scanning time [128-131].

8. Facial Nerve

The VII cranial nerve (CN VII) contains two distinct roots: a motor root to the muscles of the face and scalp (including platysma, buccinator, stapedius, stylohyoid, and posterior belly of the digastric), and a mixed motor-sensory root to the salivary glands and to taste receptors of the tongue. Facial nerves also carry special visceral efferent motor fibers (SVE). It can be divided in multiple segments [146, 147]:

1) Intra-axial segment: the facial nucleus is located antero-laterally in the pontine tegmentum and nerve fibers run postero-laterally, turning around abducens nucleus to exit at the lateral aspect of the ponto-medullary junction. Facial colliculus is a bulge on the IV ventricle floor representing the nerve turn around abducens nucleus, and it is clearly visible on MRI except in cases of nerve hypo/aplasia [148].
2) Cisternal segment: on MR high resolution T2w imaging (CISS sequences, see Paragraph 1.2), the cisternal segment is depicted running from ponto-medullary junction to the porus acusticus, crossing CPA anteriorly located to the eighth cranial nerve [147, 149].
3) Intra-temporal segment: the seventh cranial nerve crosses the petrous bone entering the IAC and exiting through stylomastoid foramen in the extra-cranial soft tissues [147]. It can be further subdivided in 4 segments:
    a) Intra-canalicular segment: CISS imaging perfectly resolves IAC content (CN VII-VIII and their divisions); facial nerve is antero-superiorly located in the IAC. At the fundus, it is separated from the inferiorly running cochlear nerve

by crista falciformis and from the posteriorly running superior vestibular nerve by Bill's bar, both visible on HRCT scan [149-151].

b) Labyrinthine segment: it is the narrowest (<0.7 mm diameter) and shortest part of the bony facial canal running antero-laterally from the fundus to the geniculate fossa, superiorly to the cochlea. Great superficial petrosal nerve (GSPN) is the first facial branch and it exits from the geniculate ganglion carrying the preganglionic parasympathetic fibers of the superior salivary nucleus through Vidian canal to the pterygopalatine ganglion and then to the lacrimal gland [147, 152].

c) Tympanic segment: from the geniculate fossa, the nerve makes a 75° turn and runs adjacent to the tympanic cavity directing posteriorly to the second (or posterior) genu. This segment runs inferiorly to the lateral semicircular canal, helpful landmark, and superiorly to the stapes, located immediately before the second genu [149, 153].

d) Mastoid segment: at the pyramidal process, the nerve makes a 95°-125° turn (second genu) directing inferiorly to the stylomastoid foramen. The mastoid segment has a vertical orientation, posteriorly to the tympanic cavity. Two branches arise from this segment, stapedius nerve superiorly and chorda tympani inferiorly, respectively carrying motor and special sensory (taste), and parasympathetic (to salivary glands) fibers [147].

4) Extracranial segment through the stylomastoid foramen, the nerve enters the parotid glands where it divides in many branches to temporofacial and cervicofacial territories [147].

Sensory and parasympathetic components are provided by nervus intermedius (Wrisberg nerve). General visceral efferent parasympathetic motor fibers arise in the superior salivary nucleus and emerge from the ponto-medullary junction as a distinct nerve from facial division. It joins motor root either as it emerges from the ponto-medullary junction or at the meatus of the IAC. Occasionally, it can be depicted by using CISS sequences as a 5th thin nerve along the acoustic canal [146, 149-154].

A small component of general sensory afferent fibers arise from geniculate ganglion to supply trigeminal (CN V_3) innervation of the concha, the EAC and the external surface of the tympanic membrane [146].

The major blood supply of intra-temporal facial nerve is the middle meningeal artery (superficial petrosal and stylomastoid branches), except for the intra-canalicular segment which is in the anterior-inferior cerebellar artery (AICA) territory (labyrinthine branch) [146].

The facial nerve can be affected by many different pathologies (Table 8) [155] resulting in weakness or paralysis and dystonias or spasm [156, 157].

Table 8. Classification of facial nerve lesions

Aetiology	Lesions	Preferred imaging modality	Distinguishing features
Tumours	Schwannoma	MRI	Enhancing lesions extending into the geniculate ganglion (along the course of the facial nerve).
	Perineural tumor spread	MRI	Extension of a known tumor along the course of facial nerve from mastoid segment.
Infectious	Ramsay Hunt Syndrome	MRI	Abnormal enhancement of facial nerve with classic clinical features (otalgia, vesicles, and facial paralysis).
	Lyme Disease	MRI	Abnormal enhancement of facial nerve with white matter lesions, meningeal enhancement, and classical clinical symptoms (erythema migrans, radiculoneuritis, and arthritis).
	Otitis media	CT	Middle ear opacification causing facial nerve canal erosion.
	Cholesteatoma	CT	Middle ear opacification causing facial nerve canal erosion.
Idiopathic	Bell palsy	MRI (atypical cases)	Abnormal facial nerve enhancement with suggestive clinical symptoms.
	Sarcoidosis	MRI	Abnormal facial nerve enhancement with basal cisterns leptomeningeal and dural enhancement.
Traumatic	Temporal bone fracture	CT	Fracture extending to the facial nerve canal.
Vascular	Hemifacial spasm	MRI	Vascular loop at the root extizone of the facial nerve.
	Hemangioma or venous malformations	MRI/CT	Enhancing lesion at the geniculate ganglion with bony spicules.
Congenital	Moebius	MRI	Absent or hypotrophic facial colliculi, cisternal/intra-canalicular facial segment hypo/aplasia.
	Aberrant course	CT	Variable intra-temporal segments course.
Pontine lesions	Infarct	MRI	Intra-axial T2 hyperintense lesion with diffusion restriction in acute phase.
	Multiple sclerosis	MRI	Multiple T2 hyperintense lesions satisfying revisited McDonald's criteria.
	Cavernous hemangioma	MRI	"Popcorn"-like appearance on T2 with susceptibility artefacts on T2*.

8.1. Facial Paralysis

Depending on which facial nerve segment is involved, different clinical manifestations are recognized. The most critical step is discerning central to peripheral facial palsy. Timing of the onset, patient age and associated symptoms can narrow the differential diagnosis and can guide the choice of the imaging modality and treatment [155-157].

8.1.1. Central Facial Palsy

Among central processes affecting the seventh cranial nerve, cerebrovascular accidents (CVAs) are by far the most frequent [158]. Middle cerebral artery (MCA) or anterior cerebral artery (ACA) stroke can cause contralateral facial paralysis, sometimes sparing the forehead region, in relation to the mixed contra/ipsilateral innervation. Stroke is a time-critical illness and it should be recognized promptly for treatment. Pontine infarcts instead cause an ipsilateral paresis of the face; they usually are lacunar infarcts representing approximately 7% of all ischemic strokes and caused by basilar perforating arteries occlusion. Depending on the blood supplying perforating arteries, pontine infarcts can be distinguished in ventral (anteromedial and anterolateral pontine arteries) and tegmental (short circumferential arteries), with different associated symptoms [159, 160]. MRI with DWI sequence is the gold-standard neuroradiological diagnostic tool for stroke imaging [160].

Brain tumors (primary or metastatic), multiple sclerosis and tumor-like lesions, as cavernous hemangiomas, should be also included as causes of facial central paralysis if located in or by the pons. Whole-brain MRI scan is required in central lesions [147].

However, lesions affecting the facial nerve distal to the decussation in the caudal pons can mimic peripheral facial palsy, despite the lesion etiology [161].

8.1.2. Peripheral Facial Palsy

The most common cause of peripheral facial paralysis is Bell's palsy. Imaging studies are not indicated in the early phase of the disease. If full recovery does not occur after 9 months from the onset, MR imaging is recommended. An earlier imaging study is also indicated if it is associated with other neurological signs or a parotid mass. On MR imaging, abnormal facial nerve enhancement after Gd administration is present; sometimes, mainly during the acute phase, the nerve is swollen, and it can mimic a schwannoma [162]. If the patient does not progressively recover, follow-up MRI is recommended [163].

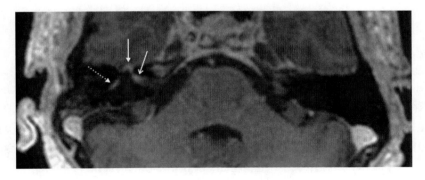

Figure 41. Facial nerve neuritis in a patient with varicella zoster virus reactivation; axial MPR from a 3D T1-weighted fast spoiled gradient echo showing enhancement of the labyrinthine (empty head arrow), tympanic/geniculate ganglion (arrow) and mastoid (dotted arrow) segments of the facial nerve.

Facial nerve enhancement is also present in other inflammatory or infectious diseases that should be included in the imaging-based differential diagnosis checklist even if clinical signs and symptoms should always guide imaging features [150]. Neurosarcoidosis has many different features on a brain MRI, but it is usually characterized by dural and leptomeningeal involvement at the level of basal cisterns, showing bright enhancement after contrast administration [164]. Ramsay Hunt syndrome and Lyme disease are infections of the CNS, respectively caused by Varicella-Zoster virus reactivation (Figure 41) and Borrelia burgdorferi. Ramsay Hunt syndrome is usually clinically evident (otalgia, vesicles and facial paralysis), but if MR imaging is acquired, enhancement of the facial nucleus could be observed in association with facial nerve enhancement. Lyme disease is also usually clinically diagnosed, but a whole-brain MRI scan is recommended due to the CNS involvement for that meningoencephalitis [165-167].

Facial nerve enhancement could even be present in facial nerve involvement by pathologies of adjacent structures, such as otitis media, malignant otitis externa, bone fractures or cholesteatoma. Considering that these diseases are used to primarily affect the temporal bone, a CT scan is adequate for the diagnosis [168, 169].

8.1.3. Facial Nerve Tumors

Many different neoplastic processes can affect facial nerves; CN VII schwannomas can affect any portion along the course of the nerve. They usually develop at the geniculate ganglion, but also along the tympanic or mastoid segment. They are well-circumscribed soft tissue masses, scalloping the adjacent bone structure, with avid enhancement after Gd administration except for cystic changes [170]. The most frequent site of origin of hemangiomas is the perigeniculate region, followed by IAC; this kind of lesions arise from the vascular plexus surrounding the facial nerve, and demonstrate a typical CT scan appearance with bony spicules and progressive avid Gd enhancement on MRI as for any venous malformation [170, 171].

Most commonly CN VII is infiltrated or compressed by lesions arising in the IAC (schwannomas, lipomas, choristomas, hemangiomas), in the middle ear (cholesteatomas, adenomas, paragangliomas, paragangliomas), in the parotid (tumors), or in the EAC (carcinomas) [168, 169].

Parotid tumors, especially adenoid cystic carcinoma (70-75%), frequently shows perineural tumoral spread (PTS); on MRI imaging, the facial nerve is swollen, clearly hyperintense on T2 fat saturated sequences due to edema, and avidly enhances after Gd administration. Conversely to inflammatory disease, PTS starts from extra-temporal segment and could eventually cause enlargement of the bony facial canal [172].

8.1.4. Congenital Malformations

Congenital malformation of the facial nerve can be clinically asymptomatic, but in some cases it determines long-standing facial weakness from childhood [148]. In aural atresia, second genu, mastoid segment and stylomastoid foramen can be displaced anteriorly and laterally [173]. Congenital inner ear malformation can be associated with an aberrant course of facial nerve, most frequently the labyrinthine segment (Figure 17), but also tympanic or mastoid depending on the associated malformations, especially of EAC or ossicular chain [152]. In congenital malformations of temporal bone, an HRCT scan is actually always recommended before surgical intervention [174, 175].

Congenital facial paralysis is also caused by abnormalities of facial nucleus in a variety of syndromes, including Moebius, DiGeorge, Goldenhar, Charge, trisomy 13, and trisomy 18. On MR imaging, CISS sequences (see paragraph 1.2) can easily demonstrate the hypo/aplasia of the nerve in the IAC or the brainstem abnormalities [147-150].

Bony dehiscence of the facial nerve usually occurs at the tympanic segment at the oval window level, predisposing the nerve to damaging from inflammatory processes of the middle ear, cholesteatoma or otologic surgery. High resolution CT scan is indicated in these cases [176].

8.2. Facial Dystonias

MR imaging is indicated in hemifacial spasm or twitching to exclude vascular encroaching of the cisternal segment; when a loop of the AICA, PICA, basilar artery or vertebral artery encroaches on the nerve transitional zone (TZ), the result could be an involuntary, unilateral, sudden contraction of facial muscles. The CN VII TZ is the zone of transition between central and peripheral myelination, which is located at 1-2 mm from the brainstem nerve root exit zone (REZ) [1]. Volumetric heavily T2-weighted (CISS) imaging is the gold-standard in demonstrating neural-vascular conflicts. MRI is recommended [147, 170].

REFERENCES

[1] Dahmani-Causse, M., Marx, M., Deguine, O., Fraysse, B., Lepage, B. and Escudé, B. (2011). Morphologic examination of the temporal bone by cone beam computed tomography: comparison with multislice helical computed tomography. *Eur Ann Otorhinolaryngol Head Neck Dis,* 128(V):230-235.

[2] Ruivo, J., Mermuys, K., Bacher, K., Kuhweide R., Offeciers E. and Casselman, JW. (2009). Cone beam computed tomography, a low-dose imaging technique in

the postoperative assessment of cochlear implantation. *Otol Neurotol*, 30 (III):299-303.

[3] Kurzweg, T., Dalchow, CV., Bremke, M., Majdani, O., Kureck, I., Knecht, R., Werner, J.A. and Teymoortash, A. (2010). The value of digital volume tomography in assessing the position of cochlear implant arrays in temporal bone specimens. *Ear Hear*, 31(III):413-419.

[4] Zou, J., Koivisto, J., Lähelmä, J., Aarnisalo, A., Wolff, J. and Pyykkö, I. (2015). Imaging Optimization of Temporal Bones with Cochlear Implant Using a High-resolution Cone Beam CT and the Corresponding Effective Dose. *Ann Otol Rhinol Laryngol*, 124(VI):466-473.

[5] Peltonen, L., Aarnisalo, A. A., Käser, Y., Kortesniemi, M. K., Robinson, S., Suomalainen, A., Jero, J. (2009). Cone-beam computed tomography: a new method for imaging of the temporal bone. *Acta Radiol*. 50(5):543-8.

[6] Buric, N., Jovanovic, G., and Tijanic, M. (2013). Usefulness of cone-beam CT for presurgical assessment of keratoma (cholesteatoma) of the maxillary sinus, *Head & Neck,*; 35(VII), E221-E225.

[7] Rafferty, M.A., Siewerdsen, J.H., Chan, Y., Daly, M.J., Moseley, D.J., Jaffray, D.A. and Irish, J.C.(2006). Intraoperative cone-beam CT for guidance of temporal bone surgery. *Otolaryngol Head Neck Surg,*134(V):801-808.

[8] Redfors, Y.D., Gröndahl, H.G., Hellgren, J., Lindfors, N., Nilsson, I., and Möller, C. (2012). Otosclerosis: Anatomy and pathology in the temporal bone assessed by multi-slice and cone-beam CT. *Otology & Neurotology*, 33:922-927.

[9] Liktor, B., Révész, P., Csomor, P., Gerlinger, I., Sziklai, I. and Karosi, T. (2014). Diagnostic value of cone-beam CT in histologically confirmed otosclerosis. *Eur Arch Otorhinolaryngol*, 271:2131-2138.

[10] Miracle, A.C. and Mukherji, S.K. (2009). Conebeam CT of the head and neck, part 1: physical principles. *AJNR Am J Neuroradiol*, 30(VI):1088-1095.

[11] Miracle, A.C. and Mukherji, S.K. (2009). Conebeam CT of the head and neck, part 2: clinical applications. *AJNR Am J Neuroradiol*, 30(VII):1285-1292.

[12] Juliano, A.F., Ginat, D.T. and Moonis, G. (2013). Imaging review of the temporal bone: part I. Anatomy and inflammatory and neoplastic processes. *Radiology*, 269(I):17-33.

[13] Juliano, A.F., Ginat, D.T. and Moonis, G.(2015). Imaging Review of the Temporal Bone: Part II. Traumatic, Postoperative, and Noninflammatory Nonneoplastic Conditions. *Radiology*, 276(III):655-672.

[14] Juliano, A.F., Ting, E.Y., Mingkwansook, V., Hamberg, L.M. and Curtin, H.D. (2016). Vestibular Aqueduct Measurements in the 45° Oblique (Pöschl) Plane. *AJNR Am J Neuroradiol*, 37(VII):1331-1337.

[15] Marsot-Dupuch K. and Meyer, B. (2001). Cochlear implant assessment: imaging issues. *Eur J Radiol*, 40(II):119-132.

[16] Bonneville, F., Savatovsky and J., Chiras, J. (2007). Imaging of cerebellopontine angle lesions: an update. Part 1: enhancing extra-axial lesions. *Eur Radiol*, 17(X):2472-2482.

[17] Bonneville, F., Savatovsky and J., Chiras, J. (2007). Imaging of cerebellopontine angle lesions: an update. Part 2: intra-axial lesions, skull base lesions that may invade the CPA region, and non-enhancing extra-axial lesions. *Eur Radiol*, 17(XI):2908-2920.

[18] Verbist, B.M.(2012). Imaging of sensorineural hearing loss: a pattern-based approach to diseases of the inner ear and cerebellopontine angle. *Insights Imaging*, 3(II):139-53.

[19] Martines, F., Dispenza, F., Gagliardo, C., Martines, E. and Bentivegna, D. (2011). Sudden sensorineural hearing loss as prodromal symptom of anterior inferior cerebellar artery infarction. *ORL J Otorhinolaryngol Relat Spec*, 73(III):137-40.

[20] Chavhan, G.B., Babyn, P.S., Jankharia, B.G., Cheng, H.L. and Shroff, M.M.(2008). Steady-state MR imaging sequences: physics, classification, and clinical applications. *Radiographics*, 28(IV):1147-1160.

[21] Baráth, K., Huber, A.M., Stämpfli, P., Varga, Z. and Kollias, S. (2011). Neuroradiology of cholesteatomas. *AJNR Am J Neuroradiol.* 32(II):221-229.

[22] Yeakley, J.W and Jahrsdoerfer, R.A. (1996). CT evaluation of congenital aural atresia: what radiologists and surgeons need to know. *J Comp Ass Tomogr*, 20:724-731.

[23] Langman, J. (1981). Ear In: *Medial Embriology*, 4th edn. Williams & Wilkins, Baltimore, pp 303-304.

[24] Grandis, J. R., Curtin, H. D., Yu, V.L. (1995). Necrotizing (malignant) external otitis: prospective comparison of CT and MR imaging in diagnosis and follow-up. *Radiology*, 196(2):499-504.

[25] Jee, W.H., Choi, K.H., Choe, B.Y., Park, J.M. and Shinn, K.S. (1996). Fibrous dysplasia: MR imaging characteristics with radiopathologic correlation. *AJR Am J Roentgenol*, 167:1523-1527.

[26] Kemink, J.L. and Gaham, M.D. (1982). Osteomas and esostoses of the external auditory canal-medial and surgical manegement. *J Otolaryngol*, 11:101-106.

[27] Heilbrun, M. E., Salzman, K. L., Glastonbury, C. M., Harnsberger, H. R., Kennedy, R. J., Shelton, C. (2003). External auditory canal cholesteatoma: clinical and imaging spectrum. *Am J Neuroradiol.*, Apr;24(4):751-6.

[28] Persaud, R. A., Hajioff, D., Thevasagayam, M. S., Wareing, M. J., Wright, A. (2004). Keratosis obturans and external ear canal cholesteatoma: how and why we should distinguish between these conditions. *Clin Otolaryngol Allied Sci.*, 29(6):577-81. Gillespie, M.B., Francis, H.W., Chee, N. and Eisele, D.W. (2001). Squamous cell carcinoma of the temporal bone: a radiographic-pathologic correlation. *Arch Otolaryngol head NeckSurg*, 127:803-807.

[29] Breau, R.L., Gardner, E.K. and Dornhoffer, J.L. (2002). Cancer of the external auditory canal and temporal bone. *Curr Oncol* Rep, 4:76-80.
[30] Luers, J.C. and Hüttenbrink, K.B. (2016). Surgical anatomy and pathology of the middle ear. *J Anat.* 228(II):338-353.
[31] Skrzat, J., Kozerska, M., Wroński, S., Tarasiu, J. and Walocha, J. (2015). Volume rendering of the tympanic cavity from micro-CT data. *Folia Med Cracov,* 55(IV):81-89.
[32] Bartel-Friedrich, S. and Wulke, C. (2007). Classification and diagnosis of ear malformations. *GMS Current Topics in Otorhinolaryngology – Head and Neck Surgery,* Vol. 6, ISSN 1865-1011.
[33] Esteves, S.D., Silva, A.P., Coutinho, M.B., Abrunhosa, J.M. and Almeida e Sousa, C. (2014). Congenital defects of the middle ear uncommon cause of pediatric hearing loss. *Braz J Otorhinolaryngol,* 80(III):251-256.
[34] Zeifer, B., Sabini, P. and Sonne, J. (2000). Congenital absence of the oval window: radiologic diagnosis and associated anomalies. *AJNR Am J Neuroradiol,* 21(II):322-327.
[35] Teunissen, B. and Cremers, CW. (1991). Surgery for congenital stapes ankylosis with an associated congenital ossicular chain anomaly. *Int J Pediatr Otorhinolaryngol*, 21(III):217-226.
[36] Kösling, S., Schneider-Möbius, C., König, E. and Meister, E.F. (1997). Computertomographie bei Kindern und Jugendlichen mit Verdacht auf eine Felsenbeinmissbildung. *Radiologe,* 37:971–976.
[37] Heikkinen, T. and Chonmaitree, T. (2003). Importance of Respiratory Viruses in Acute Otitis Media. *Clin Microbiol Rev,* 16(II): 230–241.
[38] Trojanowska, A., Drop, A., Trojanowski, P., Rosińska-Bogusiewicz, K., Klatka, J., and Bobek-Billewicz, B. (2012). External and middle ear diseases: radiological diagnosis based on clinical signs and symptoms. *Insights Imaging*, 3(I): 33–48.
[39] Maroldi, R., Farina, D., Palvarini, L., Marconi, A., Gadola, E., Menni, K. and Battaglia, G. (2001). Computed tomography and magnetic resonance imaging of pathologic conditions of the middle ear. *Eur J Radiol,*40(II):78-93.
[40] Rettig, E. and Tunkel, D.E. (2014). Contemporary concepts in management of acute otitis media in children. *Otolaryngol Clin North Am,* 47(V):651-672.
[41] Anbarasu, A., Chandrasekaran, K. and Balakrishnan, S. (2012). Soft tissue attenuation in middle ear on HRCT: Pictorial review. *Indian J Radiol Imaging,* 22(IV):298-304.
[42] Saat, R., Laulajainen-Hongisto, A.H., Mahmood, G., Lempinen, L.J., Aarnisalo, A.A., Markkola and A.T., Jero, J.P. (2015). MR imaging features of acute mastoiditis and their clinical relevance. *AJNR Am J Neuroradiol.* 36(II):361-7.

[43] Platzek, I. Kitzler, H. H., Gudziol, V. Laniado, M., Hahn G. (2014). Magnetic resonance imaging in acute mastoiditis. *Acta Radiol Short Rep*.3(2):2047981614523415.

[44] Morris, P. (2012). Chronic suppurative otitis media. *BMJ Clin Evid.* 6;2012. pii: 0507.

[45] Silva, M.N., Muller, S., Selaimen, F.A., Oliveira, D.S., Rosito, L.P. and Costa, S.S.(2013). Tomographic evaluation of the contralateral ear in patients with severe chronic otitis media. *Braz J Otorhinolaryngol,* 79(IV):475-479.

[46] Swartz, J.D., Wolfson, R.J., Marlowe, F.I. and Popky, G.L. (1985). Postinflammatory ossicular fixation: CT analysis with surgical correlation. *Radiology.* 154(III):697-700.

[47] Viswanatha, B., Sarojamma and Roopashree T,J. (2013). Mastoid cholesteatoma: a result of metaplasia. *Indian J Otolaryngol Head Neck Surg.* 65(III):665-669.

[48] Dubach, P. and Häusler, R. (2008). External auditory canal cholesteatoma: reassessment of and amendments to its categorization, pathogenesis, and treatment in 34 patients. *Otol Neurotol*, 29:941–948.

[49] De Foer, B., Vercruysse, J.P., Bernaerts, A., Meersschaert, J., Kenis, C., Pouillon, M., De Beuckeleer, L., Michiels, J., Bogaerts, K., Deckers, F., Somers, T., Hermans, R., Offeciers, E. and Casselman, J.W. (2010). Middle ear cholesteatoma: non-echo-planar diffusion-weighted MR imaging versus delayed gadolinium-enhanced T1-weighted MR imaging--value in detection. *Radiology.* 255(III):866-872.

[50] Wallis, S., Atkinson, H. and Coatesworth, A.P.(2015). Chronic otitis media. *Postgrad Med.* 127(IV):391-395.

[51] Smith, J.A. and Danner, C.J. (2006). Complications of chronic otitis media and cholesteatoma. *Otolaryngol Clin North Am,* 39(VI):1237-1255.

[52] Penido Nde, O., Toledo, R.N., Silveira, P.A., Munhoz, M.S., Testa, J.R. and Cruz, O.L.(2007). Sigmoid sinus thrombosis associated to chronic otitis media. *Braz J Otorhinolaryngol,* 73(II):165-170.

[53] Chatterjee, P., Khanna, S. and Talukdar, R. (2015). Role of High Resolution Computed Tomography of Mastoids in Planning Surgery for Chronic Suppurative Otitis Media. *Indian J Otolaryngol Head Neck Surg,* 67(III):275-80.

[54] Khater, N. H., Fahmy, H. S., El Shahat, H. M., Kater, A. M. (2015). Chronic inflammatory middle ear disease: Postoperative CT and MRI findings. *The Egyptian Journal of Radiology and Nuclear Medicine*, 46(III):629-638.

[55] Williams, M.T. and Ayache, D. (2004). Imaging of the postoperative middle ear. *Eur Radiol*, 14(III):482-495.

[56] Toyama, C., da Costa-Leite, C., Filho, I.S.B., de Brito-Neto R.V., Bento, R.F., Cerri, G.G. and Gebrim, E.M.M.S. (2008). The role of magnetic resonance imaging

in the postoperative management of cholesteatomas. *Braz J Otorhinolaryngol,* 74(V):693-696.

[57] Dündar, Y., Akcan, F.A., Dilli A, Tatar E, Korkmaz H, Özdek A. (2015). Does Diffusion-Weighted MR Imaging Change the Follow-Up Strategy in Cases with Residual Cholesteatoma? *J Int Adv Otol.* 11(1):58-62.

[58] House, J.W. Otosclerosis. In: Cummings, C.W., Fredickson, J.M., Harker, L.A., Krause, C.J., Schuller, D.E., eds. *Otolaryngology Head and Neck Surgery.* 3rd. ed. St. Louis, MO; Mosby: 3126–3135.

[59] Levin, G., Fabian, P. and Stahle, J. (1988). Incidence of otosclerosis. *Am J Otol,* 9(IV):299–301.

[60] Purohit, B., Hermans, R. and Op de beeck, K.(2014). Imaging in otosclerosis: A pictorial review. *Insights into Imaging,* 5(II):245-252.

[61] Rudic, M., Keogh, I., Wagner, R., Wilkinson, E., Kiros, N., Ferrary, E., Sterkers, O., Bozorg-Grayeli, A., Zarkovic, K. and Zarkovic, N. (2015). The pathophysiology of otosclerosis: Review of current research. *Hearing Research,* 330: 51-56.

[62] Chole, R.A. and McKenna, M. Pathophysiology of otosclerosis. *Otology & Neurotology*: official publication of the American Otological Society, American Neurotology Society [and] European Academy of Otology and Neurotology. 22 (II): 249-257.

[63] Niedermeyer, H.P. and Arnold, W. (2002). Etiopathogenesis of otosclerosis. *ORL,* 64:114–119.

[64] Schwartz, J.D. and Mukherji, S.K. (2009): The Inner Ear and Otodystrophies. In: Swartz, J.D., Loevner, L.A. (eds.) *Imaging of the Temporal Bone*, 4th edn. Thieme, New York, pp 298.

[65] Chadwell, J.B., Halsted, M.J., Choo, D.I., Greinwald, J.H. and Benton, C. (2004). The cochlear cleft. *AJNR Am J Neuroradiol,* 25:21–24.

[66] Lagleyre, S., Sorrentino, T., Calmels, M.N., Shin, Y.J., Escudé, B., Deguine, O. and Fraysse, B. (2009). Reliability of high-resolution CT scan in diagnosis of otosclerosis. *Otol neurotol,* 30(VIII):1152–1159.

[67] Rangheard, A.S., Marsot-Dupuch, K., Mark, A.S., Meyer, B. and Tubiana, J.M. (2001). Postoperative complications in otospongiosis: usefulness of MR imaging. *AJNR Am J Neuroradiol,* 22(VI):1171–1178.

[68] Kenna, M.A. (1990). Embriology and developmental anatomy of the ear. In: Bluestone, C.D., Stool, S.E., Scheetz, M.D. (eds.) *Pediatric Otolaryngology.* Philadelphia: WB Saunders: 77-87.

[69] Parry, D.A., Booth, T. and Roland, P.S. (2005). Advantages of magnetic resonance imaging over computed tomography in preoperative evaluation of pediatric cochlear implant candidates. *Otol Neurotol,* 26(V): 976–982.

[70] Casselman, J.W., Offeciers, E.F., De Foer, B., Govaerts, P., Kuhweide, R. and Somers, T. (2001). CT and MR imaging of congenital abnormalities of the inner ear and internal auditory canal. *Eur J Radiol,* 40(II): 94–104.

[71] Brookhauser PE. (1993). Genetic hearing loss. In: Johnson, J.T., Kohut, R.I., Pillsbury, H.C., Tardy, M.E. (eds.) *Head and Neck Surgery Otolaringology.* Philadelphia: Lippicott:1754-1766.

[72] Lalwani, A.K., Castelein, C.M. (1999). Cracking the auditory genetic code: nonsyndromic hereditary hearing impairment. *Am J Otol* Jan, 20:115–132.

[73] Varsha, M. J., Shantanu K. G. and Ravi, K. K. (2012). Jitender R, E. C. Vinay Kumar. CT and MR Imaging of the Inner Ear and Brain in Children with Congenital Sensorineural Hearing Loss. *RadioGraphics*, 32:683–698.

[74] Jackler, R.K., Luxford, W.M. and House, W.F. (1987). Congenital malformations of the inner ear: a classification based on organogenesis. *Laryngoscope,* 97: 2-14.

[75] Sennaroglu, L. and Saatci, I. (2002). A new classification for cochleovestibular malformations. *Laryngoscope,* 112: 2230-41.

[76] Ozgen, B., Oguz, K.K., Atas, A. and Sennaroglu, L. (2009). Complete labyrinthine aplasia: clinical and radiological findings with review of the literature. *AJNR Am J Neuroradiol*, 30: 774-780.

[77] Sennaroglu, L. (2016). Histopathology of inner ear malformations: Do we have enough evidence to explain pathophysiology? *Cochlear Implants Int;* 17:3-20.

[78] Sennaroğlu, L. and Bajin, M.D. (2017). Classification and Current Management of Inner Ear Malformations. *Balkan Med J*, 34:397-411.

[79] Sennaroglu, L. and Saatci, I. (2004). Unpartitioned versus incompletely partitioned cochleae: radiologic differentiation. *Otol Neurotol,* 25:520-529.

[80] Lo, W.W. (1999). What is a 'Mondini' and what difference does a name make? *AJNR Am J Neuroradiol,* 20:1442-1444.

[81] Nance, W.E., Setleff, R., McLeod, A., Sweeney, A., Cooper, C. and McConnell, F. (1971). X-linked mixed deafness with congenital fixation of the stapedial footplate and perilymphatic gusher. *Birth Defects Orig Artic Ser,* 7:64-69.

[82] Sennaroglu, L., Sarac, S. and Ergin, T. (2006). Surgical results of cochlear implantation in malformed cochlea. *Otol Neurotol*, 27:615-623.

[83] Huang, B.Y., Zdanski, C. and Castillo, M. (2012). Pediatric Sensorineural Hearing Loss, Part 2: *Syndromic and Acquired Causes AJNR Am J Neuroradiol*, 33:399–406.

[84] Choo, D.I., Tawfik, K.O., Martin, D.M. and Raphael, Y. (2017). Inner ear manifestations in CHARGE: Abnormalities, treatments, animal models, and progress toward treatments in auditory and vestibular structures. *Am J Med Genet.* 175(C):439–449.

[85] McKenna, M.J. (1997). Measles, mumps, and sensorineural hearing loss. *Ann NY Acad Sci,* 830:291–298.

[86] Hegarty, J. L., Patel, S., Fischbein, N., Jackler, R.K., Lalwani, A.K. (2002). The value of enhanced magnetic resonance imaging in the evaluation of endocochlear disease. *Laryngoscope*, 112(1):8-17.

[87] Lemmerling, M. M., De Foer, B., Verbist, B. M., VandeVyver, V. (2009). Imaging of inflammatory and infectious diseases in the temporal bone. *Neuroimaging Clin N Am,* 19:321–337.

[88] Waltzman, S. B., Fisher, S. G., Niparko, J. K., Cohen, N. L. (1995). Predictors of postoperative performance with cochlear implants. *Ann Otol Rhinol Laryngol Suppl,* 165:15–18.

[89] Digge, P., Solanki, R. N., Shah, D. C., Vishwakarma. R., Kumar, S. (2016). Imaging Modality of Choice for Pre-Operative Cochlear Imaging: HRCT vs. MRI Temporal Bone. *Journal of Clinical and Diagnostic Research.* 10(X): TC01-TC04.

[90] Young, J., Ryan, M, E. and Young, N. M. (2014). Preoperative Imaging of Sensorineural Hearing Loss in Pediatric Candidates for Cochlear Implantation. *RadioGraphics,* 34:E133–E149.

[91] Young, N. M., Kim, F. M., Ryan, M. E., Tournis, E., Yaras, S. (2012). Pediatric cochlear implantation of children with eighth nerve deficiency. *Int J Pediatr Otorhinolaryngol*, 76(X):1442–1448.

[92] Bonneville, F., Sarrazin, J. L., Marsot-Dupuch, K., Iffenecker, C., Cordoliani, Y. S., Doyon, D., Bonneville, J. F. (2001). Unusual lesions of the cerebellopontine angle: a segmental approach. *Radiographics*, 21:419–438.

[93] Sarrazin, J.L. (2006). Infratentorial tumors. *J Radiol*, 87:748–763.

[94] Hentschel, M.A., Kunst, H.P.M., Rovers, M.M., Steens, S.C.A. (2018). Diagnostic accuracy of high-resolution T2-weighted MRI vs contrast-enhanced T1-weighted MRI to screen for cerebellopontine angle lesions in symptomatic patients. *Clinical Otolaryngology,* 43:805–811.

[95] Salzman, K. L., Davidson, H. C., Harnsberger, H. R., Glastonbury, C. M., Wiggins, R. H., Ellul, S., Shelton, C. (2001). Dumbbell schwannomas of the internal auditory canal. *AJNR Am J Neuroradiol*, 22:1368–1376.

[96] Gagliardo, C., Martines, F., Bencivinni, F., La Tona, G., Lo Casto, A. and Midiri, M. (2013). Intratumoral haemorrhage causing an unusual clinical presentation of a vestibular schwannoma. *Neuroradiol J.* 26(I):30-34.

[97] Guermazi, A., Lafitte, F., Miaux, Y., Adem, C., Bonneville, J. F., Chiras, J. (2005). The dural tail sign-beyond meningioma. *Clin Radiol*, 60:171–188.

[98] Gomez-Brouchet, A., Delisle, M. B., Cognard, C., Bonafe, A., Charlet, J. P., Deguine, O., Fraysse, B. (2001). Vestibular schwannomas: correlations between magnetic resonance imaging and histopathologic appearance. *Otol Neurotol*, 22:79–86.

[99] Papanagiotou, P., Grunwald, I. Q., Politi, M., Struffert, T., Ahlhelm, F., Reith, W. (2006).Vascular anomalies of the cerebellopontine angle. *Radiologe*, 46:216–223.

[100] Liu, P., Saida, Y., Yoshioka, H. and Itai, Y. (2003). MR imaging of epidermoids at the cerebellopontine angle. *Magn Reson Med Sci*, 2:109–115.

[101] Ikeda, H., Deinsberger, W. and Boker, D.K. (2000). Petroclival arachnoid cyst presenting with spontaneous intracystic haemorrhage-case presentation. *Acta Neurochir (Wien)*, 142:1317–1318.

[102] Scangas, G., Remenschneider, A. and Santos, F. (2015) Lipochoristoma of the Internal Auditory Canal. *J Neurol Surg Rep*, 76(I): e52–e54.

[103] Sade, B., Mohr, G. and Dufour, J.J. (2005). Cerebellopontine angle lipoma presenting with hemifacial spasm: case report and review of the literature. *J Otolaryngol*, 34:270–273.

[104] Wu, S.S., Lo, W.W., Tschirhart, D.L., Slattery, W.H. 3rd, Carberry, J.N. and Brackmann, D.E. (2003). Lipochoristomas (lipomatous tumors) of the acoustic nerve. *Arch Pathol Lab Med*, 127(XI):1475-1479.

[105] Mohanty, P. P., Pasricha, R., Datta, N. R., Jain, M. (2003). Primary chondroid chordoma of the petrous part of the temporal bone. *Clin Oncol (R Coll Radiol)*, 15:365–366.

[106] Currey, J.D. (2003). How well are bones designed to resist fracture? *J Bone Miner Res*, 18:591–598.

[107] Gagliardo, C., La Tona, G., Iovane, A. (2014). "Trauma cranico nello sport" in "Principi di diagnostica per immagini in medicina dello sport"; Iovane, A.; Solarino, M.; Sutera, R.; Edises, ISBN: 9788879598132 January 2014.

[108] Saraiya, P.V. and Aygun, N. (2009) Temporal bone fractures. *Emerg Radiol*, 16:255–265.

[109] Zarandy M. M., Rutka, J. (2010). *Diseases of the Inner Ear* doi: 10.1007/978-3-642-05058-9_5, © Springer-Verlag Berlin Heidelberg 2010.

[110] Gurdjian, E.S., Lissner, H.R. (1946). Deformation of the skull in head injury studied by "stress coat" technique: quantitative determinations. *Surg Gynecol Obstet*, 83:219–233

[111] Ishman, S.L. and Friedland, D.R. (2004). Temporal bone fractures: traditional classification and clinical relevance. *Laryngoscope*, 114(X):1734-1741.

[112] Dahiya, R., Keller, J.D., Litofsky, N.S., Bankey, P.E., Bonassar, L.J. and Megerian, C.A. (1999). Temporal bone fractures: otic capsule sparing versus otic capsule violating clinical and radiographic considerations. *J Trauma*, 47(VI):1079–1083.

[113] Sudhoff, H., Linthicum and F.H. Jr. (2003). Temporal bone fracture and latent meningitis: temporal bone histopathology study of the month. *Otol Neurotol* 24(III):521-522.

[114] Gross, M., Yaacov, A.B. and Eliashar, R. (2003). Cochlear involvement in a temporal bone fracture. *Otol Neurotol*, 24(VI): 958–959.

[115] Lancaster, J.L., Alderson, D.J. and Curley, J.W. (1999). Otological complications following basal skull fractures. *J R Coll Surg Edinb*, 44(II):87–90.

[116] Nosan, D.K., Benecke, J.E. Jr and Murr, A.H.(1997). Current perspective on temporal bone trauma. *Otolaryngol Head Neck Surg*, 117(I):67–71.
[117] Zayas, J. O., Feliciano, Y. Z., Hadley, C. R., Gomez, A. A., Vidal, J. A. (2011). Temporal bone trauma and the role of multidetector CT in the emergency department. *RadioGraphics,* 31:1741–1755.
[118] Lourenco, M.T., Yeakley, J.W. and Ghorayeb, B,Y. (1995). The "Y" sign of lateral dislocation of the incus. *Am J Otol,* 16(III):387-392.
[119] Jäger, L., Strupp, M., Brandt, T., Reiser, M. (1997) Imaging of labyrinth and vestibular nerve. *Nervenarzt,* 86:443–458.
[120] Maillot, O., Attyé, A., Boyer, E., Heck, O., Kastler, A., Grand, S., Schmerber, S. and Krainik, A. (2016). Post traumatic deafness: a pictorial review of CT and MRI findings. *Insights Imaging,* 7(III):341-50.
[121] Holland, N.J. and Weiner, G.M. (2004). Recent developments in Bell's palsy. *BMJ*, 329:553–557.
[122] Chan, E.H., Tan, H.M., Tan, T.Y. (2005). Facial palsy from temporal bone lesions. *Ann Acad Med Singapore*, 34:322–329.
[123] Brodie, H.A. and Thompson, T.C. (1997). Management of complications from 820 temporal bone fractures. *Am J Otol,* 18:188–197.
[124] Delgado-Almandoz, J.E., Kelly, H.R., Schaefer, P.W., Lev, M.H., Gonzalez, R.G. and Romero, J.M. (2010). Prevalence of traumatic dural venous sinus thrombosis in high-risk acute blunt head trauma patients evaluated with multidetector CT venography. *Radiology,* 255(II):570-577.
[125] Ghuman, M.S., Salunke, P., Sahoo, S.K. and Kaur, S. (2016). Cerebral venous sinus thrombosis in closed head trauma: A call to look beyond fractures and hematomas! *Journal of Emergencies, Trauma, and Shock.* 9(I):37-38.
[126] Leonetti, J.P., Shownkeen, H. and Marzo, S.J. (2001). Incidental petrous apex findings on magnetic resonance imaging. *Ear Nose Throat J* 80(IV):200-2, 205-6.
[127] Chapman, P. R., Shah, R., Curé, J. K., Bag, A. K. (2011) Petrous Apex Lesions: Pictorial Review, *AJR Am J Roentgenol,* 196: WS26-WS37.
[128] Arriaga, M.A. and Brackmann, D.E. (1991) Differential diagnosis of primary petrous apex lesions. *Am J Otol,* 12(VI):470-474 *Am J Otol* May; 13(III):297.
[129] Radhakrishnan, R., Son, H.J. and Koch, B.L. (2014). Petrous apex lesions in the pediatric population *Pediatr Radiol,* 44(III):325-339; quiz 323-324.
[130] Isaacson, B. (2015). Cholesterol granuloma and other petrous apex lesions, *Otolaryngol Clin N Am,* 48(2):361-373.
[131] Larson, T.L., Wong, M.L. (1992). Primary mucocele of the petrous apex: MR appearance. *AJNR Am J Neuroradiol,* 13(I):203-204.
[132] Fitzgerald, D.C. (2001). Nasopharyngeal abscess and facial paralysis as complications of petrous apicitis: a case report *Ear Nose Throat J*, 80(V):305-307.

[133] Nelson, J.J., Goyal, P. (2012). Extraorbital pseudotumor of the petrous apex: biopsy via a transnasal endoscopic approach *Ear Nose Throat J,* 91(IV):E6-9.

[134] Kim, B. J., Lee, E. J., Chang, H. W., Jung, H. R., Kim, E., Sohn, S. I., Kim, S. P. (2014). Aneurysmal bone cyst in the temporal bone and complete resection with preoperative embolization. A case report. *Interv Neuroradiol,* 31; 20(V):609-613.

[135] Bialer, O. Y., Rueda, M. P., Bruce, B. B., Newman, N. J., Biousse, V., Saindane, A. M. (2014). Meningoceles in idiopathic intracranial hypertension *AJR Am J Roentgenol,* 202(3):608-613.

[136] Van Es, S., North, K.N., McHugh, K. and De Silva, M. (1996), MRI findings in children with neurofibromatosis type 1: a prospective study *Pediatr Radiol,* 26(VII):478-487.

[137] Mafee, M. F., Kumar, A., Heffner, D.K. (1994). Epidermoid cyst (cholesteatoma) and cholesterol granuloma of the temporal bone and epidermoid cysts affecting the brain. *Neuroimaging Clin N Am,* 4(III):561-578.

[138] Zivković, N., Marković, M., Mihajlović, G., Jovanović, M. (2014). Surgical treatment of intradiploic epidermoid cyst treated as depression. *Srp Arh Celok Lek,* 142(I-II):67-71.

[139] Bacciu, A., Di Lella, F., Pasanisi, E., Gambardella, I., Saccardi, M. S., Bacciu, S., Vincenti, V. (2014). Open vs closed type congenital cholesteatoma of the middle ear: two distinct entities or two aspects of the same phenomenon? *Int J Pediatr Otorhinolaryngol,* 78(XII):2205-2209.

[140] Makarem, A.O., Hoang, T.A., Lo, W.W., Linthicum F.H. Jr and Fayad, J.N. (2010). Cavitating otosclerosis: clinical, radiologic, and histopathologic correlations *Otol Neurotol,* 31(III):381-384.

[141] Moe, K.S., Li, D., Linder, T.E., Schmid, S. and Fisch, U. (1999), An update on the surgical treatment of temporal bone paraganglioma. *Skull Base Surg,* 9(III):185-194.

[142] Martucci, V.L., Pacak, K. (2014). Pheochromocytoma and paraganglioma: diagnosis, genetics, management, and treatment. *Curr Probl Cancer,* 38(I):7-41.

[143] Corrales, C. E., Fischbein, N., Jackler R. K. (2015). Imaging innovations in temporal bone disorders *Otolaryngol Clin North Am,* 48(II):263-280.

[144] Szymańska, A., Szymański, M., Czekajska-Chehab, E., Szczerbo-Trojanowska, M. (2015) Non-paraganglioma tumors of the jugular foramen – Growth patterns, radiological presentation, differential diagnosis. *Neurol Neurochir Pol,* 49(III):156-163.

[145] Naidich, Th. P., Duvernoy, H. M., Delman, B. N., Sorensen, A. G., Kollias, S. S., Haacke, E. M. (2009) *Duvernoy's atlas of the brainstem and cerebellum.* Springer.

[146] Borges, A. (2015). Pathology of the facial nerve. In: Lemmerling, M., de Foer, B. (eds.), Temporal bone imaging. *Medical Radiology* (Diagnostic Imaging). p257-306. Springer

[147] Verzijl, H. T., Valk, J., de Vries, R., Padberg, G. W. (2005). Radiologic evidence for absence of the facial nerve in Möbius syndrome. *Neurology*, 64:849-855.
[148] Veillon, F. Ramos-Taboadaa, L.,Abu-Eida, M., Charpiotb, A. Riehma, S. (2010). Imaging of the facial nerve. *Eur J Radiol*, 74(II):341-348.
[149] Borges, A., Casselman, J. (2007). Imaging the cranial nerves: Part I: methodology, infectious and inflammatory, traumatic and congenital lesions. *Eur Radiol*, 17(VIII):2112-2125.
[150] Ünel, S., Yilmaz, M., Albayram, S., Işık, Z., Ceyhan, E., Isildak, H., Teixido, M., Savas, Y. and Kiris, A. (2012). Anastomoses of the Vestibular, Cochlear, and Facial Nerves. *J Craniofac Surg*, 23(V):1358-1361.
[151] Jin, A., Xu, P., Qu, F. (2018). Variations in the labyrinthine segment of facial nerve canal revealed by high-resolution computed tomography. *Auris Naus Larynx*, 45(II):261-264.
[152] Alicandri-Ciufelli, M., Fermi, M., Bonali, M., Presutti, L., Marchioni, D., Todeschini, A. and Anschuetz, L. (2018). Facial sinus endoscopic evaluation, radiologic assessment, and classification. *Laryngoscope*, [Epub ahead of print].
[153] Burmeister, H. P., Baltzer, P. A., Dietzel, M., Krumbein, I., Bitter, T., Schrott-Fischer, A., Guntinas-Lichius, O., Kaiser, W. A. (2001). Identification of the nervus intermedius using 3T MR imaging. *Am J Neuroradiol*, 32(III):460-464.
[154] Singh, A.K., Bathla, G., Altmeyer, W., Tiwari, R., Valencia, M.P., Bazan, C. and Tantiwongkosi, B. (2015). Imaging Spectrum of Facial Nerve Lesions. *Current Problems in Diagnostic Radiology*, 44(I): 60-75.
[155] Lorch, M., Teach, S.J. (2010). Facial nerve palsy: etiology and approach to diagnosis and tratment. *Pediatr Emerg Care*, 26(X):763-769 quiz 770-773.
[156] Gupta, S., Mends, F., Hagiwara, M., Fatterpekar, G. and Roehm, P.C. (2013). Imaging the Facial Nerve: A Contemporary Review. *Radiology research and practice*, 2013: 248039.
[157] Thömke, F., Urban, P. P., Marx, J. J., Mika-Grüttner, A., Hopf, H. C. (2002). Seventh nerve palsies may be the only clinical sign of small pontine infarctions in diabetic and hypertensive patients. *J Neurol*, 249(XI):1556-1562.
[158] Kobayashi, J., Ohara, T., Minematsu, K., Nagatsuka, K. and Toyoda, K. (2014). Etiological mechanisms of isolated pontine infarcts based on arterial territory involvement *J Neurol Sci*, 339(I-II):113-117.
[159] Wilson, L. K., Pearce, L. A., Arauz, A., Anderson, D. C., Tapia, J., Bazan, C., Benavente, O. R., Field, T. S., SPS3 Investigators. (2016). Morphological classification of penetrating artery pontine infarcts and association with risk factors and prognosis: The SPS3 trial. *Int J Stroke*, 11(IV):412-419.
[160] Park, J.H., Yoo, H.U. and Shin, H.W. (2008). Peripheral type facial palsy in a patient with dorsolateral medullary infarction with infranuclear involvement of the caudal pons *J Stroke Cerebrovasc Dis* 17(V):263-265.

[161] Lanser, M.J., Jackler, R.K. (1991). Gadolinium magnetic resonance imaging in Bell's palsy. *Western Journal of Medicine* 154(VI):718–719.

[162] Alaani, A., Hogg, R., Saravanappa, N. and Irbing, R.M. (2005), An analysis of diagnostic delay in unilateral facial palsy. *J Larungol Otol,* 119(III):184-188.

[163] Smith, J.K., Matheus, M.G. and Castillo, M. (2004). Imaging manifestations of neurosarcoidosis. *Am J Roentgenol,* 182:289-295.

[164] Kuya, J., Kuya, K., Shinohara, Y., Kunimoto, Y., Yazama, H., Ogawa, T. and Takeuchi, H. (2017). Usefulness of high-resolution 3D multi-sequences for peripheral facial palsy differentiation between Bell's palsy and Ramsay *Hunt syndrome. Otol Neurotol,* 38(X):1523-1527.

[165] Labin, E., Tore, H., Alkuwaiti, M. and Streib, C. (2017). Teaching NeuroImages: Classic Ramsay Hunt syndrome and associated MRI findings. *Neurology,* 89(VII):e79-e80.

[166] Ebner, D., Smith, K., DeSimone, D. and Sohail, M.R. (2010). Cranial neuropathy and severe pain due to early disseminated Borrelia burgdorferi infection. *BMJ Case Rep,* 23;2018.

[167] Burmeister, H. P., Baltzer, P. A., Klingner, C. M., Pantel, M., Kaiser, W.A. (2010). CT and MR Imaging of the facial nerve. *HNO* 58(V):433-442.

[168] Petrus, L.V., Lo, W.W. (1997) The anterior epitympanic recess: CT anatomy and pathology. *Am J Neuroradiol,* 18(VI):1109-1114.

[169] Borges, A. and Casselman, J., (2007). Imaging the cranial nerves: Part II: primary and secondary neoplastic conditions and neurovascular conflicts. *Eur Radiol,* 17(IX):2332-2344.

[170] Yue, Y., Jin, Y., Yang, B., Yuan, H., Li, J. and Wang, Z. (2015). Retrospective case series of the imaging findings of facial nerve hemangioma. *Eur Arch Otorhinolaryngol,* 272(IX):2497-2503.

[171] Ojiri, H. (2006). Perineural spread in head and neck malignancies. *Radiat Med,* 24:1-8.

[172] Zhao, S., Han, D., Wang, Z., Li, J., Qian, Y., Ren, Y., Dong, J. (2015). An imaging study of the facial nerve canal in congenital aural atresia. *Ear Nose Throat J,* 94(X-XI):E6-13.

[173] Song, J. J., Park, J. H., Jang, J. H., Lee, J. H., Oh, S. H., Chang, S. O., Kim, C. S. (2012) Facial nerve aberrations encountered during cochlear implantation. *Acta Otolaryngol,* 132(VII):788-794.

[174] Vincenti, V., Di Lella, F., Falcioni, M., Negri, M. and Zanetti, D. (2018) *Cochlear implantation in children with CHARGE syndrome: a report of eight cases.* 275(VIII):1987-1993.

[175] Kozerska, M., Skrzat, J., Spulber, A., Walocha, J., Wronski, S. and Tarasiuk, J. (2017), Micro-CT study of the dehiscences of the tympanic segment of the facial canal. *Surg Radiol Anat,* 39(IV):375-382.

ATLAS

Imaging Based Atlas of the Hearing System

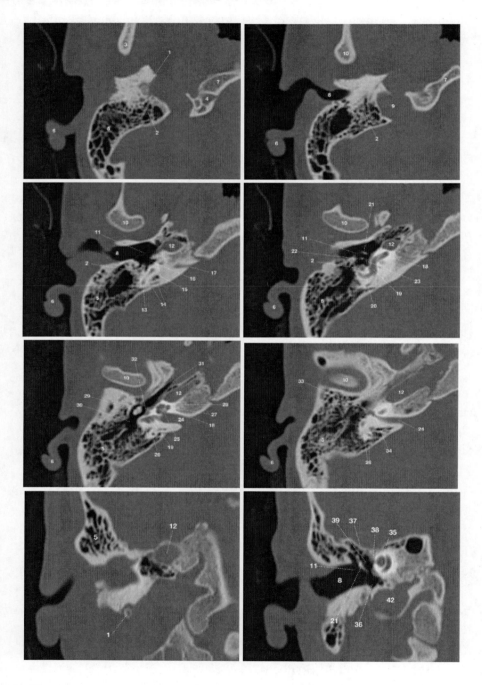

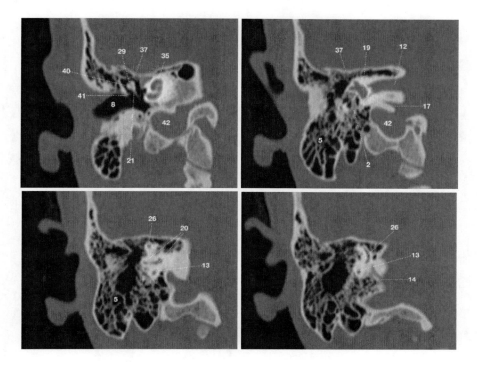

Atlas legend:

1) styloid process
2) facial nerve (mastoid segment)
3) condyloid process
4) hypoglossal canal
5) mastoid cells
6) pinna
7) C1 (atlas) anterior arch
8) external auditory channel (EAC)
9) jugular foramen
10) condylar process
11) tympanic membrane
12) internal carotid artery (ICA)
13) posterior semicircular canal (PSCC)
14) vestibular aqueduct
15) sinus tympani
16) round window niche
17) cochlear aqueduct
18) basal turn cochlea
19) vestibule
20) lateral semicircular canal (LSCC)
21) malleus
22) incus (short process)
23) stapes
24) internal auditory channel (IAC)
25) modiolus
26) superior semicircular canal (SSCC)
27) middle turn cochlea
28) apical turn cochlea
29) incudomalleolar joint
30) aditus ad antrum
31) Eustachian tube entrance
32) facial nerve (tympanic segment)
33) geniculate ganglion
34) facial nerve (labyrinthine segment)
35) cochlea
36) hypo tympanum
37) tegmen tympani
38) tensor tympani muscle
39) tensor tympani tendon
40) Prussak's space
41) scutum
42) jugular bulb.

Section 2. Sensorineural Hearing Loss: Pathology

In: Sensorineural Hearing Loss
Editors: F. Dispenza and F. Martines

ISBN: 978-1-53615-048-3
© 2019 Nova Science Publishers, Inc.

Chapter 6

AGE-RELATED HEARING LOSS

*Rocco Bruno, MD, Bruno Galletti, MD, Pietro Abita, MD,
Giuseppe Impalà, Francesco Freni, MD, PHD
and Francesco Galletti, MD, PHD*

University of Messina, Department of Human Pathology,
Adult and Developmental Age "G. Barresi", Messina, Italy

ABSTRACT

Age-related hearing loss (ARHL, also known as presbycusis) is a hearing loss linked to ageing in which there is a typical deterioration in the ability to understand verbal messages, caused by physiological ageing processes of the whole auditory system, from the peripheral receptors up to the central processing centres (Central Auditory Processing, CAP).

This chronic health condition affects approximately one-third of the population. The incidence among the elder patients (over 80 years old) reaches the 80%, and over 90% of hearing loss in the elderly is caused by presbycusis.

ARHL is classicaly defined as a progressive, bilateral and symmetrical hearing loss primarily observed in the high frequency region, associated with a deterioration in detection, localization of sound and verbal discrimination, especially in a competitive environment (for example, in the presence of background noise).

Four categories of risk factors associated with ARHL were identified in humans: genetic predisposition, environment, health co-morbidities and cochlear and CAP ageing. For these reasons ARHL can be defined ad a multifactorial disorder.

By analyzing human temporal bones, it could be distinguished six distinct forms of ARHI, with different pathologic changes correlated with a different audiologic pattern. According to this classification presbycusis can be divided into: Sensory presbycusis, Neural presbycusis, Strial presbycusis, Cochlear conductive presbycusis, Indeterminate presbycusis, Mixed presbycusis.

This chapter aims to give an overview of the scientific findings related to Age-related hearing impairment that is a complex disorder.

Keywords: age related hearing loss; presbyacusis; hearing impairment

DEFINITION

Age-related hearing loss (ARHL, also known as presbycusis) is a hearing loss linked to ageing in which there is a typical deterioration in the ability to understand verbal messages, caused by physiological ageing processes of the whole auditory system, from the peripheral receptors up to the central processing centres (Central Auditory Processing, CAP).

It is defined as a progressive, bilateral and symmetrical hearing loss primarily observed in the high frequency region, associated with a deterioration in detection, localization of sound and verbal discrimination, especially in a competitive environment (for example, in the presence of background noise) [1].

EPIDEMIOLOGY

AHRI is a chronic health condition that affects approximately one-third of the population. The incidence among the elder patients (over 80 years old) reaches the 80%, and over 90% of hearing loss in the elderly is caused by presbycusis [2]. The alteration in perception of pure tones already occurs in younger adults (approx. 30 years old), involving the acute frequencies (>10 kHz), which are not commonly examined in the classical tonal audiometric examination. This leads to the idea that a damage in perception of high frequency sounds has already taken place once the diagnosis of ARHL has been made with a conventional pure tone audiometry [3].

Epidemiological studies have confirmed two kinds of modifications in the auditory thresholds, involving different parts of the spectral frequencies: the decline in the higher frequencies (6-12,5 kHz) seems to have an early outset (beginning even at 31 years old) and a rapid growth while for the low and middle frequencies (up to 4kHz) the decline seems to have a late outset and a slower growth [4, 5].

The elaboration of data taken by the National Health and Nutrition Examination Survey (NHANES) demonstrates that the prevalence of ARHL is two times higher in men compared to women for frequencies between 0,5-8 kHz, especially after 50 years old, probably because of the protective role played by female hormones. From the same study emerged that in black individuals the prevalence of ARHL is lower than the one registered for white individuals, suggesting a protective role played by melanocyte function. Further studies are necessary to confirm this link, tough [3, 5].

CAUSES AND RISK FACTORS

ARHL is an inevitable hearing impairment associated with reduction of communicative skills related to ageing. Even if the development of this pathology is, as remarked before, inevitable, many Authors have found factors that can affect the extent of hearing loss.

Yamasoba et al. [6] identified four categories of risk factors associated with ARHL in humans: genetic predisposition, environment, health co-morbidities and cochlear and CAP ageing. For these reasons ARHL can be defined ad a multifactorial disorder.

1. Genetics

Contributions of the genetic factors to ARHL in humans have been well documented, despite the genetic mechanisms underlying the development of this pathology are not yet fully known.

Genome wide association studies have reported a strong link between ARHL and single nucleotide polymorphisms (SNPs) located in GRM7, a gene encoding metabotropic glutamate receptor type 7 protein (mGluR7) [7, 8].

A number of genes and mutations responsible for monogenic non-syndromic hearing loss are linked to ARHL, including: SNPs in 13-kb region in the middle of the KCNQ4, a gene which encodes a voltage-gated K-channel found in both outer and inner hair cells of cochlea [9]; 35delG heterozygosis mutation of GJB2, a gene that encodes gap junction proteins expressed in the inner ear (Connexin 26) [10-14]; mutation in GRHL2, a gene that encodes a transcription factor expressed in cells lining cochlear duct [15]; mutation in MYO6, a gene that encodes myosin VI found in inner ear hair cells [16]. It is known that genes that are linked to oxidative stress such as mutant allele (NAT2*6A), an isoform of N-acetyltransferases which encodes metabolism of reactive oxygen species [17, 18] and Glutathione S-transferases (GSTs) which encodes synthesis of glutathione antioxidant enzymes [19] are linked with the development of ARHL.

Furthermore it is necessary to mention, as possible responsible for presbycusis, mutations in mitochondrial DNA (deletion of 4,977bp of mitochondrial DNA and haplogroups U and K of mitochondrial DNA) [20, 21], and genes coding for Apolipoprotein E [22] and Endothelin-1 [23].

All the findings made on human DNA have been sustained over time by the initial discovery of analogous genes and alleles mutated in laboratory animals, especially in mice of the "inbred" strain.

In fact, in some studies on animal models, there have been identified some genes called AHL (age-hearing loss) that seems to contribute to the onset of ARHL: AHL2 on chromosome 5; AHL1, AHL4 and AHL5 on chromosome 10; AHL8 on chromosome 11; AHL3 on chromosome 17; AHL6 on chromosome 18 [24].

2. Environmental Factors

A variety of environmental risk factors such as exposure to industrial chemicals, occupational and recreational noise exposure are reported to be associated with ARHL [25-27]. Synergistic effects of simultaneous exposure to industrial chemicals and noise has a greater effect on ARHL than the impact of either one of the agents acting on its own [28-31].

3. Health Co-Morbidities

Several diseases and drugs have been associated over time with an increased probability of developing ARHL. The best known associations are between ARHL and type 2 diabetes mellitus, cardiovascular diseases, atherosclerosis, smoking, and the use of ototoxic drugs such as platinum-derived chemotherapeutics, loop diuretics, anti-inflammatory drugs and aminoglycoside antibiotics [5].

4. Ageing of the Auditory System

The inner ear is more prone to age-related changes than both the external and middle ear [32].

The first Author who managed to describe the damages caused by ageing on the inner hear, basing his discoveries on underlying case history information, audiometric configurations, and temporal bone analyses, was Harold Friederick Schuknecht [33-36]. He divided ARHL into four distinct classes:

- *Sensory:* loss of hair cells - inner (IHCs) and outer (OHCs) - and supporting cells - rod cells, Deiters, Hensen and Claudius cells. It is distinguished by a sharp drop in the audiometric track on the high frequencies and a bad speech discrimination in noisy environment. The otoacoustic emissions are absent. It is the most common form, typically linked to exposure to noise and environmental factors. It is also called *sociocusis*;

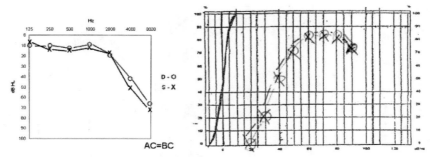

- *Neural:* linked to the loss of afferent neurons of the spiral ganglion, associated with a normal Organ of Corti. The audiogram is distinguished with a falling curve on the high frequencies, typically differentiated from the sensory form due to the bad speech discrimination;

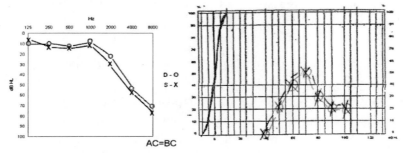

- *Metabolic or strial:* linked to atrophy of cochlear lateral wall and Stria vascularis. The audiogram is characterized by a pantonal hearing loss or with a slight fall on the higher frequencies with a good speech discrimination. The otoacoustic emissions are present. It is thought to be the form strongly correlated to genetic causes, since it is present in about 50% of the sisters, 40% in mother-daughter and about 30% in the siblings;

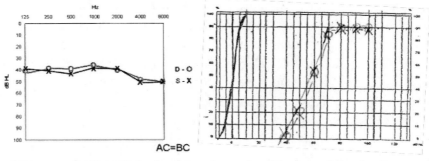

- *Cochlear conductive:* linked to atrophy and stiffening of the basilar membrane. The audiogram shows a typical and gradual descent on the high frequencies, with good verbal discrimination and with present otoacoustic emissions. It seems to be the least frequent form of the four, less probable from an etiopathogenetic point of view.

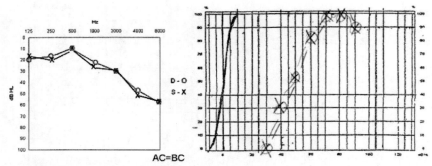

Later Shucknecht added two more categories to the four described above:

- *Mixed:* consisting of a mixture of pathological characteristics;
- *Indeterminate:* consisting of none of the aforementioned pathological characteristics.

In spite of the valuable contribution of Schuknecht in defining the pathophysiological mechanisms underlying ARHL, the above classification has been recently overcome due to the difficulties encountered in recognizing the different forms in a strict way. Nowadays it is common to use a much simpler distinction, based on the anatomical region in which the damage is established: we, then, recognize a *peripheral ARHL* (in which the hearing loss is caused by damages in the peripheral auditory system) and a *central ARHL* (in which hearing problems originate from a CAP dysfunction). The two nosological entities, however, may not present themselves exclusively, acting synergistically in the development of the pathology.

Peripheral ARHL

Peripheral ARHL includes all those forms characterized by an altered morphology of the audiogram with less or none deterioration in speech recognition. These forms are caused by damages to the structures of the inner ear, markedly against outer hair cells (progressive deterioration and decrease in the number of OHCs), stria vascularis (loss of cells and deterioration of its capillaries), spiral ganglion (deterioration of its neurons), lamina spiralis (reduction of the number of nerve fibers at this level) and internal auditory artery (hypertrophy of its elastic lamina) [34, 37-42]. The cause of all these damages has been proven to be oxidative stress: in fact, it has been demonstrated that an increased production of toxic catabolites (following, for example, noise exposure, use of ototoxic drugs, etc.) together with their inadequate disposal (as a result of mitochondrial dysfunction due to ageing) can damage the microstructures of the inner ear causing their death. Even alterations of the cochlear vascularization have been proven to be responsible for the damaging of inner ear's structures [43-53].

As far as we know, there are two different measurable alterations in a cochlea suffering from aging processes: the decrease of the electrical potential of endolymph (due to decreased expression of specific electrolytes transportation enzymes) and the increase in the threshold of the cochlear nerve compound action potential (due to the asynchrony of discharge of the single fibers that compose it [38].

Central ARHL

Central ARHL includes all those forms in which the main characteristic is an altered speech discrimination together with a partially conserved tonal auditory threshold. These forms originate from an alteration of the cortical networks and connections, resulting in a reduction of cortical plasticity, a physiological phenomenon due to ageing. In central ARHL what is typically altered is the Central Auditory Processing (CAP). CAP dysfunction is indeed occupying more and more importance in the establishment of the late phases of ARHL, while it is thought that the alterations of the peripheral auditory function are the *primum movens* in the development of the initial phases of presbycusis [54-57].

The three fundamental key points analyzed in Literature nowadays are:

1. What kind of alterations we find at various levels of the auditory path and how they affect the perception of complex stimuli, such as speech;
2. If and how these alterations are the effect of a peripheral system depletion, or if and how they run independently of it;
3. If and how there are correlations between ARHL, cognitive impairment and dementia.

I. The main alterations of central processing found in the latest studies are related to three main parameters: deficiency of temporal processing of complex stimuli, lesser ability to encode the signal in presence of noise and decline in spectral resolution. The first of the three seem to be the parameter that contributes most to the deterioration of all those skills useful to understand complex stimuli, such as speech.

As a consequence of aging, in fact, we can find at various levels of the auditory path: a decline in inhibitory neurotransmission mediated by glycine in cochlear nuclei, especially in the dorsal portion, as reported in the strain of aged Fischer-344 rats [58]; a marked decline of GABA-mediated inhibitory impulses together with a prevalence of the excitatory area over the inhibitory one in the inferior colliculus, as reported in various strains of aged rats [59, 60]; a 45% reduction of GABA receptors in the medial geniculate nucleus reported in aged rats [61]; decline in number of SMI-32-immunoreactive neurons and levels of non-phosphorylated neuro-filament proteins [62]. Human studies have found a deterioration in GABA-mediated inhibitory neurotransmission (both presynaptic and post-synaptic) in the primary auditory cortex and a deterioration of the Startle reflex evaluated through pre-pulse inhibition [63-65]. All these changes influence the temporal processing of acoustical stimuli and are reported to be contributing to central ARHL. The alterations of the remaining parameters (decline in spectral resolution and lesser ability to encode the signal in presence of noise) seems to be mainly caused by a deterioration of the capacity of fine tuning of the neuronal populations present in the primary auditory cortex (fine-tuned receptive fields) [66-68]. There is therefore a lower capacity in the primary auditory cortex to execute a fine spectral processing of complex signals, which leads to a lower capacity to encode properly a signal in the presence of background noise (poorly-tuned receptive fields).

It is also thought that age-associated changes in calcium binding proteins (parvalbumin, calbindin, calretinin) disrupt the calcium homeostasis and could lead to impaired synaptic transmission, reduced neural plasticity, and degeneration of neurons reported in ARHL [69-73]. Thanks to the advent of new imaging methods (PET and functional MRI) it was possible to show as a consequence of aging a reduction in both gray and white matter volumes, associated with cortical thinning. Alterations in the above mentioned neural networks are implicated in impaired cognitive functions such as verbal recognition memory, episodic visuospatial memory, learning and association ability, working memory and executive functions as well as attention switching [74-77].

II. An alteration of the central auditory system alone is extremely rare, whilst seems much more common an alteration of both the peripheral and central auditory system at the same time [78]. In addition, it appears that CAP alterations depend also on the reduction of peripheral inputs. (e.g., the deterioration of glycine-mediated neurotransmission at the level of cochlear nuclei found in the Fischer-344 rats [58], the evidence of a tonotopic reorganization of the primary auditory cortex found in animals, which follows the peripheral/cochlear hearing loss) [79, 80]. Even peripheral decline (e.g., different kind of glial alteration found in the strain of C57BL/6J mice) [81] and aging itself (documented as anatomical modifications in the whole brain) have been seen to be responsible for the alterations in CAP [78].

III. Increasing evidence has linked ARHL to more rapid progression of cognitive decline and incidental dementia, in an escalating form that can lead also to Alzheimer's disease (AD) - the most common form of dementia [2, 3, 57]. As far as we know it has not been yet discovered the keystone to explain whether the hearing impairment determines the development of dementia (due to the degradation of sensory inputs sent from the periphery to the central nervous system) or if cognitive decline leads to an altered capacity of auditory discrimination, especially in noisy environments (leading the elderly to further isolate themselves, worsening their dementia).

From an analysis of epidemiological and clinical evidences, four hypothesis have been theorized to explain the link between ARHL and cognitive impairment [2]:

1. *Cognitive load on perception hypothesis:* cognitive decline may reduce the cognitive resources that are available for auditory perception, increasing the effects of hearing loss;
2. *Degradation of audiological information hypothesis:* when the inputs are poor, either through degraded stimuli (e.g., in noisy environment) or impaired perception, additional cognitive resources are required to understand the signal. Therefore, this cognitive resources will not be available for cognitive roles.
3. *Sensory deprivation hypothesis:* described by Lin and colleagues [82-84], it suggests that hearing loss causes a cognitive decline that is permanent or potentially remediable after rehabilitation (e.g., with the use of hearing aids). It has been theorized that an impaired perception could lead to worsening cognition over time and social isolation, which in turn leads to cognitive decline.
4. *Common cause hypothesis:* according to this hypothesis numerous factors that act synergistically with each other are responsible for cognitive decline in the elderly. These include cardiovascular diseases, diabetes and tissue damage caused by increased Reactive Oxygen Species (ROS) production.

Although none of the four hypotheses is able to clarify the causal link between ARHL and cognitive decline [3], it has emerged that CAP dysfunction can be considered an important and early risk factor in determining the future onset of cognitive impairment up to Alzheimer's dementia [54].

ARHL AND FRAILTY

In addition to the close connection between ARHL and cognitive impairment, ARHL is also considered an important marker for frailty in older age. Frailty reflects a nonspecific state of vulnerability and multisystem physiological change that predisposes an individual to adverse health outcomes such as disability, falls, institutionalization, hospitalization and death [85], and is of high importance in the clinical care of the older population. Thus, psychological, cognitive and social factors contribute to define this condition.

The recruitment of cognitive areas which are not directly responsible for speech encoding causes neural resources to be sacrificed. Alterations in the above mentioned neural networks are implicated in impaired cognitive functions such as verbal recognition memory, episodic visuospatial memory, learning and association ability, working memory and executive functions, and attention switching [3, 54]. Moreover, it is thought that hearing loss is associated with a 20% increased risk of mortality compared with normal hearing [86].

DIAGNOSIS

The most important part in the diagnosis of ARHL is the anamnesis. Investigating the life of the patient, asking if there has ever been a chronic exposition to noise, a genetic susceptibility or a history of chronic illnesses linked to presbycusis, associated with tinnitus (a condition often related to hearing loss) is the cornerstone for a correct diagnosis.

After asking for the medical history it is necessary to submit the patient to different kind of audiological exams, which often have limitations in implementation due to the reduction of the level of attention and cooperation from the patient, which can trigger any anxiety states, further affecting the success of the examination. It will be necessary, therefore, to put the patient at ease, explaining in a clear and comprehensible way each task and the manner in which it must be completed.

During the course of the examinations it is important to take into account that the laxity of the tissues of the auricle and the ear canal, physiological in the elderly, can facilitate, collapsing, a reduction of the auditory acuity [1, 2].

Pure Tone Audiometry

It's the screening test for the evaluation of auditory acuity. It allows to highlight the presence of a hearing loss that is characteristically sensorineural, bilateral and symmetrical with a typical saving of the lower frequencies and a fall on the medium/higher frequencies. The magnitude of this loss depends significantly on the age of the patient and the amount of risk factors present in the medical history.

Speech Audiometry

Speech audiometry refers to procedures that use speech stimuli to assess auditory function. The goal of speech audiometry is to quantify a patient's ability to understand everyday communication. Speech audiometry testing can be done in isolation or with acoustic interferences which can be differentiated into two main groups: a kind of background noise which is similar to the primary signal (e.g., cocktail party) and another kind constituted by pure noise, different from the primary signal (e.g., pink noise).

Results from speech recognition tests in quiet testing condition and in background noise should be evaluated in relation to the pure-tone thresholds. Underperformance in speech recognition in comparison with expectations based on peripheral hearing function suggests central auditory processing dysfunction [54]. If word-recognition scores equal or exceed those that might be expected from the audiogram, then suprathreshold speech recognition ability is thought to be normal for the degree of hearing loss. If word recognition scores are poorer than would be expected, then suprathreshold ability is abnormal for the degree of hearing loss. Abnormal speech recognition is often the result of cochlear distortion or retrocochlear disorder.

The typical pattern of ARHL in speech detection threshold demonstrates what is called "rollover", in which speech recognizing function declines substantially as speech intensity increases beyond the level producing the maximum performance score. In other words, as speech intensity level increases, performance rises to a maximum level then declines or "rolls over" sharply as intensity increases. This rollover effect is commonly observed when the site of hearing loss is retrocochlear, in the auditory nerve or the auditory pathways in the brainstem [87].

Redundancy and Sensitized Speech Measures (SSM)

There is a great deal of redundancy associated with our ability to hear and process speech communication. Intrinsically, the central auditory nervous system has a rich system of anatomic, physiologic, and biochemical overlap. Among other functions, such intrinsic redundancy permits multisensory processing and simultaneous processing of different auditory signals. Another aspect of intrinsic redundancy is that the nervous system can be altered substantially by neurologic disorder and still maintain its ability to process information. Extrinsically, speech signals contain a wealth of information due to phonetic, phonemic, syntactic, and semantic content and rules. Such extrinsic redundancy allows us to hear only part of a speech segment and still understand what is being said. Extrinsic redundancy increases as the content of the speech signal increases.

The issue of redundancy plays a role in the selection of speech materials. If you are trying to assess the effects of a cochlear hearing impairment on speech perception, then signals that have reduced redundancy should be used. If you are trying to assess the effects of a disorder of the central auditory nervous system on speech perception, the situation becomes more difficult. The solution to assessing central auditory nervous system disorders is to reduce the extrinsic redundancy of the speech information enough to reveal the reduced intrinsic redundancy caused by neurologic disorder [87, 88].

Thanks to the use of sensitized speech measures it is possible to evaluate CAP and any of its dysfunction (CAPD) establishing critical listening conditions, as described above. The most diffused SSM tests in the last few years are based on:

- the administration of phrases with a verbal competitive signal characterized by continuous speech, presented ipsilaterally or contralaterally to the primary signal (SSI-ICM: synthetic sentence identification with ipsilateral competing message,

SSI-CCM: synthetic sentence identification with contralateral competing message);
- the administration of phrases in presence of a competitive noise, generally consisting of pink noise (SPIN: speech in noise perception);
- the administration of verbal signal idegraded in its spectral component ("distorted voice") or temporal component (by introducing interruptions - "interrupted voice" - or compressing the times - "accelerated voice").

It is not yet clear whether these tests specifically identify CAPD or are significantly influenced by alterations in cognitive abilities, often present in several individuals affected by ARHL with concomitant cognitive impairment, dementia and/or AD (Alzheimer's disease) [89].

Tympanometry

This test provides a valuable aid in the topodiagnosis of ARHL, excluding a transmission deficit in the middle ear (presence of type A tympanograms), and evaluating the presence (with recruitment) or absence of the cocleo-stapedial reflexes [1].

Otoacoustic Emissions

Not necessary for the diagnosis of ARHL in the typical audiological examination. They may be useful in objecting a damage of OHCs in case of peripheral receptor damage [1].

PREVENTION AND REHABILITATION

It is impossible to counteract the aging processes which lead to ARHL. As for the prevention of the pathology it is therefore important to avoid a rapid progression of the deterioration in the auditory system.

As it could be imagined, the main prevention for ARHL is avoiding all those conditions in which the ear can suffer from chronic acoustic stress (e.g., use of headphones and earphones at high volume, attendance of discos, lack of soundproofing in the workplace, exposition to noise in the city environment, hobbies related to auditory stress such as hunting, etc.) and preventing all of those diseases capable of altering the auditory function (ischemic heart disease, strokes, hyperlipidemia, diabetes mellitus, etc.).

The first and fundamental tool of prevention in the diagnosis of ARHL is the periodic control of the auditory function, in order to recognize at an early stage the moment in which the hearing loss begins to determine a deficit in personal and communicative skills of an individual.

There are conflicting opinions concerning therapeutic strategies for ARHL. On the basis of its etiopathogenesis, however, it has been advised the use of substances with antioxidative powers (such as A, B, C, E vitamins, selenium, N-acetylcysteine, methionine, etc.) to contrast the damages made by ROS in the inner ear.

Nowadays the pivotal tool for an early diagnosis of ARHL is still the pure tone audiometry. Every adult over 65 years old should undergo annually to this exam, especially when predisposing factors are documented in his medical history. The mail goal of an early diagnosis lies on the possibility to establish a rapid therapeutic-rehabilitative strategy, counteracting the evolution of the pathology and the social isolation, which can eventually lead to cognitive impairment and dementia.

Hearing Aids (HAs) are the most valid and effective instrument in the field of auditory rehabilitation in ARHL. Different studies, in fact, prove that the use of HAs influence significantly in a positive way the quality of life in those who wear them [90]. HAs exploit the functional residues of the organ of Corti amplifying, transducing and sending sounds directly to the tympanic membrane. They can be useful when the hearing loss is not susceptible to medical and/or surgical intervention. For a documentable benefit from the use of HAs there must be an average pure tone threshold higher than 55dB SPL on 500, 1000, 2000 and 4000 frequencies, together with an identification greater than 60% of the words in closed lists and a recognition of more than 40% of the words in open lists without the help of labiolecture in speech audiometry with an emission of 65dB SPL.

HAs are chosen on the basis of the characteristics of each patient (grade of hearing loss, expectancies and necessities). These modern digital amplification systems are completely innovative and allow, thanks to better sound processing and division of the frequency spectrum into multiple channels, to have excellent results in those hearing losses where personalization and fine adjustment are fundamental for a good hearing rehabilitation.

Clinical trials have demonstrated that hearing loss has a negative impact on working memory, which is important for speech understanding especially in difficult or noisy environments. Other trials proved that the use of hearing aids in the earliest stages of ARHL can improve a person's performances on auditory memory tests [90].

Conventional HAs come in several styles and with a range of functionality. The most common styles of hearing aids are known as behind-the-ear (BTE) and in-the-ear (ITE) hearing aids. A radical change in terms of hearing rehabilitation in ARHL was the birth of Open Fitting (OF) coupling system. Thanks to the OF system the ear is left open and the snail is replaced by a small silicone dome that can be pierced or "tulip-shaped"; it is supported by a small tube that can be empty or more frequently traveled by an electric wire if the receiver is in the ear canal and not in the body of the HA. This has allowed a greater miniaturization and camouflage of the prosthesis, together with a greater tolerability and acceptance by the patient, as well as a better hearing quality thanks to the reduced effects of autofonia and occlusion of the external auditory canal [88].

Despite the high incidence of ARHL, the percentage of hearing impaired elderly who use hearing aids is relatively low (it is estimated, in fact, that only 20% of patients who need acoustic amplification regularly use HAs). This is mostly due to cultural and mental status, degree of socialization, education and/or family situation. In this regard, in the context of rehabilitation, a careful counseling activity aimed at patients and their relatives is very important, purposing to encourage the acceptance and adaptation of HAs, encouraging their use. In fact, elderly patients must be gradually educated to amplified hearing, giving them the opportunity to hear again sounds they were no longer used to hear [88].

The main limitation of HAs is in all those severe and profound hearing losses whose gain from the use of HAs is not able to activate the analyzing processes necessary for speech understanding. In these cases, after a careful evaluation of the patient and his life expectancy, and if there are no general medical contraindications, it will be possible to restore hearing thanks to Cochlear Implantation (CI). While in the past CI was not recommended for older patients, to date the outlook has completely changed. In fact, the majority of elderly patients using cochlear implants have demonstrated, both through subjective and objective assessments, a marked improvement in the ability to discriminate speech versus preoperative assessments, as well as an overall satisfaction and better hearing performance even compared to patients who have undergone surgery for CI at a younger age [2, 91, 92].

Given these considerations, counteracting ATHL since the earliest symptoms is very important, both from a prosthetic and an implantological point of view.

Future perspectives in the field of audiological rehabilitation in the elderly are focusing on the possibility of developing a "hybrid" prosthetic system, able to stimulate the ear either by direct acoustic stimulation (as with the HA) or by electromagnetic stimulation (CI). This solution would be particularly indicated in all patients presenting a pure tone threshold rapidly falling on the higher frequencies with partial or total preservation of the lower frequencies. Other interesting research cues are oriented towards the discovery of one or more drugs able to prevent the death of acoustic receptors, hindering the worsening of ARHL or even exploiting stem cells in order to restore a "physiological hearing" [1, 93].

REFERENCES

[1] Fortunato, S., Forlì, F., Guglielmi, V., De Corso, E., Paludetti, G., Berrettini, S., Fetoni, A.R. (2016) A review of new insights on the association between hearing loss and cognitive decline in ageing. *Acta Otorhinolaringol Ital*; 36: 155-166.

[2] Jayakody, D.M.P., Friedland, P.L., Martins, R.N., Sohrabi, H.R. (2018) Impact of aging on the auditory system and related cognitive functions: a narrative review. *Front Neurosci*; 12 (125).

[3] Lee, J., Dhar, S., Abel, R., Banakis, R., Grolley, E., Lee, J. (2012) Behavioral hearing thresholds between 0.125 and 20 kHz using depth-compensated ear simulator calibration. *Ear Hear*; 33: 315.

[4] Agrawal, Y., Platz, E.A., Niparko, J.K. (2008) Prevalence of hearing loss and differences by demographic characteristics among US adults: data from the National Health and Nutrition Examination Survey, 1999-2004. *Arch Intern Med*; 168: 1522-1530.

[5] Yamasoba, T., Lin, F.R., Someya, S., Kashio, A., Sakamoto, T., Kondo, K. (2013) Current concepts in age-related hearing loss: epidemiology and mechanistic pathways. *Hear Res*; 303: 30-38.

[6] Friedman, R.A., Van Laer, L., Huentelman, M.J., Sheth, S.S., Van Eyken, E., Corneveaux, J.J. (2009) GRM7 variants confer susceptibility to age-related hearing impairment. *Hum Mol Genet*; 18: 785-796.

[7] Newman, D.L., Fisher, L.M., Ohmen, J., Parody, R., Fong, C.T., Frisina, S.T. (2012) GRM7 variants associated with age-related hearing loss based on auditory perception. *Hear Res*; 294: 125-132.

[8] Van Eyken, E., Van Laer, L., Fransen, E., Topsakal, V., Lemkens, N., Laureys, W. (2006) KCNQ4: a gene for age-related hearing impairment? *Hum Mutat*; 27: 1007-1016.

[9] Van Eyken, E., Van Laer, L., Fransen, E., Topsakal, V., Hendrickx, J.J., Demeester, K. (2007) The contribution of GJB2 (Connexin 26) 35delG to age-related hearing impairment and noise-induced hearing loss. *Otol Neurotol*; 28: 970-975.

[10] Amorini, M., Romeo, P., Bruno, R., Galletti, F., Di Bella, C., Longo, P., Briuglia, S., Salpietro, C., Rigoli, L. (2015) Prevalence of Deafness-Associated Connexin-26 (GJB2) and Connexin-30 (GJB6) Pathogenic Alleles in a Large Patient Cohort from Eastern Sicily. *Ann Hum Genet*. Jun 19.

[11] Lin, Y.H., Wu, C.C., Hsu, C.J., Hwang, J.H., Liu, T.C. (2011) The grainyhead-like 2 gene (GRHL2) single nucleotide polymorphism is not associated with age-related hearing impairment in Han Chinese. *Laryngoscope*; 121: 1303.

[12] Martines, F., Salvago, P., Bartolotta, C., Cocuzza, S., Fabiano, C., Ferrara, S., La Mattina, E., Mucia, M., Sammarco, P., Sireci, F., Martines, E. (2015) A genotype–

phenotype correlation in Sicilian patients with GJB2 biallelic mutations. *European Archives of Oto-Rhino-Laryngology*, 272 (8), pp. 1857-1865.

[13] Bartolotta, C., Salvago, P., Cocuzza, S., Fabiano, C., Sammarco, P., Martines, F. (2014) Identification of D179H, a novel missense GJB2 mutation in a Western Sicily family. *European Archives of Oto-Rhino-Laryngology*, 271 (6), pp. 1457-1461.

[14] Salvago, P., Martines, E., La Mattina, E., Mucia, M., Sammarco, P., Sireci, F., Martines, F. (2014) Distribution and phenotype of GJB2 mutations in 102 Sicilian patients with congenital non syndromic sensorineural hearing loss. *International Journal of Audiology*, 53 (8), pp. 558-563.

[15] Oonk, A.M.M., Leijendeckers, J.M., Lammers, E.M., Weegerink, N.J.D., Oostik, J., Beynon, A.J. (2013) Progressive hereditary hearing impairment caused by aMYO6 mutations resembles presbyacusis. *Hear Res*; 299: 88-98.

[16] Van Eyken, E., Van Camp, G., Fransen, E., Topsakal, V., Hendrickx, J.J., Demeester, K. (2017) Contribution of the N-acetyltransferase 2 polymorphism NAT2*6° to age-related hearing impairment. *J Med Genet*; 44: 570.

[17] Ünal, M., Tamer, L., Dogruer, Z.N., Yildirim, H., Vayisoglu, Y., Çamdeviren, H. (2005) N-acetyltransferase 2 gene polymorphism and presbycusis. *Laryngoscope*; 115: 2238-2241.

[18] Ates, A., Ünal, M., Tamer, L., Derici, E., Karakas, S., Ercan, B. (2005) Glutathione S-transferase gene polymorphism in presbycusis. *Otol Neurotol*; 26: 392-397.

[19] Bai, U., Seidman, M.D., Hinojosa, R., Quirk, W.S. (1997) Mithochondrial DNA deletions associated with aging and possibly presbycusis: a human archival temporal bone study. *Am J Otol*; 18: 449.

[20] Manwaring, N., Jones, M.M., Wang, J.J., Rochtchina, E., Howard, C., Newall, P. (2007) Mitochondrial DNA aplogroups and age-related hearing loss. *Arch Otolaryngol Head Neck Surg*; 133: 929-933.

[21] O'Grady, G., Boyles, A.L., Speer, M., Deruyter, F., Strittmatter, W., Worley, G. (2007) Apolipoprotein E alleles and sensorineural hearing loss. *Int J Audiol*; 46: 183.

[22] Uchida, Y., Sugiura, S., Nakashima, T., Ando, F., Shimokata, H. (2009) Endothelin-1 gene polymorphism and hearing impairment in elderly Japanese. *Laryngoscope*; 119: 938-943.

[23] Fetoni, A.R., Picciotti, P.M., Paludetti, G., Troiani, D. (2011) Pathogenesis of presbycusis in animal models: a review. *Exp Gerontol*; 46(6): 413-425.

[24] Campo, P., Morata, T.C., Hong, O. (2013) Chemical exposure and hearing loss. *Dis Month*; 59:119.

[25] Fransen, E., Topsakal, V., Hendrickx, J.J., Van Laer, L., Huyghe, J.R., Van Eyken, E. (2008) Occupational noise, smoking and a high body mass index are risk factors for age-related hearing imparment and moderate alcohol consumption is protective:

a European population-based multicenter study. *J Assoc Res Otolaryngol*; 9: 264-276.

[26] Clark, W.W. (1991) Noise exposure from leisure activities: a review. *J Acoust Soc Am*; 90: 175.

[27] Sliwinska-Kowalska, M., Zamyslowska-Szmytke, E., Szymczack, W., Kotylo, P., Fiszer, M., Wesolowsky, W. (2004) Effects of co-exposure to noise and mixture of organic solvents on hearing in dockyard workers. *J Occup Environ Med*; 46: 30-38.

[28] Chang, S., Chen, C., Lien, C., Sung, F. (2006) Hearing loss in workers exposed to toluene and noise. *Environ Health Perspect*; 114: 1283.

[29] Fuente, A., McPherson, B. (2006) Organic solvents and hearing loss: the challenge for audiology. *Int J Audiol*; 45: 367.

[30] Dispenza, F., De Stefano, A., Costantino, C., Marchese, D., Riggio, F. (2013) Sudden sensorineural hearing loss: Results of intratympanic steroids as salvage treatment. *American Journal of Otol – Head and Neck Medicine and Survey;* 34(4), 296-300.

[31] Dispenza, F., Mazzucco, W., Bianchini, S., Mazzola, S., Bennici, E. (2015) Management of labyrinthine fistula in chronic otitis with cholesteatoma: case series; *Euromediterranean Biomedical Journal* 10(21), 255-261.

[32] Gordon-Salant, S. (2010) *The Aging Auditory System,* Ed. Springer-Verlag, USA 2010.

[33] Schuknecht, H.F. (1974) *Pathology of the Ear.* Cambridge, MA: Harvard University Press 1974.

[34] Schuknecht, H.F., Gacek, M.R. (1993) Cochlear pathology in presbycusis. *Ann Otol Rhinol Laryngol*; 102, 1-16.

[35] Schuknecht, H.F., Watanuki, K., Takahashi, T., Belal, A.A. Jr., Kimura, R.S., Jones, D.D., Ota, C.Y. (1974) Atrophy of the stria vascularis, a common cause for hearing loss. *Laryngoscope*; 84 (10): 1777-1821.

[36] Schuknecht, H.F. (1964) Further observations on the pathology of presbycusis. *Arch Otolaryngol*; 80: 369-382.

[37] Buckiova, D., Popelar, J., Syka, J. (2007) Aging cochleas in the F-344 rat: morphological and functional changes. *Exp Gerontol*; 42: 629-638.

[38] Gates, G.A., Mills, J.H. (2005) Presbycusis. *Lancet*; 366: 1111-1120.

[39] Gratton, M.A., Shulte, B.A. (1995) Alterations in microvasculature are associated with atrophy of the stria vascularis in quiet-aged gerbils. *Hear Res*; 82: 44-52.

[40] Hinojosa, R., Nelson, E.G. (2011) Cochlear nucleus neuron analysis in individuals with presbycusis. *Laryngoscope*; 121: 2641–2648.

[41] Mills, J.H., Konrad-Martin, D., Leek, M., Hood, L.J. (2006) Roundtable discussion: pathophysiology of the aging auditory system. *Semin Hear*; 27: 237–242.

[42] Belal, A. (1975) Presbycusis: physiological or pathological. *J. Laryngol. Otol*; 89: 1011–1025.

[43] Henderson, D., Bielefeld, E.C., Harris, K.C., Hu, B.H. (2006) The role of oxidative stress in noise-induced hearing loss. *Ear Hear*; 27: 1-19.

[44] Tabuki, K., Nishimura, B., Nakamagoe, M., Hayashi, K., Nakayama, M., Hara, A. (2011) Ototoxicity: mechanism of cochlear impairment and its prevention. *Curr Med Chem*; 18: 4866-4871.

[45] Cannizzaro, E., Cannizzaro, C., Plescia, F., Martines, F., Sole, L., Pira, E., Lo Coco, D. (2014) Exposure to ototoxic agents and hearing loss: A review of current knowledge. *Hearing, Balance and Communication*; 12: 166-175.

[46] Martines, F., Ballacchino, A., Sireci, F., Mucia, M., La Mattina, E., Rizzo, S. (2016) Audiologic profile of OSAS and simple snoring patients: the effect of chronic nocturnal intermittent hypoxia on auditory function. *European Archives of Oto-Rhino-Laryngology*; 273: 1419-1424.

[47] Martines, F., Messina, G., Patti, A., Battaglia, G., Bellafiore, M., Messina, A., Rizzo, S., Salvago, P., Sireci, F., Traina, M., Iovane, A. (2015) Effects of tinnitus on postural control and stabilization: A pilot study. *Acta Medica Mediterranea*; 31: 907-912.

[48] Ferrara, S., Salvago, P., Mucia, M., Ferrara, P., Sireci, F., Martines, F. (2014) Follow-up after pediatric myringoplasty: Outcome at 5 years. *Otorinolaringologia*; 64: 141-146.

[49] Rizzo, S., Bentivegna, D., Thomas, E., La Mattina, E., Mucia, M., Salvago, P., Sireci, F., Martines, F. (2016) Sudden sensorineural hearing loss, an invisible male: State of art. *Hearing loss: etiology,management and societal implications*, 75-86.

[50] Cheng, A.G., Cunningham, L.L., Rubel, W.E. (2005) Mechanism of hair cell death and protection. *Curr Opin Otolaryngol Head Neck Surg*; 13: 343-348.

[51] Someya, S., Prolla, T.A. (2010) Mitochondrial oxidative damage and apoptosis in age-related hearing loss. *Mech Ageing Dev*; 131: 480-486.

[52] Wen, J., Duan, N., Wang, Q., Jing, G.X., Xiao, Y. (2017) Protective effect of propofol on noise-induced hearing loss. *Brain Res*; 1657: 95-100.

[53] Nomiya, R., Nomiya, S., Kariya, S., Okano, M., Morita, N., Cureoglu, S. (2008) Generalized arteriosclerosis and changes of the cochlea in young adults. *Otol Neurotol*; 29: 1993-1997.

[54] Panza, F., Solfrizzi, V., Logroscino, G. (2015) Age-related hearing impairment – a risk factor and frailty marker for dementia and AD. *Nat Rev Neurol*; 11: 166-175.

[55] Martines, F., Maira, E., Ferrara, S. (2011) Age-related hearing impairment (ARHI): A common sensory deficit in the elderly. *Acta Medica Mediterranea*, 27 (1), 47-52.

[56] Salvago, P., Rizzo, S., Bianco, A., Martines, F. (2017) Sudden sensorineural hearing loss: is there a relationship between routine haematological parameters and audiogram shapes? *International Journal of Audiology*; 56(3): 148-153.

[57] Ballacchino, A., Salvago, P., Cannizzaro, E., Costanzo, R., Di Marzo, M., Ferrara, S., La Mattina, E., Messina, G., Mucia, M., Mulè, A., Plescia, F., Sireci, F., Rizzo, S., Martines, F. (2015) Association between sleep-disordered breathing and hearing disorders: Clinical observation in Sicilian patients. *Acta Medica Mediterranea*; 31(3): 607-614.

[58] Caspary, D.M. (2005) Age-related changes in the inhibitory response properties of dorsal cochlear nucleus output neurons: role of inhibitory inputs. *J. Neurosci*; 25: 10952-10959.

[59] Burianova, J., Ouda, L., Profant, O., Syka, J. (2009) Age-related changes in GAD levels in the central auditory system of the rat. *Exp. Gerontol*; 44: 161–169.

[60] Simon, H., Frisina, R.D., Walton, J.P. (2004) Age reduces response latency of mouse inferior colliculus neurons to AM sounds. *J Acoust Soc Am*; 116: 469–477.

[61] Richardson, B.D., Ling, L.L., Uteshev, V.V., Caspary, D.M. (2013) Reduced GABA(A) receptor-mediated tonic inhibition in aged rat auditory thalamus. *J Neurosci*; Jan 16;33(3):1218-27a.

[62] Burianova, J., Ouda, L., Syka, J. (2015) The influence of aging on the number of neurons and levels of non-phosporylated neurofilament proteins in the central auditory system of rats. *Front Aging Neurosci*; 7: 27.

[63] Gao, F., Edden, R.A.E., Li, M., Puts, N.A.J., Wang, G., Liu, C. (2013) Edited magnetic resonance spectroscopy detects an age-related decline in brain GABA levels. *Neuroimage*; 78: 75-82.

[64] Gao, F., Wang, G., Ma, W., Ren, F., Li, M., Dong, Y. (2015) Decreased auditory GABA+ concentrations in presbycusis demonstrated by edited magnetic resonance spectroscopy. *Neuroimage*; Feb 1;106:311-6.

[65] Koch, M. (2005) The neurobiology of startle. *Prog Neurobiol*; 59: 107-128.

[66] Turner, J.G. (2005) Effects of aging on receptive fields in rat primary auditory cortex layer V neurons. *J Neurophysiol*; 94: 2738–2747.

[67] Juarez-Salinas, D.L., Engle, J.R., Navarro, X.O., Recanzone, G.H. (2010) Hierarchical and serial processing in the spatial auditory cortical pathway is degraded by natural aging. *J Neurosci*; 30: 14795–14804.

[68] Hughes, L.F., Turner, J.G., Parrish, J.L., Caspary, D.M. (2010) Processing of broadband stimuli across A1 layers in young and aged rats. *Hear Res*; 264: 79-85.

[69] Verkhratsky, A., Toescu, E.C. (1998) Calcium and neuronal ageing. *Trends Neurosci*; 21: 2–7.

[70] Idrizbegovic, E., Bogdanovic, N., Willott, J.F., Canlon, B. (2004) Age related increases in calcium-binding protein immunoreactivity in the cochlear nucleus of hearing impaired C57BL/6J mice. *Neurobiol Aging*; 25: 1085-1093.

[71] Ouda, L., Burianova, J., Syka, J. (2012) Age-related changes in calbindin and calretinin immunoreactivity in the central auditory system of the rat. *Exp Gerontol*; 47: 497–506.

[72] Engle, J.R., Gray, D.T., Turner, H., Udell, J.B., Recanzone, G.H. (2014) Age related neurochemical changes in the rhesus macaque inferior colliculus. *Front Aging Neurosci*; 6: 73.

[73] Gray, D.T., Rudolph, M.L., Engle, J.R., Recanzone, G.H. (2013) Parvalbumin increases in the medial and lateral geniculate nuclei of aged rhesus macaques. *Front Aging Neurosci*; 5: 69.

[74] Husain, F.T., Medina, R.E., Davis, C.W., Szymko-Bennett, Y., Simonyan, K., Pajor, N.M. (2011) Neuroanatomical changes due to hearing loss and chronic tinnitus: a combined VBM and DTI study. *Brain Res*; 1369: 74-88.

[75] Boyen, K., Langers, D.R.M., de Kleine, E., Van Dijk, P. (2013) Gray matter in the brain: differences associated with tinnitus and hearing loss. *Hear Res*; 295: 67-78.

[76] Eckert, M.A., Cute, S., Vaden, K., Kuchinsky, S., Dunho, J. (2012) Auditory cortex signs of age-related hearing loss. *J Assoc Res Otolaryngol*; 13: 703-713.

[77] Chang, Y., Lee, S., Lee, Y., Hwang, M., Bae, S., Kim, M. (2004) Auditory neural pathway evaluation on sensorineural hearing loss using diffusion tensor imaging. *Neuroreport*; 15: 1669-1703.

[78] Ouda, L., Profant, P., Syka, J. (2014) *Age-related changes in the central auditory system*. Springer-Verlag 2014.

[79] Willott, J.F., Aitkin, L.M., McFadden, S.L. (1993) Plasticity of auditory cortex associated with sensorineural hearing loss in adult C57BL/6J mice. *J Comp Neurol*; 329: 402-411.

[80] Robertson, D., Irvine, D.R.F. (1989) Plasticity of frequency organization in auditory cortex of guinea pigs with partial unilateral deafness. *J Comp Neurol*; 282: 456-471.

[81] Tremblay, K.L., Burkhard, R.F. (2012) *Hearing Across the Lifespan - Assessment and Disorders*. San Diego, CA: Plural Publishing, Inc 2012.

[82] Lin, F.R., Metter, E.J., O'Brien, R.J. (2011) Hearing loss and incident dementia. *Arch Neurol*; 68: 214-20.

[83] Lin; F.R. (2011) Hearing loss and cognition among older adults in the United States. *J Gerontol A Biol Sci Med Sci*; 66: 1131-6.

[84] Lin, F.R., Yaffe, K., Xia, J. (2013) Hearing loss and cognitive decline in older adults. Health ABC Study Group. *JAMA Intern Med*; 173: 293-9.

[85] Fried, L.P. (2001) Frailty in older adults: evidence for a phenotype. *J Gerontol A Biol Sci Med Sci*; 56: M146–M156.

[86] Genther, D.J., Betz, J., Pratt, S. (2000) Association of hearing impairment and mortality in older adults. *J Gerontol A Biol Sci Med Sci*; 55: M10-16.

[87] Stach, B.A. (2010) *Clinical Audiology: An Introduction*, II Ed. Delmar, Cengage Learning; Canada, 2010.

[88] Prosser, S., Martini, A. (2013) *Argomenti di Audiologia*. Omega Edizioni, Torino, 2013.

[89] Humes, L.E. (2012) Central presbycusis: a review and evaluation of the evidence. *J Am Acad Audio*; 23: 635-666.

[90] Doherty, K.A. (2015) The benefit of amplification on auditory working memory function in middle-aged and young-older hearing impaired adults. *Front Psychol* 2015.

[91] Di Nardo, W., Anzivino, R., Giannantonio, S. (2014) The effects of cochlear implantation on quality of life in the elderly. *Eur Arch Otorhinolaryngol*; 271: 65-73.

[92] Lin, F.R., Albert, M. (2014) Hearing loss and dementia – who is listening? *Aging Ment Health*; 18: 671-673.

[93] Vaisbuch, Y. (2018) Age-Related Hearing Loss: Innovations in Hearing Augmentation. *Otolaryngol Clin North Am* 2018.

Chapter 7

TRAUMATIC SENSORINEURAL HEARING LOSS

Michele Cassano, MD, Valeria Tarantini, MD,
Eleonora M. C. Trecca, MD, Antonio Moffa, MD
and Gianluigi Grilli, MD

Department of Otorhinolaryngology, University of Foggia,
Foggia, Italy

ABSTRACT

Sensorineural hearing loss (SNHL) is a common consequence after head trauma. Head injury may cause temporal bone fracture that can result in damage to the otic capsule, petrous pyramid, and/or other middle and/or inner ear structures. The pathophysiology of hearing loss following temporal bone fractures has been largely attributed to the mechanical forces that grossly disrupt the fragile *structures of the middle and inner ear. Another proposed mechanism is endolymphatic hydrop resulting from obstruction of the endolymphatic duct by the temporal bone fracture.

However, remains a subset of patients who had traumatic brain injury with hearing loss without temporal bone fractures. There are different mechanisms that can cause such SNHL: disruption of the membranous labyrinth, avulsion or trauma to the cochlear nerve, interruption of the cochlear blood supply, hemorrhage into cochlea, and perilymphatic fistulae.

Prompt evaluation of patient, early diagnosis and early treatment improves the prognosis. CT can detect pneumolabyrinth and signs of perilymphatic fistulae but fails to detect subtle lesions within the inner ear, such as labyrinthine haemorrhage or localized brain axonal damage along central auditory pathways, which are better detected by MRI.

Treatment can be based upon etiology. If no definitive or treatable etiology is found, treatment is done as in Ideopathic sudden sensorineural hearing loss. Oral corticosteroid therapy is among the few treatment modalities that have gained acceptance. Intratympanic injection of dexamethasone is shown to effectively improve hearing in

---

Corresponding Author's Email: michele.cassano@unifg.it

patients with severe or profound SNHL after treatment failure with standard therapy. Cochlear implants have been demonstrated to be effective in restoring hearing in cases of bilateral profound SNHL after traumatic injury, although traumatic and anatomical limitations may make some patients unsuitable for cochlear implantation.

Keywords: sensorineural hearing loss, traumatic sensorineural hearing loss, temporal bone fracture

INTRODUCTION

Head injuries are sustained by 5% of the population annually. Sensorineural hearing loss (SNHL) is very common following traumatic head injury with the incidence ranging from 7% to 50% [1]. Hearing impairment can be due to central or peripheral causes with middle ear or cochlea being the most common site of peripheral injury. The most pronounced injury is fracture of temporal bone but even labyrinthine concussion is frequent [2].

Since the injury occurs to the ear that contains both hearing and vestibular apparatus, generally SNHL is also associated with tinnitus, dizziness or vertigo [3].

In some patients deterioration of hearing and vestibular functions occurs immediately after head injury and it may be transient or permanent. In other patients the symptoms may not manifest until a few weeks post trauma. In some cases patients can show facial nerve palsy or perilymphatic fistula.

A prompt diagnosis is necessary to establish the best treatment and improve the prognosis.

PATHOPHYSIOLOGY

Traumatic brain injuries (TBIs) are leading cause of morbidity and mortality worldwide. TBI is defined as a disruption in normal brain function caused by external forces, either direct or transmitted including falls, motor vehicle collisions, sport-related injuries, abuse/assault, and a strike by a blunt object or pressure blasts [4, 5]. Regardless of its cause, brain injury can result in physical, cognitive and behavioral impairments, leading to temporary or permanent dysfunction [6]. Patients with TBI can appear with significant central and peripheral neurological deficits. Auditory dysfunction after TBI has been well described in literature [7]. In order to better understand the mechanism underlying the traumatic sensorineural hearing loss, TBI can be classified into:

1. TBI with temporal bone fracture
2. TBI without temporal bone fracture

TBI with Temporal Bone Fracture

The temporal bone forms a part of the lateral skull base and houses the hearing and balance organs; it also brings the facial nerve from the brainstem to the facial soft tissues. The bone itself is subdivided into four parts: the mastoid process, the tympanic portion, the squamous and the petrous apex [8]. Temporal bone fractures have traditionally been classified as either longitudinal, transverse, and/or mixed according to the long axis of the fracture line considering the long axis of the petrous bone (Table 1) [9]. Longitudinal fractures are generally the most common of the two types and result from laterally derived blow. The fracture lines run parallel and extend through the petrosquamous suture line and continue anteriorly to the otic capsule. This results in a haemotympanum and ossicular disruption causing a conductive hearing loss (CHL) in the patient. The facial nerve (FN) could be involved in approximately 15%–20% of these fractures. Transverse skull base fractures are commonly caused by direct trauma delivered to the back of the head. The fracture line begins at the jugular foramen and extends across the petrous pyramid to the area of the foramen spinosum and foramen lacerum. Transverse fractures can lead to SNHL and vertigo. 50% of patients experience facial nerve palsy [10]. Increasing data demonstrate that the majority of these fractures do not fit easily into one these categories but have mixed features.[2] Moreover, this fracture classification does not provide useful prognostic information with regards to neurotologic deficits [11]. In 1994, a simpler method of classifying fractures proposed by Kelly and Tami [12], is to separate fractures into otic capsule disrupting or otic capsule sparing (Table 1). Their classification has proven more predictive of clinical outcomes [13].

Fractures that disrupt the otic capsule will almost always result in a sensorineural hearing loss (SNHL) and are associated with a much higher incidence of facial nerve paralysis, nerve disruption, cerebrospinal fluid (CSF) leaks, and intracranial complications as compared with otic capsule sparing fractures. Blows to the occipital region usually cause otic capsule disrupting fractures. This kind of fractures runs from the foramen magnum across the petrous pyramid to the otic capsule. They will commonly pass through the jugular foramen, internal auditory canal, and foramen lacerum. These fractures rarely involve the ossicular chain or external auditory canal (EAC).

Otic capsule sparing fractures usually cause a conductive or mixed hearing loss and they are normally caused by a blow to the temporoparietal region and involve the squamous temporal bone and posterosuperior wall of the EAC. They pass through the mastoid air cells and middle ear, fracture the tegmen mastoideum and tegmen tympani, and then continue anterolaterally to fracture the tegmen in the region of the facial hiatus [11].

Table 1. Classification schemes and complications by TBI with temporal bone fracture

Classification scheme	Fracture class	Complications
Traditional classification (In relation to the petrous bone axis)	Longitudinal	Hemotympanum, ossicular disruption, CHL, FN palsy (15-20%)
	Transverse	SNHL, vertigo, FN palsy reported in 50% of patients
	Mixed	Mixed features
Alternative classification (Kelly and Tami, 1994)	Otic capsule disrupting	SNHL, higher incidence of facial nerve paralysis, nerve disruption, CSF fistula, intracranial complications
	Otic capsule sparing	Conductive or mixed hearing loss

There are other pathogenic mechanisms producing SNHL in temporal bone fractures: the cochlear nerve may be avulsed or directly injured by fractures that extend across or along the internal auditory canal [14, 15]; vascular vasospasm, thrombosis or hemorrhage into the inner ear may result in SNHL [14, 16]; the fracture line may extend across the vestibular acqueduct, resulting in occlusion and secondary endolymphatic hydrop [14, 17].

TBI without Temporal Bone Fracture

While hearing loss following temporal bone fracture is common, few data exist on auditory dysfunction in patients with TBI without temporal bone fracture. Among possible causes are considered trauma to peripheral pathway (labyrinthine concussion) or even direct damage to the central auditory system [18, 19]. Labyrinthine concussion may be described as perceptive deafness and vertigo resulting from a blow to the head without fracture of bony labyrinth capsule. A head injury can lead to either an isolated damage to the otolith organs (vestibular labyrinthine concussion) or injuries to the labyrinth of the inner ear without damage to the otic capsule or intralabyrinthine limiting membranes (cochlear labyrinthine concussion) [20, 21]. The underlying pathology was thought to be due to damage from the acceleration/deceleration forces on the inner ear. The nature of the injury is a tearing or rupture of the sensory cells from their supporting cell attachments on the basilar membrane induced by the excessive displacement of the basilar membrane. In less severe instances, separations of the Hensen cell tight cell junctions at the reticular lamina are created which also leads to an intermixing of cochlear fluids and the eventual loss of sensory cells [22]. It is also speculated that high-pressure waves caused by a blow to the head is directly transmitted to the cochlea by bone conduction [23-25].

Regarding damage to the central auditory system, there are two primary damage categories: injury to the brainstem such as the inferior colliculi [26, 27] and injury to the brain such as temporal bone contusion [28].

Perilymphatic Fistula with Pneumolabyrinth

A perilymphatic fistula (PLF) is an abnormal connection between the inner ear and middle ear or mastoid cavity secondary to a dehiscence in the otic capsule, oval or round window [29]. PLFs typically present with hearing loss and vertigo following head or ear trauma that can mimic many other otolaryngologic entities, such as labyrinthine concussion, traumatic Meniere's and cervical vertigo. Trauma is currently the most common cause of PLF, and can be associated with blunt or penetrating trauma, with or without associated temporal bone fracture [30].

Pneumolabyrinth describes a condition of acute inner ear dysfunction associated with perilymphatic fistula and the presence of air within the labyrinth. Symptoms associated with pneumolabyrinth include acute hearing loss, vertigo and pressure sensation in the affected ear. These symptoms presumably reflect changes in resonance of basilar membrane motion, impaired transduction, and pressure changes within the labyrinth [31]. The pathophysiology of symptoms produced by pneumolabyrinth is due to the presence of air on the ear membrane potential generation. This could be due to entry of air through an apical opening thereby increasing the threshold of the action potential (CAP) of the auditory nerve [31, 32]; perfusion of scala tympani with air causing immediate and drastic decrease of the cochlear microphonics (CM) and compound action potential with relatively little effect on endocochlear direct current potential (endocochlear potential) [31, 33]; with air perfusion of the scala vestibule, CM potentials were more drastically attenuated than with similar air applied to the scala tympani, suggesting a poorer prognosis with fistula of the oval window compared with that of the round window [31, 34].

DIAGNOSIS

Clinical Evaluation (Table 2)

The otologic evaluation should include inspection of the mastoid prominence for Battle sign, which is an ecchymosis over the mastoid prominence related to emissary vein disruption seen in lateral skull base fractures and, specifically, temporal bone fractures [35].

Table 2. Diagnostic protocol

Diagnostic levels	Examination	
Clinical assessment	History	Past medical history, onset of facial palsy, trauma mechanism, audiological and/or neurological symptoms
	Clinical examination	• Inspection of the mastoid prominence (Battle sign) • Inspection of the ear canal/tympanic membrane
	Cranial nerve examination	• Functional status of the FN
	Auditory testing	• Pure tone and speech audiometry • ABR
	Vestibular testing	• ENG/VNG • Romberg sign, gait ataxia and moving platform posturography
Radiological evaluation	CT	• Temporal bone fractures and ossicular injuries • Perilymphatic fistula
	MRI	• Detection of inner ear hemorrhage • Post-traumatic lesions of the brain parenchyma

The ear canal must be inspected and assessed for the most common findings associated with traumatic brain injuries including tympanic membrane perforation, bloody otorrhea and hemotympanum [9, 35-37]. In temporal bone fractures it is possible to find external ear canal stenosis, brain herniation and fracture of the roof of the EAC.

Traumatic perilymphatic fistula is suspected in cases of cerebrospinal fluid otorrhea. In otic capsule-sparing fractures, the CSF usually leaks through a fracture of the tegmen tympani or mastoideum into the epitympanum, antrum, and mastoid air cell tract. It can present as clear otorrhea if the tympanic membrane is disrupted or as rhinorrhea if the tympanic membrane is intact. In otic capsule-disrupting fractures, CSF will flow from the posterior fossa into the middle ear through the otic capsule.

It is essential that the functional status of the facial nerve have to be recorded as soon as possible during the initial general clinical examination because a nerve injury could lead to a prompt surgical treatment.

Early audiometric testing is recommended for evaluating the baseline post-injury hearing status [38].

TBI can be associated with conductive, sensorineural or mixed hearing loss that can be assessed with a pure tone and a speech audiometry. In otic capsule-violating fractures, severe to profound SNHL can be immediately apparent. Otic capsule- sparing fractures can manifest both sensorineural and conductive hearing loss. Conductive losses are caused by initial hemotympanum or effusion, and permanent deficits are caused by disruption of the ossicular chain, which occurs in approximately 20% of patients [39]. The most common injuries of the ossicular chain include subluxation of the incudo-stapedial (IS) joint (82%), dislocation of the incus (57%), and fracture of the stapes crura (30%) [40]. A subsequent full audiological examination should be performed three to six weeks post-injury, to allow sufficient time for the resolution of haemotympanum, because the presence of middle ear fluid (CSF or blood) results in a conductive loss.

In labyrinthine concussion, sensorineural hearing loss particularly affected high frequencies with recruitment [21]. When present, the most common pattern of hearing loss is similar to that of a noise-induced hearing loss, with a loss that is most apparent at 4 kHz [41, 42].

The use of auditory brain-stem response (ABR) has been reported as the standard to evaluate comatose patients [43]. Indeed the ABR grading system is a sensitive index of brainstem dysfunction and the presence or prolongation of V wave and I-V interwave latency even in one ear is of good prognostic value in the comatosed patient [43]. Also Testing DPOAE may help in detecting sub-clinical injuries to cochlea. Distortion product oto-acoustic emissions assessment at 3000 and 4000 Hz has a higher predictive value in assessing outer hair cell damage [44].

The presence and type of nystagmus should be noted. Electronystagmography/video nystagmography (ENG/VNG) can aid in categorization of vestibular injury. Romberg sign, gait ataxia and moving platform posturography are helpful to quantify balance deficits [45, 46]. The most common type of vertigo associated with head trauma is benign paroxysmal positional vertigo (BPPV). Most post-traumatic vertigo and nystagmus resolve spontaneously in the first 4 to 6 weeks after injury.

Radiological Evaluation (Table 2)

Radiological evaluation is important in patients with post-traumatic hearing loss. The adequacy and selection of the imaging technique with correct interpretation is crucial for diagnosis and prognosis, enabling the selection of the appropriate treatment [47].

Computed Tomography (CT) is the first choice technique and will allow the detection of alterations that cause conductive hearing loss. It allows radiologists to examine the complex anatomy of the temporal bone with sub-millimetric resolution and it is capable of revealing a broad spectrum of ossicular lesions that may not be apparent on clinical findings alone. Virtual otoscopy with 3-D reconstructions of CT images can provide a different view on ossicular chain anomalies in traumatic conditionsn [48]. In the case of sensorineural hearing loss, CT can detect pneumolabyrinth and signs of perilymphatic fistulae but fails to detect subtle lesions within the inner ear, such as labyrinthine haemorrhage or localized brain axonal damage along central auditory pathways [49] In these cases, Magnetic Resonance Imaging (MRI) with 3D-FLAIR acquisition is very important in the detection of inner ear haemorrhage and post-traumatic lesions of the brain parenchyma that may lead to auditory neuropathy.

The potential lesions that cause post-traumatic hearing loss are discussed below and the most suitable radiological examination will be suggested.

Temporal Bone Fractures and Ossicular Injuries

CT is the modality of choice for evaluating temporal bone fractures (Figure 1). The fractures investigated include fracture line's direction (longitudinal, trasverse or mixed), the affected portion (fractures that involve the petrous apex and those that spare the petrous apex)[50] and the otic capsule involvement (otic capsule violating or otic capsule sparing).

One of the most complex spaces of the temporal bone is the middle ear cavity. Within this space resides the ossicular chain constituted by three ossicles - the malleus, the incus, and the stapes - linked together by two articulations: the incudo- malleolar joint and the incudo-stapedial joint. The incus is the heavier ossicle, with a body and two processes of differing length. The body articulates with the head of the malleus, and the short process is directed posterolaterally while the thin long process runs inferiorly in parallel to the malleus handle. Laterally, the tympanic membrane and the malleus handle close the middle ear cavity. The head of the malleus is better observed on the upper axial slices at the incudo- malleolar joint. The lower slices show the lenticular process of the incus articulating with the head of the stapes. This is connected to the footplate via the neck, from which the anterior crus and posterior crus emerge [49].

Ossicular chain disruption is usually seen with longitudinal fractures or otic capsule–sparing fractures of the temporal bone. CT findings of ossicular injury may be difficult to evaluate due to hemotympanum. Ossicular dislocation is more common than ossicular fracture. There are five types of dislocations: incudo-stapedial joint separation, incudo-malleal joint separation, incus dislocation, incudo-malleal complex dislocation, and stapedio-vestibular dislocation [48].

Stapedio-vestibular dislocation is often associated with cochleovestibular symptoms including SNHL, tinnitus and acute vestibulopathy because the injury of the annular ligament or stapes footplate may cause a perilymphatic fistula. Transverse reconstruction of CT in the plane of the oval window and coronal reconstruction can show the medial displacement of the stapes footplate and the distal portion of both stapedial crura within the vestibule due to injury to the annular ligament.

Isolated ossicular fractures are less frequent than joint luxation and may involve any one part of the chain. Injuries to the stapes may be difficult to diagnose at the early stages due to hemotympanum and they are more frequently associated with severe high frequency hearing loss. Fracture of the footplate occurs secondary to a transverse fracture passing through the oval window, and may cause a perilymphatic fistula with pneumolabyrinth [49].

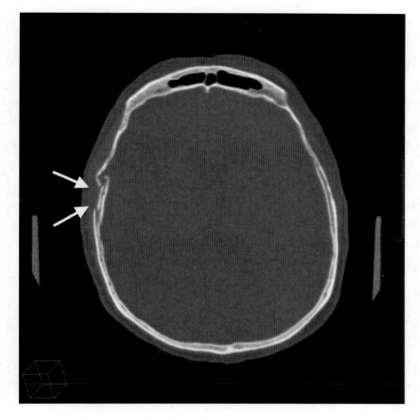

Figure 1.CT scan showing a right temporal bone fracture.

Labyrinthine Concussion

This injury of the membranous labyrinth without bone fracture is difficult to evaluate with CT [47]. MRI can demonstrate hemolabyrinth; in the T1-weighted sequences. It presents as an intrinsic hyperintensity due to its methaemoglobin content [49-53], although the 3D-FLAIR sequence is more useful because of its greater sensitivity to detect subtle changes in the signal of the lymphatic fluid (blood alters the composition of the perilymph) [54]. Non-enhanced FLAIR acquisition may reveal a hypersignal inside the cochlea, vestibule or both [25].

Perilymphatic Fistula

A perilymphatic fistula is a direct connection between the middle ear and inner ear cavities. There are two zones of weakness between these two cavities: the oval window and the round window. The oval window is affected either by a footplate fracture or by a lesion to the annular ligament, which may be isolated or associated with stapedio-vestibular disarticulations or stapes dislocation (external or internal). When the round window is affected, the fracture line can be seen around the edges of the window. The radiologist must examine CT scan thoroughly to identify the fracture line in the axial and coronal planes [49]. A pneumolabyrinth or pneumocochlea can be seen in the absence of temporal bone fracture [55]. CT can help identify the possible fracture trace and the pneumolabyrinth. Other possible specific signs are the intravestibular displacement of the plate and the presence of opacity at the site of the oval window [56]. When the exact site of bony defect is not identified, CT cisternography with intrathecal contrast can be used. Intrathecal fluorescein is a highly sensitive and specific test used typically when the other methods have failed to locate the fistula. There are occasional reports of neurotoxicity, seizures, and paraparesis, but these complications are infrequent and occur at higher doses of fluorescein than is recommended [11]. MRI can detect perilymph in the middle ear, although it is difficult to differentiate it from the hemotympanum.

Endolymphatic Hydrops

It is a post-traumatic dilatation of the endolymphatic space. In a normal patient, the endolymphatic duct is observed in MRI as a hypointense laminar structure due to its lack of contrast uptake, while the perilymphatic space show contrast uptake and is hyperintense. The saccule and the utricle are individualized and have a rounded shape. To look for a post-traumatic endolymphatic hydrops, it is necessary to perform the FLAIR sequence 4 hours after contrast media injection, to identify a dilatation of the endolymphatic duct that completely obliterates the vestibular ramp and a dilatation of the saccule and the utricle that completely fills the vestibule [47].

Injury to the Central Auditory Pathways

The central auditory pathway should be assessed along its whole length: cochlea, cochlear nerve, cochlear nucleus, inferior colliculus, medial geniculate body and auditory cortex.

It is important to distinguish injuries that occur along the central auditory pathways before the decussation into the superior olivary nucleus that may lead to asymmetrical SNHL, from those potentially responsible for associated auditory neuropathy [57]. The lesions that may lead to SNHL may be secondary to axonal injury, contusion or hemorrhage. Cochlear nerves could be injured by a superficial leptomeningeal hemosiderosis that may be seen after head trauma [58]. The diagnosis of hemosiderosis often relies on MRI with susceptibility-weighted imaging. Theoretically, isolated injury of the thalamus, auditory radiations, or auditory cortex could alter auditory function.

Isolation of auditory radiations requires advanced diffusion techniques, such as MR tractography, while the auditory cortex can be visualized with functional MRI [59, 60]. Post-traumatic cerebral contusion located along the Heschl's gyrii may be responsible for SNHL. New MR techniques such as susceptibility-weighted imaging or track-weighted imaging will likely prove useful in the assessment of focal brain lesions after trauma, including mild traumatic brain injury.

Labyrinthitis Ossificans

When a temporal bone fracture involves the inner ear structures (usually an otic capsule–violating fracture), labyrinthitis ossificans can result, in which the fluid-filled lumen of the otic capsule is replaced by bone (or fibrous tissue at the early stages) [61, 62]. Clinically, this is associated with profound sensorineural hearing loss and loss of vestibular function. On high-spatial-resolution CT images, osseous attenuation is noted within the inner ear. The corresponding MR images show loss of fluid signal intensity within the membranous labyrinth and enhancement on gadolinium- enhanced images. Heavily T2-weighted high-spatial-resolution sequences are most sensitive for detection at its earliest (fibrous) stage. MR findings precede CT changes by many months, as the earlier fibrous stage prior to ossification may not be detectable on CT images but may be seen on MR images as loss of fluid signal intensity in the membranous labyrinth [63].

TREATMENT

The prognosis for patients with post-traumatic brain injury SNHL is very poor. Cochlear implants (Table 3) have been demonstrated to be effective to restore hearing in cases of bilateral profound SNHL after traumatic injury, given that the functions of the cochlear nerve and brain are intact [64], although traumatic and anatomical limitations may make some patients unsuitable for cochlear implantation.

There are several factors to be considered before performing cochlear implantation in patients with profound hearing loss caused by bilateral temporal bone fractures. The decision to proceed with cochlear implantation after trauma is very difficult and the proper timing of the operation is still controversial.

Temporal bone fracture may result in destruction and degeneration of hair cells, supporting cells, and ganglion cells [65]. It is intuitive that implantation shortly after trauma would provide less time for spiral ganglion cell loss and would increase the chance of successful rehabilitation. On the other hand, surgical intervention that is too early can preclude the opportunity for natural restoration of hearing. Regular audiometric examination must be performed to confirm that the hearing level has been fixed.

In case of labyrinthine concussion, hemorrhage in the inner ear causes a hyperplastic inflammatory response leading to degeneration of neural elements, eventual fibrosis and new bone formation [66]. Labyrinthitis ossificans as a result of TB fractures and secondary infection may also inhibit successful insertion of the electrode array. The most frequent site of ossification appears to be the basal turn of the scala tympani [67, 68]. It is likely that the sooner cochlear implantation is performed after injury, the less time there is for cochlear osteoneogenesis and, therefore, the greater the likelihood for successful electrode insertion. When there is a significant time delay between the initial CT scan and the time of cochlear implantation, repeat imaging is beneficial to rule out labyrinthitis ossificans and other structural abnormalities that may inhibit successful placement of electrodes. Preoperative CT and high-resolution T2 MRI are useful methods to determine the patency of the cochlea [69, 70]. The possibility of retrocochlear lesions (auditory nerve, brain) should be considered. If a patient has bilateral fractures through the internal auditory canal, brain stem implantation (Table 3) may be an option for aural rehabilitation instead of cochlear implantation [71]. Results of cochlear implantation in patients with auditory cortex injuries are equivocal. Cognitive, behavioral and communicative deficits, including aphasia, should all be evaluated to determine the aural rehabilitation method. Promontory stimulation testing can be beneficial to confirm the presence of functioning eighth nerve. Although unilateral cochlear implantation generally provides good speech understanding in quiet conditions, unilateral cochlear implantation patients frequently report difficulties in understanding speech and localizing sound in noisy environments. Bilateral cochlear implantation has several advantages over unilateral implantation including improvement in speech perception in noisy environments and improved sound localization by head shadow, binaural squelch and binaural summation effects. In patients deafened by bilateral temporal bone fractures, bilateral cochlear implantation may be a better method for aural rehabilitation than unilateral cochlear implantation [69, 72].

There is no standard treatment protocol for management of sensorineural hearing loss in the immediate post trauma time [73-76]. Treatment options for SNHL depend on the severity of hearing loss and presence of associated complications.

In case of labyrinthine concussion or otic capsule sparing temporal bone fractures with mild symptoms associated, conservative treatment with high-dose corticosteroids (Table 3) is suggested [9].

Most cases of CSF leak occur in the first week after trauma and close spontaneously with conservative medical management (strict bed rest, elevation of bed by 30°, and avoidance of straining) [63]. If the CSF leak fails to respond, exploratory surgery is suggested. Fat and perichondrium are commonly used for repair [77]. Also temporalis fascia and muscle are used for fistula repair [14]. Repair of the fistula, even if done relatively late, markedly reduces vestibular symptoms and improves low and middle frequency sensorineural hearing.

The indications for early surgical intervention (Table 3) in patients with TBI include facial paralysis, persisting cerebrospinal fluid leakage and vestibular symptomatology (with severe symptoms such as intractable nausea and vomiting), recurrent meningitis [9, 29]. Observation and high- dose steroids can manage incomplete facial paralysis, with surgical exploration considered only if an evident bone fragment is seen impinging the facial nerve canal. Early complete paralysis may predicate the need for urgent surgical exploration. The perigeniculate area is more susceptible to injury due to traction from the greater superficial petrosal nerve [79-82].

Table 3. Treatment

Treatment		Indications
Conservative treatment	High-dose corticosteroids	• Labyrinthine concussion • Otic capsule sparing temporal bone fractures • Mild symptoms associated • Incomplete FN paralysis
Early surgical intervention		• FN paralysis • Persisting cerebrospinal fluid leakage • Vestibular symptomatology (with severe symptoms such as intractable nausea and vomiting) • Recurrent meningitis
Aural rehabilitation	• Cochlear implants • Brainstem implantation	• Bilateral profound SNHL after traumatic injury • Possibility of retro-cochlear lesions (auditory nerve, brain)

REFERENCES

[1] Fitzgerald, D. C. (1996). Head trauma: hearing loss and dizziness. *J Trauma* 40(3): 488-496.

[2] Dahiya. R., Keller, J. D., et al. (1999). Temporal bone fractures: otic capsule sparing versus otic capsule violating clinical and radiographic considerations. *J Trauma;* 47: pp 1079-83.

[3] Folmer, R. L., Griest, S. E. (2003). Chronic tinnitus resulting from head or neck injuries. *Laryngoscope*; 113(5):821-7.

[4] Najem, D., Rennie, K., Ribecco-Lutkiewicz, M., Ly, D., Haukenfrers, J., Liu, Q., Nzau, M., Fraser, D., Bani, M. (2018). Traumatic Brain Injury: Classification, Models and Markers. *Biochem Cell Biol.* 25. doi: 10.1139/bcb-2016-0160.

[5] Taylor, C. A., Bell, J. M., Breiding, M. J., Xu, L. (2017). Traumatic brain injury–related emergency department visits, hospitalizations, and deaths—United States, 2007 and 2013. *MMWR Surveill Summ*; 66(9):1-16.

[6] Reis, C., Wang, Y., Akyol, O., Ho, W. M., Ii, R. A., Stier, G., Martin, R, and Zhang, J. H. (2015). What's new in traumatic brain injury: update on tracking, monitoring and treatment. *Int. J. Mol. Sci.* 16(6): 11903–11965.

[7] Segal, S., Eviatar, E., Berenholz, L., Kessler, A., Shlamkovitch, N. (2002). Dynamics of sensorineural hearing loss after head trauma. *Otol Neurotol*; 23: 312-5.

[8] Honeybrook, A., Patki, A., Chapurin, N., Woodard, C. (2017). Hearing and Mortality Outcomes following Temporal Bone Fractures. *Craniomaxillofac Trauma Reconstr*; 10:281–285.

[9] Cannon, C. R., Jahrsdoerfer, R. A. (1983). Temporal bone fractures: review of 90 cases. *Arch Otolaryngol*; 109:285–8.

[10] Kanavati, O., Salamat, A. A., Tan, T. Y., Hellier, W. (2015). Bilateral temporal bone fractures associated with bilateral profound sensorineural hearing loss. *Postgrad Med J*; 0:1–2.

[11] Ghorayeb, B. Y., Yeakley, J. W. (1992). Temporal bone fractures: longitudinal or oblique? The case for oblique temporal bone fractures. *Laryngoscope*; 102(2):129–134.

[12] Kelly, K. E., Tami, T. A. Temporal bone and skull base trauma. In: Jackler RK, Brackmann DE, eds. *Neurotology*. St Louis: Mosby, 1994;1127–47.

[13] Brodie, H. A., Thompson, T. C. (1997). Management of complications from 820 temporal bone fractures. *Am J Otol*; 18(2):188–197.

[14] Lyos, A. T., Marsh, M. A., Jenkins, H. A., et al. (1995). Progressive hearing loss after transverse temporal bone fracture. *Arch Otolaryngol Head Neck Surg*; 121:795Y9.

[15] Ward, P. H. (1969). The histopathology of auditory and vestibular disorders in head trauma. *Ann Otol Rhinol Laryngol.*; 78: 227-238.

[16] Schuknecht, H. F. (1969). Mechanism of inner ear injury from blow to the head. *Ann Otol Rhinol Laryngol.*; 78: 253-262.

[17] Rizvi, S. S., Gibbin, K. P. (1979). Effect of transverse temporal bone fracture on the fluid compartment of the inner ear. *Ann Otol Rhinol Laryngol.*; 88: 741-748.

[18] Chen, J. X., Lindeborg, M., Herman, S. D., Ishai, R., Knoll, R. M. et al. (2018). Systematic review of hearing loss after traumatic brain injury without associated temporal bone fracture. *Am J Otolaryngol.*; 39 (3): 338-344.

[19] Makishima, K., Snow, J. B. (1975). Pathogenesis of hearing loss in head injury: Studies in man and experimental animals. *Arch Otolaryngol*; 101:426–432.

[20] Brusis, T. (2011). Sensorineural hearing loss after dull head injury or concussion trauma. *Laryngorhinootologie*; 90 (2): 73-80.

[21] Chiaramonte, R., Bonfiglio, M., D'Amore, A., et al. (2013). Traumatic Labyrinthine Concussion in a Patient with Sensorineural Hearing Loss. *The Neuroradiology Journal* 26: 52-55.

[22] Patterson Jr., J. H., Hamernik, R. P. (1997). Blast overpressure induced structural and functional changes in the auditory system. *Toxicology;* 121:29-40.

[23] Schuknecht, H. F., Davison, R. C. (1956). Deafness and vertigo from head injury. *AMA Arch Otolaryngol*; 63:513–528.

[24] Choi, M. S., Shin, S. O., Yeon, J. Y., Choi, Y. S., Kim, J., Park, S. K. (2013). Clinical Characteristics of Labyrinthine Concussion. *Korean J Audiol*; 17:13. doi:10.7874/kja.2013.17.1.13.

[25] Ulug, T., Ulubil, S. A. (2006). Contralateral labyrinthine concussion in temporal bone fractures. *J Otolaryngol*; 35: 380-3.

[26] Hu, C. J., Chan, K. Y., Lin, T. J., Hsiao, S. H. (1997). Traumatic brainstem deafness with normal brainstem auditory evoked potentials. *Neurology*; 48:1448–51.

[27] Jani, N. N. (1991). Deafness after bilateral midbrain contusion: a correlation of magnetic resonance imaging with auditory brain stem evoked responses. *Neurosurgery*; 29:106–9.

[28] Fujimoto, C., Ito, K., Takano, S., Karino, S. (2007). Successful cochlear implantation in a patient with bilateral progressive sensorineural hearing loss after traumatic subarachnoid hemorrhage and brain contusion. *Ann Otol Rhinol Laryngol*; 116:897–901.

[29] Prisman E., Ramsden, J. D., et al. (2011). Traumatic Perilymphatic Fistula with Pneumolabyrinth: Diagnosis and Management. *Laryngoscope*, 121:856–859.

[30] Kim. S. H., Kazahaya, K., Handler, S. D. (2001). Traumatic perilymphatic fistulas in children: etiology, diagnosis and management. *International Journal of Pediatric Otorhinolaryngology*; 60.147–153.

[31] Lao W. W., Niparko, J. K. (2007). Assessment of Changes in Cochlear Function with Pneumolabyrinth After Middle Ear Trauma. *Otology & Neurotology* 28(8):1013-1017.

[32] Nishioka, I., Yanagihara, N. (1986). Role of air bubbles in the perilymph as a cause of sudden deafness. *Am J Otol*; 7:430-8.

[33] Kobayashi, T., Itoh, Z., Sakurada, T., et al. (1990). Effect of perilymphatic air perfusion on cochlear potentials. *Acta Otolaryngol* (Stockholm); 110:209-16.

[34] Kobayashi, T., Sakurada, T., Ohyama, K., et al. (1993). Inner ear injury caused by air intrusion to the scala vestibule of the cochlear. *Acta Otolaryngol* (Stockholm); 113:725-30.

[35] Diaz R. C., Cervenka, B., Brodie, H. A. (2016). Treatment of Temporal Bone Fractures. *J Neurol Surg B*; 77:419–429.

[36] Ferrara, S., Salvago, P., Mucia, M., Ferrara, P., Sireci, F., Martines, F. (2014). Follow-up after pediatric myringoplasty: Outcome at 5 years. *Otorinolaringologia*; 64: 141-146.

[37] Martines, F., Bentivegna, D., Maira, E., Marasà, S., Ferrara, S. (2012). Cavernous haemangioma of the external auditory canal: Clinical case and review of the literature. *Acta Otorhinolaryngol Ital;* 32(1): 54-57.

[38] Song, S. W., Jun, B. C., Kim, H. (2017). Clinical features and radiological evaluation of otic capsule sparing temporal bone fractures. *The Journal of Laryngology & Otology*, 131, 209–214.

[39] Yoganandan, N., Pintar, F. A., Sances, A. Jr, et al. (1995). Biomechanics of skull fracture. *J Neurotrauma*; 12(4):659–668.

[40] Hough, J. V. D., Stuart, W. D. (1968). Middle ear injuries in skull trauma. *Laryngoscope*; 78(6):899–937.

[41] Flint, P., Haughey, B., et al. Etiology of Sensorineural Hearing Loss. In: *Cummings otolaryngology head & neck surgery*. Elsevier; 2004. 5th edition, Chap.149.

[42] Bamiou, D. E., Davies, R. A., Mckee, M., et al. (1999). The effect of severity of unilateral vestibular dysfunction on symptoms, disabilities and handicap in vertiginous patients. *Clin Otolaryngol Allied Sci.*; 24 (1): 31-38.

[43] Abd al-Hady, M. R., Shehata, O., el-Mously, M., Sallam, F. S. (1990). Audiological findings following head trauma. *J Laryngol Otol.*; 104(12):927-36.

[44] Emerson, L. P., Mathew, J., Balraj, A., Job, A., Singh, P. R. (2011). Peripheral Auditory Assessment in Minor Head Injury: A Prospective Study in Tertiary Hospital. *Indian J Otolaryngol Head Neck Surg*; 63(1):45–49.

[45] Thomas, E., Martines, F., Bianco, A., Messina, G., Giustino, V., Zangla, D., Iovane, A., Palma, A. (2018). Decreased postural control in people with moderate hearing loss. *Medicine* (Baltimore); 97(14): e0244.

[46] Martines, F., Messina, G., Patti, A., Battaglia, G., Bellafiore, M., Messina, A., Rizzo, S., Salvago, P., Sireci, F., Traina, M., Iovane, A. (2015). Effects of tinnitus on postural control and stabilization: A pilot study. *Acta Medica Mediterranea*; 31: 907-912.

[47] Mazón M., Pont, E., Albertz, N., Carreres-Polo, J., Más-Estellés, F. (2018). Imaging of post-traumatic hearing loss. *Radiología*; 60,(2),119-127.

[48] Fatterpekar, G. M., Doshi, A. H., Dugar, M. et al. (2006). Role of 3D CT in the evaluation of the temporal bone. *Radiographics* 26(Suppl 1): S117–S132.

[49] Maillot, O., Attyé, A., Boyer, E., Heck, O., Kastler, A., Grand, S., et al. (2016). Post traumatic deafness: a pictorial review of CT and MRI findings. *Insights Imaging*; 7:341-50.

[50] Ishman, S. L., Friedland, D. R. (2004). Temporal bone fractures: traditional classification and clinical relevance. *Laryngoscope*; 114(10): 1734–1741.

[51] Meriot, P., Veillon, F., Garcia, J.F., et al. (1997). CT appearances of ossicular injuries. *RadioGraphics*; 17(6):1445–1454.

[52] Park, G. Y., Choi, J. E., Cho, Y-S. (2014). Traumatic ossicular disruption with isolated fracture of the stapes suprastructure: comparison with incudostapedial joint dislocation. *Acta Otolaryngol* 134:1225–1230.

[53] Petrovic, B. D., Futterer, S. F., Hijaz, T., Russell, E. J., Karagianis, A. G. (2010). Frequency and diagnostic utility of intralabyrinthine FLAIR hyperintensity in the evaluation of internal auditory canal and inner ear pathology. *Acad Radiol.*; 17:992-1000.

[54] Sugiura, M., Naganawa, S., Sato, E., Nakashima, T. (2006). Visualization of a high protein concentration in the cochlea of a patient with a large endolymphatic duct and sac, using three-dimensional fluid- attenuated inversion recovery magnetic resonance imaging. *J Laryngol Otol* 120:1084–1086.

[55] Lee, E. J., Yang, Y. S., Yoon, Y. J. (2012). Case of bilateral pneumolabyrinth presenting as sudden, bilateral deafness, without temporal bone fracture, after a fall. *J Laryngol Otol* 126:717–720.

[56] Herman, P., Guichard, J. P., Van den Abbeele, T., Tan, C. T., Bensimon, J. L., Marianowski, R., et al. (1996). Traumatic luxation of the stapes evidenced by high-resolution CT. *AJNR Am J Neuroradiol.*;17:1242-4.

[57] Hattiangadi, N., Pillion, J. P., Slomine, B. et al. (2005). Characteristics of auditory agnosia in a child with severe traumatic brain injury: a case report. *Brain Lang* 92:12–25.

[58] Sydlowski, S. A., Levy, M., Hanks, W. D. et al. (2013). Auditory profile in superficial siderosis of the central nervous system: a prospective study. *Otol Neurotol* 34:611–619.

[59] Javad, F., Warren, J. D., Micallef, C. et al. (2014). Auditory tracts identi- fied with combined fMRI and diffusion tractography. *Neuroimage* 84:562–574.

[60] Profant, O., Škoch, A., Balogová, Z. et al. (2014). Diffusion tensor imaging and MR morphometry of the central auditory pathway and auditory cortex in aging. *Neuroscience* 260:87–97.

[61] Juliano, A. F., Ginat, D. T., Moonis, G. (2013). Imaging review of the temporal bone: part I. anatomy and inflammatory and neoplastic processes. *Radiology*; 269(1):17–33.

[62] Aralaşmak, A., Dinçer, E., Arslan, G., Cevikol, C., Karaali, K. (2009). Posttraumatic labyrinthitis ossificans with perilymphatic fistulization. *Diagn Interv Radiol*; 15(4):239–241.

[63] Juliano, A. F., Ginat, D. T., Moonis, G. (2015). Imaging review of the temporal bone: part II. Traumatic, Postoperative, and Noninflammatory Nonneoplastic Conditions. *Radiology* 276(3):655-72.

[64] Shin, J. H., Park, S., Baek, S. H., et al. (2008). Cochlear implantation after bilateral transverse temporal bone fractures. *Clin Exp Otorhinolaryngol*; 1:171-3.

[65] Nadol Jr, J. B., Young, Y. S., Glynn, R. J. (1989). Survival of spiral ganglion cells in profound sensorineural hearing loss: implications for cochlear implantation. *Ann Otol Rhinol Laryngol*; 98:411-6.

[66] Morgan, W. E., Coker, N. J., Jenkins, H. A. (1994). Histopathology of temporal bone fracture. Implications for cochlear implantation. *Laryngoscope* 104(4):426-32.

[67] Camilleri, A. E., Toner, J. G., Howarth, K. L., Hampton, S., Ramsden, R. T. (1999). Cochlear implantation following temporal bone fracture. *J Laryngol Otol*; 113:454–457.

[68] Vermeire, K., Brokx, J. P. L., Dhooge, I., Van de Heyning, P. H. (2012). Cochlear implantation in posttraumatic bilateral temporal bone fracture. *ORL*; 74: 52-56.

[69] Chung, J. H., Shin M. C., Min H. J., Park C. W., Lee S. H. (2011). Bilateral cochlear implantation in a patient with bilateral temporal bone fractures. *American Journal of Otolaryngology–Head and Neck Medicine and Surgery* 32:256–258.

[70] Seidman, D. A., Chute, P. M., Parisier, S. (1994). Temporal bone imaging for cochlear implantation. *Laryngoscope*; 104:562-5.

[71] Simons, J. P., Whitaker, M. E., Hirsch, B. E. (2005). Cochlear implantation in a patient with bilateral temporal bone fractures. *Otolaryngol Head Neck Surg*; 132:809-11.

[72] Brown, K. D., Balkany, T. J. (2007). Benefits of bilateral cochlear implantation: a review. *Curr Opin Otolaryngol Head Neck Surg*; 15:315-8.

[73] Rizzo, S., Bentivegna, D., Thomas, E., La Mattina, E., Mucia, M., Salvago, P., Sireci, F., Martines, F. (2016). Sudden sensorineural hearing loss, an invisible male: State of art. *Hearing loss: etiology, management and societal implications*, 75-86.

[74] Salvago, P., Rizzo, S., Bianco, A., Martines, F. (2017). Sudden sensorineural hearing loss: is there a relationship between routine haematological parameters and audiogram shapes? *International Journal of Audiology*; 56(3): 148-153.

[75] Martines, F., Salvago, P., Ferrara, S., Mucia, M., Gambino, A., Sireci, F. (2014). Parietal subdural empyema as complication of acute odontogenic sinusitis: A case report. *Journal of Medical Case Reports*, 8 (1).

[76] Dispenza, F., De Stefano, A., Costantino, C., Marchese, D., Riggio, F. (2013). Sudden Sensorineural Hearing Loss: results of intratympanic steroids as salvage treatment. *Am J Otolaryngol*; 34:296-300.

[77] Yanagihara, N., Nishioka, I. (1987). Pneumolabyrinth in perilymphatic fistula: report of three cases. *Am J Otol*; 8:313-8.

[78] Dispenza, F., Mazzucco, W., Bianchini, S., Mazzola, S., Bennici, E. (2015). Management of labyrinthine fistula in chronic otitis with cholesteatoma: case series. *EuroMediterranean Biomedical Journal* 10(21): 255-261.

[79] Coker, N. J. (1991). Management of traumatic injuries to the facial nerve. *Otolaryngol Clin North Am*; 24(1):215–227.

[80] Lambert, P. R., Brackmann, D. E. (1984). Facial paralysis in longitudinal temporal bone fractures: a review of 26 cases. *Laryngoscope*; 94(8):1022–1026.

[81] Saraiya, P. V., Aygun, N. (2009). Temporal bone fractures. *Emerg Radiol*; 16(4):255–265.

[82] Dispenza, F., Battaglia, A. M., Salvago, P., Martines, F. (2018). Determinants of failure in the reconstruction of the tympanic membrane: a case-control study. *Iranian Journal of Otorhinolarhingology*, 30(6): 341-346.

Chapter 8

ADVANCED OTOSCLEROSIS

Nicola Quaranta[1], MD, Vito Pontillo[1], MD and Francesco Dispenza[2], MD, PhD

[1]Otolayngology Unit, Department of Basic Medical Science,
Neuroscience and Sensory Organs, University of Bari Aldo Moro, Bari, Italy
[2]Istituto Euromediterraneo di Scienza e Tecnologia – IEMEST, Palermo, Italy

ABSTRACT

Otosclerosis is characterized by a continuous and aberrant process of osteolysis and osteogenesis of the endochondral bone of the otic capsule, most commonly involving the fissula ante fenestram (fenestral otosclerosis) and resulting in a conductive hearing loss. As it undergoes a maturation process, the sclerotic bone may invade deeper into the labyrinth, resulting in retrofenestral otosclerosis and gradually leading to severe mixed hearing loss and then to profound sensorineural hearing loss. This cochlear involvement of otosclerosis audiologically reflects as advanced otosclerosis (AO) and can be defined by audiometric and radiological criteria.

Treatment for AO has evolved over the past 20 years with the improvement in hearing aid devices and the availability of cochlear impants (CI) as an alternative surgical option.

Most authors suggest treating AO with stapes surgery and postoperative amplification by hearing aids.

Cochlear implants have become available in the last 20 years and, since their introduction, many otosclerotic patients have undergone implantation with good hearing and communicative outcomes. Cochlear Implantation in otosclerosis poses some surgical problems, mainly related to cochlear obliteration and facial nerve stimulation. For cases of unsuccessful stapedotomy, the results obtained by a salvage CI are as good as those of CI when no prior stapedectomy was performed.

Keywords: advanced otosclerosis, stapes surgery, stapedectomy, cochlear implantation, CI

INTRODUCTION

Otosclerosis is a rather hereditary disease that usually develops in the post-lingual period, specifically between the second and the fifth decade of life [1]. It is characterized by a continuous and aberrant process of osteolysis and osteogenesis of the endochondral bone of the otic capsule [2, 3]. The most common site of involvement is the fissula ante fenestram (fenestral otosclerosis), which results in conductive hearing loss due to stapes footplate fixation [4, 5]. Hearing loss is initially observed at low frequencies and later also at higher frequencies [6]. As it undergoes a maturation process, the sclerotic bone can increase in size and depth and may invade deeper into the labyrinth, resulting in retrofenestral otosclerosis; this process gradually leads to severe mixed hearing loss and then to profound sensorineural hearing loss (SNHL) [5]. This cochlear involvement of the disease affects about 10% [7] of patients with otosclerosis and, from an audiological point of view, is defined as advanced otosclerosis (AO). Shea et al. [8] estimated that 1.6% of patients with otosclerosis may then evolve to profound SNHL.

DEFINITION

There is no universally accepted definition for advanced otosclerosis. "Far-Advanced Otosclerosis" (FAO) was first described by House and Sheehy [9] in 1961 and was defined by an air conduction (AC) threshold worse than 85 dB and a bone conduction (BC) threshold beyond the measurement limits of the standard clinical audiometers available at that time. In the modern era, the criteria for diagnosing FAO have considerably changed since the availability of more powerful audiometers with higher detection limits. Merkus et al. [10] have therefore proposed that speech discrimination scores (SDS) are more likely to be used than pure-tone thresholds and the term "far advanced otosclerosis" should be no longer applicable. Some Authors prefer to use the term "advanced otosclerosis" instead of far advanced otosclerosis, and define it as a SNHL with decreased speech recognition abilities or with an AC threshold higher than 85 dB and even a poor/unmeasurable BC threshold [5].

Iurato et al. [11] in 1992 described very far-advanced otosclerosis (VFAO) in patients with undetectable air and bone conduction levels with standard clinical audiometers, resulting in a "blank audiogram." Calmels and colleagues [12] recently described VFAO as a condition characterized by dissyllabic word discrimination lower than 30% at 70 dB SPL in the best aided condition and a blank audiogram.

PATHOGENESIS

The mechanisms leading to SNHL have been widely studied and many theories have been proposed:

- Siebenmann [13] suggested that *toxic substance released* by the otospongiotic foci into the inner ear fluids could impair the function of the cochlea. These hypothesis has been corroborated by the findings of electron microscopy, that showed the presence of lysosomes at the margins of the advancing otospongiotic foci [14, 15].
- Ruedi [16] described *venous shunts* between the otospongiotic foci and vessels of the cochlea. It is suspected that these shunts might produce venous congestion, interfering with the normal metabolism of the cochlea, resulting in hypoxia and degeneration of the spiral ligament, hence producing hearing loss.
- *Atrophy and hyalinization of the spiral ligament, and of the stria vascularis* have been found in patients with advanced otosclerosis, but the mechanism that produces them is uncertain [17].
- Linthicum et al. [18, 19] proposed the invasion of the cochlear walls by the otospongiotic foci, causing a narrowing of the lumen of the cochlea and a *distortion of the basilar membrane*, with subsequent inhibition of the traveling wave throughout the rest of the cochlea.
- More recently, some Authors proposed that retrofenestral foci may lead to hearing loss through *disturbance of the ionic homeostasis* of the cochlea by hindering ion recycling and reducing the endocochlear potential [20, 21].

In all probability, more than one of these factors is responsible for the hearing loss in each case. The atrophy and hyalinization, which can be determined by both lytic enzymes and venous shunts, may lead both to a distortion of the basilar membrane and to an alteration of the ionic homeostasis. Detritus caused by the aberrant osteoclastic/osteoblastic activity may also alter the normal composition of perilymphatic fluids by inflammatory reactions mediated by immune complexes or by the sum of several of these factors [17, 18].

RADIOLOGIC DIAGNOSIS AND CLASSIFICATION

If it is still debated the utility of imaging in the diagnosis of otosclerosis, there is no controversy in stating that it is of essential importance when the disease progresses into AO and cochlear implantation is taken into consideration.

High-resolution CT (*HRCT*) scanning is the imaging modality of choice for assessing cochlear involvement of otosclerosis, characteristically manifesting with irregularities of the outline of the otic capsule or with the more specific presence of a lucent area in the normally homogeneously dense otic capsule. This lucent area might be presenting as a focal lucency or with the characteristic double ring/halo sign (pericochlear lucency) [22, 23, 24], emerging when the pericochlear confluent foci surround the cochlear lumen [25, 26]. Besides, HRCT can be used to assess the location and extension of hypodense lesions, helping to quantify the degree of otospongiosis and the severity of disease, which has been demonstrated to be correlated to the degree of sensorineural hearing loss [27]. Finally, HRCT might be used for preoperative evaluation of the patency of the cochlear lumen, which can be obstructed in cases of AO, and of the risk of facial nerve stimulation (FNS). These findings can help the surgeon respectively to be prepared for extra-drilling and to choose a perimodiolar electrode rather than straight electrodes in selected patients [26, 28, 29].

In case of intralabyrinthine involvement, also *MRI* can be performed to explore the cochlear status and evaluate the patency of the cochlear lumen [30], particularly on fast-spin T2-weighted scans [31], demonstrated to be even superior to CT scans in the assessment of luminal patency [32]. In cochlear otosclerosis a ring with an isointense signal is usually detected in the peri-cochlear and peri-labyrinthine area on T1-weighted images, with mild to moderate enhancement after gadolinium, related to hypervascularity and inflammatory response in cases of large otospongiotic peri-cochlear foci [31]. T2-weighted images might detect hyperintense signal as well [30, 33]. Lombardo et al. [34] demonstrated three-dimensional fluid attenuation inversion recovery sequence using 3T MRI to be useful for the demonstration of an alteration in the composition of the endocochlear fluid due to inflammation and blood-labyrinth barrier breakdown, which was demonstrated in 81,8% of their patients.

Single-photon emission computed tomography (*SPECT*) using 99-technetium-diphosphonates was proposed by Berrettini et al. [33] as a diagnostic alternative in difficult cases and for medical treatment follow-up, with high sensitivity (95.2%) and specificity (96.7%) in identifying otospongiotic foci in the otic capsule.

Many types of *radiographic grading systems* were proposed in order to describe the location and stage of otosclerosis, often in relationship with audiological findings. Valvassori [22] was the first to propose a grading system for advanced otosclerosis based on disease progression. In more recent studies, Rotteveel and colleagues [26] (Table 1), Symons and Fanning [35] (Table 2) and Kabbara and colleagues [36] (Table 3) described other classification systems based on CT evaluation of the otic capsule involvement.

Table 1. Rotteveel et al. imaging-based grading system [26]

	Otosclerotic Lesions of the Otic Capsule
Type 1	Solely fenestral involvement
Type 2	Retrofenestral (with or without fenestral involvement)
a	Double ring effect
b	Narrowed basal turn
c	Double ring effect and narrowed basal turn
Type 3	Severe retrofenestral involvement (unrecognizable otic capsule), with or without fenestral involvement

Table 2. Symons and Fanning's imaging-based grading system [35]

	Plaques Location
Grade 1	Solely fenestral involvement (spongiotic/sclerotic)
Grade 2	Patchy localized cochlear disease (with or without fenestral involvement)
a	To basal cochlear turn
b	To middle/apical turn
c	Both
Grade 3	Diffuse confluent cochlear involvement (with or without fenestral involvement)

Table 3. Kabbara's imaging-based grading system [36]

	Otosclerotic Lesions
Stage 1	Limited footplate and pericochlear lesions without endosteum involvement
Stage 2	Significant pericochlear and endosteum involvement
Stage 3	Full obliteration of the round window and/or basal turn ossification associated with pericochlear lesions

Table 4. Diagnostic clues suggested by Sheehy (1978) for advanced otosclerosis [37]

(1) positive family history for otosclerosis
(2) progressive hearing loss beginning in early adult life
(3) paracusis during the early stage of the disease
(4) past use of a bone-conduction hearing aid
(5) previous audiograms showing an airbone gap

Although the diagnostic clues suggested by Sheehy [37] (Table 4) together with instrumental imaging may help, definitive diagnosis often requires exploratory surgery [38].

TREATMENT STRATEGIES

The management of patients with AO is a real challenge. Although various methods have been used in recent years, no standard guidelines have been established. The following therapeutic options are in common use [10, 39, 40]:

A. No intervention and hearing aids with follow-up;
B. Stapes surgery and hearing aids;
C. Cochlear implantation;
D. Direct acoustic cochlear stimulation implant.

In some cases, choosing between these options can be difficult for two main factors: first, with mixed hearing loss it is not easy to predict the success rate of stapedectomy; second, otospongiotic foci around the otic capsule can lead to surgical complications and difficulties during cochlear implantation.

Hearing Aids and Follow-Up

This option can be taken into consideration in case of patients with good audiological (SDS >50%) and radiologic (Rotteveel grade 1, 2A or 2B) findings but with an air-bone gap lower than 30 dB, in which a stapes surgery would be ineffective, considering the reduced conductive component [10].

Stapes Surgery and Hearing Aids

Patients with advanced otosclerosis and no benefit from a powerful hearing aid may be suitable candidates for stapes surgery.

This indication was first discussed by House in 1960 [41]. In 1964 Sheehy stated that "there is no maximum bone conduction threshold above which stapedectomy is contraindicated" [37].

Conducting a stapedectomy with subsequent placement of a hearing aid has been widely studied, with varying audiological results: 46–100% hearing improvement, 38-75% post-operative SDS and 17–75% improvement of SDS [8, 10-12, 37, 38] (Table 5). Several Authors have stated that there are no contraindications for performing stapedectomy in any case of AO and assert that stapes surgery should be considered as first line therapy in these patients, especially in countries with limited economic resources, since even though the results should be unsatisfactory, a contralateral stapedotomy [42] or a salvage CI [6] can still be performed. Abdurehim and colleagues in their meta-analysis [3] revealed that previously failed stapedotomy does not affect the outcomes in terms of SDS after salvage CI.

Complications in patients with advanced otosclerosis are statistically different from those in patients withot AO [43]. One of the most feared complications of stapedectomy is the deterioration of sensorineural hearing loss, which can be due to several causes (among them penetration of the prosthesis into the inner ear, perylimphatic fistula or granuloma) and might thus result in a functionally deaf ear. However, the surgeon should not be excessively worried about this possibility in case of advanced otosclerosis, because he is dealing with a severe to profound HL. Furthermore, the 'second chance' of CI is still possible.

Some of the *advantages* of stapedotomy are lower cost and difficulties, local anaesthesia, fewer risks and postoperative requirements (fitting of a hearing aid) and better natural sound and music perception. However, stapedectomy does not treat the sensorineural component of mixed hearing loss and does not stop the aberrant maturation process of the otic capsule. Moreover, the outcomes are less predictable, especially if compared with CI [38]. Several Authors have tried to demonstrate the utility of different prognostic factors: it has been stated that patients with severe retrofenestral involvement and speech recognition scores of less than 30% are associated with poorer results if compared with subjects with less retrofenestral involvement and speech recognition scores of more than 50% [5]. For this reason patients should be carefully selected and each case must be assessed individually.

Controversy still exists about the possibility to perform a second stapedectomy on the opposite ear [43]. Many Authors believe that there is no real justification for this if the first stapedectomy was successful [43]. Others believe that each patient should be offered the potential benefit of binaural amplification even for a hearing loss of this severity. In conclusion, each decision should be individualized to the single subject and the final decision should be left to the patient after fully considering all the risks and benefits. In case of contralateral stapes surgery is taken into consideration, the normal protocol of delaying of 1 year the second operation for fear of SN deterioration has no reason to exist in AO, because, as already mentioned, we are dealing with patients with sever to profound HL and no apparent cochlear reserve.

Cochlear Implantation

Cochlear implantation was once considered to be contraindicated in patients affected by otosclerosis, because it was generally agreed that the pathologic process led to an inadequate number of neural elements with subsequent reduction of the electric stimulation [44].

The literature has demonstrated that treating advanced otosclerosis with CIs yield satisfactory results. This can be explained by the fact that this pathologic condition mainly affects the lateral wall of the cochlea, resulting in a degeneration of the spiral ligament and stria vascularis, but leaving the fibres of the auditory nerve uninvolved in a first period [45]; even though spiral ganglion cells are involved by the process, they have been demonstrated to be present in a sufficient number (40-85% of normal) [46] for successful electrical stimulation [47], thus not affecting the performance of the implant [24], but implying the need for higher electrical charges [48].

Several publications have reported hearing improvement in 100% of patients submitted to CI [1, 10, 12, 26, 29, 32, 35, 38, 46, 49-51] (Table 5). Moreover, a significant improvement in speech perception (34-94%) was reported after CI in studies that compared pre- and post-operative speech discrimination (SD) scores [1, 12, 29, 38, 50], with an average SDS after implantation of 45-98% [10]. In a study conducted in 2005 [49] our group found similar results, with an average postoperative SD score of 60% (using two-syllable words test) and 83% (using sentences test).

With such a high rate of success (hearing improvement of 100% vs 46-100% of stapedectomy; post-operative SD scores of 45-98% vs 38-75% of stapedectomy; improvement in SD after surgery of 34-94% vs 17-75% of stapedectomy) [10], CI should be considered the treatment of choice for these patients. However, CI undoubtedly present negative aspects. Some disadvantages of cochlear implantation include high cost, challenging programming/rehabilitation and the high rate of difficulties and complications, thus requiring experienced surgeons. Furthermore, because of the progression of otosclerosis, also late postoperative failure of the CI must be taken into account [31]: in this case reprogramming with higher stimulus levels might be required, although this can increase the risk of facial nerve stimulation.

Table 5. Audiological results after stapes surgery and cochlear implantation

	Patients Hearing Improved	Average SDS after surgery	Improvement SDS after surgery
Stapes surgery	46-100%	38-75%	17-75%
CI	100%	45-98%	34-94%
CI: cochlear implantation; SDS: Speech Discrimination Score			

The *surgical technique* is the same than in standard non-otosclerosis patients, with conventional cortical mastoidectomy and posterior tympanotomy, but continuous and aberrant production of bone in the cochlea can determinate several *difficulties* during the procedure:

- The conventional *landmarks* for CI, such as the promontory and round window niche, may be altered due to bony remodelling in otosclerosis patients, thereby making the identification of scala tympani difficult.
- *Round window and basal turn ossification* often occur in FAO, with a reported incidence of 8-89% and 10-60% respectively [10]. Placing a CI electrode in an ossified cochlea is certainly a challenge, however, is not a contraindication and does not affect the audiological results [2, 46]. A number of techniques have been proposed in order to enable full electrode insertion in these patients: in case of fenestral ossification, extra-drilling may be required to detect the lumen of the basal turn [44]; alternatively the cochleostomy can be placed 1-2 mm cranially with scala vestibuli insertion of the electrode [29, 38, 53].
- *Partial insertion or misplacement of the electrode* has been reported in 19% of patients [26, 35, 38]. Partial insertion can be caused by the obliteration of the apical regions of the scala tympani [8]. The evolution of otospongiotic lesions can lead to the creation of osteolytic cavities surrounding the cochlea, which can be confused with the opening of the basal turn, resulting in an electrode misplacement in this false lumen [26, 28] It is also possible that an electrode normally inserted in the basal turn penetrates the cochlear endosteum and enters this false lumen [54].
- It has been demonstrated that 60% of preoperative CT scans does not reveal findings consistent with otosclerosis. Therefore, the surgeon must be prepared for extra-drilling despite lack of imaging findings [32].

In otosclerosis patients CI *complications* have been described more frequently than in non-otosclerosis ones:

- *Facial nerve stimulation (FNS)* has been reported between 25 and 75% [26, 29, 55] of otosclerosis patients versus the 0.9-14.9% of the general CI population [6]. It is thought to occur because of an altered electrical impedance of the spongiotic bone: this can generate current leaks outside the cochlea, especially in case of partial electrode insertion [54-56], thus resulting in an electrical shunt with the facial nerve [25]. The bone resorption and the progressive thinning of the bone between the electrode and the facial nerve may contribute to this shunt [55, 57]. It has been suggested that the electrode design can influence the incidence of FNS, with perimodiolar (modiolar hugging) electrodes demonstrated to be a useful strategy for preventing this problem [58].

When it occurs, FNS usually appears with facial twitching, pain and paraesthesia [59] at the first connection of the CI or after an average time period of 6.8 months after implant activation [60, 61], but an onset as long as 13 years after implantation has been described [31]. Some Authors [35] have speculated that the higher incidence of FNS with straight electrodes could be explained by the fact that these devices have been in situ longer than the newer modiolar hugging electrodes.

It has been also demonstrated that the higher risk of developing FNS interests subjects with grade 3 (Rotteveel grading system) advanced otosclerosis [35]. This suggests that disease severity on CT scanning may predict cases in which FNS is more likely.

Once occurred, FNS can usually be resolved by reprogramming or deactivation of the involved electrodes [25], that usually are the most distal/apical one, the ones in close proximity to the geniculate ganglion and labyrinthine portion of the facial nerve [26, 55]. However, when many electrodes require deactivation, the performance of the CI unavoidably decreases. The "variable-mode programming," by leaving normal pulses for non-offending electrodes and setting wider pulses for the offending electrodes, may represent the right compromise between audiological performance and FNS solving [61]. Another treatment modality for refractory FNS is the injection of botulinum toxin [62]. Gold and colleagues [62] also reported the benefit of oral fluoride treatment in refractory cases. In some cases, FNS cannot be resolved through the aforementioned modalities and reimplantation may be necessary [25, 63].

- Other non-auditory stimulations were reported in the literature to be more common in patients with otosclerosis submitted to cochlear implantation: *tympanic plexus stimulation* (manifesting as otalgia) and *vestibular structures stimulation* (clinically presenting with dizziness) [64]. Other untoward symptoms described in patients with advanced otosclerosis after CI are *tinnitus*, *headaches* [32, 50] and *throat discomfort* [49]. The treatment in all cases consists in the deactivation of the offending electrodes.
- As otosclerosis progresses, demineralization can cause the formation of cavitation around the cochlea with resultant *perilymphatic gusher* during cochleostomy [36].

Direct Acoustic Cochlear Implant

The direct acoustic cochlear implant (DACI) is a new type of acoustic hearing implant designed for patients with severe to profound mixed hearing loss [65] but not yet approved by US Food and Drug Administration.

DACI transfers acoustic energy directly to the inner ear via an implantable electromagnetic transducer introduced into the oval or round window or in a surgically created 'third' window [40]. As a result, pathological outer and middle ear structures of the ear are bypassed and the amplified signal is directly provided to the cochlea. Häusler et al. [40] and Bernhard et al. [66] were the first to describe a DACI device called DACS. The successor of the DACS, the Codacs investigational device, has been demonstrated to be safe and clinically useful in the treatment of patients with severe to profound MHL due to advanced otosclerosis [67].

Several studies have stated that the outcomes in otosclerosis patients with severe to profound hearing loss treated with DACI, in terms of hearing improvement and speech intelligibility, are significantly better than in case of CI [63] or conventional hearing aids [68].

Busch and colleagues [68] defined the indication for DACI as a BC threshold between 40 and 80 dB hearing loss and AC threshold higher than 60-dB hearing loss. Larger clinic trials with this device are however required to reach definitive conclusions [6].

Treatment Strategy and Counselling

Different criteria should be considered when choosing the best treatment strategy, including rate of success, economic criteria and potential complications of each option.

Merkus and colleagues [10] proposed a *treatment algorithm* that can help the surgeon in choosing the best treatment strategy basing on SD rates and CT findings (Figure 1). First, patients are divided into 3 main groups according to their maximum SD scores, using standard speech audiometry (open-set monosyllables) [69]: group 1 SD scores are less than 30%; group 2 SD scores are 30% to 50%, and group 3 SD scores are 50% to 70%.

For group 1 patients (SDS < 30dB), who often suffer from sever SNHL, the most effective treatment has been demonstrated to be cochlear implantation, because stapedectomy does not act on the sensorineural component. Group 2 patients (SDS between 30 and 50%) might be treated with both CI and stapedectomy in relation to their CT scan Rotteveel grade. In case of severe retrofenestral otosclerosis with Rotteveel grade 2C or 3, cochlear implantation is typically recommended, because of the likely progression of cochlear damage that could make CI very difficult in future. In case of less advanced CT lesions (Rotteveel grade 1, 2A or 2B) the air-bone gaps should guide the surgeon: if the ABG is equal or greater than 30 dB, stapedotomy is recommended; if the ABG is less than 30 dB, CI still remains the best option in the Authors' opinion. Group 3 patients (SD between 50 and 70%) undergo the same management as group 2, except that in case of limited CT cochlear involvement and ABG less than 30 dB hearing aids and follow-up are recommended rather than CI.

Despite this interesting algorithm appears to be a useful to help the surgeon choose the best treatment to perform, retrospective evidence suggests that CT and audiological findings are not sensitive or specific enough to predict the outcomes of stapedotomy [36,

42]. Furthermore, it has been demonstrated that even in patients with a "blank" audiogram (unmeasurable air and bone conduction thresholds) and 0% SD, stapedectomy with a well-fitted hearing aid can still lead to acceptable outcomes in up to 30% of patients [12, 36].

Because of the advantages listed above, several Authors still recommend to consider stapes surgery with hearing aid as a first option [6]. In fact, the results of auditory stimuli appears to be better than electrical stimuli in terms of sound quality, musical appreciation and speech discrimination in loud environments [70-72]. If stapes surgery does not have a successful outcome, a cochlear implantation is still an option [6].

In addition, multiple factors must be considered in the surgical decision, such as the degree of residual hearing in the contralateral ear, the duration of hearing deprivation and the patient preference.

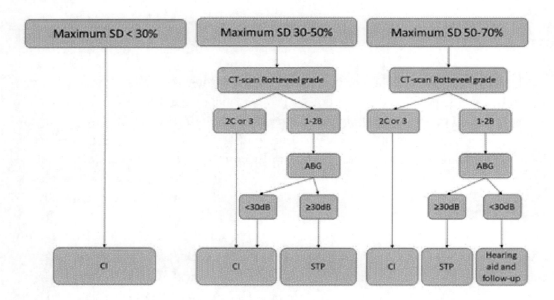

Figure 1. Algorithm guideline proposed by Merkus et al. for advanced otosclerosis.
SD: Speech Discrimination; ABG: air-bone gap; CI: cochlear implantation; STP: stapedectomy.

Careful preoperative counselling is extremely important in patients with advanced otosclerosis. Especially in cases selected for stapedectomy, patients must be aware of the risk of the procedure, of the limited goals and of the possibility, in case of failure, that a CI can be carried out in the next future. Failure is normally defined by no improvement of threshold levels or speech recognition with well fitted hearing aids at 3 months after the surgery and when the patient is not satisfied [73]. Nevertheless, patients should be informed that, since cochlear otosclerosis is an evolutive process, the results of a stapedectomy can deteriorate with time; in these cases, CI must be proposed.

Quite recent publications showed promising results with the use of high dose *third-generation bisphosphonates* in the treatment of SNHL in otosclerosis, with stabilization and up to 68% improvement of SD [74, 75]. The mechanism is thought to be linked to a reduction in osteoclast activity and, hence, of TNF-alpha diffusion to the perilymph and hair cells [74, 75]. Although more studies are necessary, this therapeutic option may decrease the number of patients requiring salvage cochlear implantation after stapedotomy and improve the long-term stability of the procedure.

CONCLUSION

Recent reviews concluded that CI leads to a statistically greater and consistent improvement in speech discrimination scores compared with stapes surgery. Stapedotomy is not universally effective; however, it yields results comparable to CI in at least half of patients.

In conclusion, stapedectomy with subsequent hearing aid adaptation should not be forgotten as a valid procedure for these patients. Each case must be thoroughly analysed and the choice of treatment should be individualized for each patient.

For cases of unsuccessful stapedectomy, the option of CI is still open, and the results obtained by a salvage CI are as good as those of CI when no prior stapedotomy was performed.

REFERENCES

[1] Rama-Lopez J, Cervera-Paz FJ, Manrique M. Cochlear implantation of patients with far-advanced otosclerosis. *Otol Neurotol* 2006;27:153-158.

[2] Castillo F, Polo R, Gutiérrez A, et al. Cochlear implantation outcomes in advanced otosclerosis. *Am J Otolaryngol* 2014;35:558-564.

[3] Dispenza F, Cappello F, Kulamarva G, De Stefano A. The discovery of stapes. *Acta Otorhinolaryngol Ital*, 2013; 33:357-359.

[4] Ferrara S, Di Marzo M, Martines F, Ferrara P. Medical and surgical update on "atelectasic - Adhesive – Tympanosclerotic" otitis media. *Otorinolaringologia* 2011; 61:11-17.

[5] Abdurehim Y, Lehmann A, Zeitouni AG. Stapedotomy vs cochlear implantation for advanced otosclerosis: systematic review and meta-analysis. *Otolaryngol Head Neck Surg* 2016;155:764-770.

[6] Eshraghi AA, Ila K, Ocak E, Telischi FF. Stapes Surgery or Cochlear Implantation? *Otolaryngol Clin N Am* 2018;51:429-440.

[7] Ramsay HA, Linthicum Jr FH. Mixed hearing loss in otosclerosis: indication for long-term follow-up. *Am J Otol* 1994;15:536-539.

[8] Shea PF, Ge X, Shea Jr JJ. Stapedectomy for far-advanced otosclerosis. *Am J Otol* 1999;20:425-429.

[9] House HP, Sheehy JL. Stapes surgery: selection of the patient. *Ann Otol Rhinol Laryngol* 1961;70:1062-1068.

[10] Merkus P, van Loon MC, Smit CF, et al. Decision making in advanced otosclerosis: an evidence-based strategy. *Laryngoscope* 2011;121:1935-1941.

[11] Iurato S, Ettorre GC, Onofri M, et al. Very far-advanced otosclerosis. *Am J Otol* 1992;13:482-487.

[12] Calmels MN, Viana C, Wanna G, Marx M, James C, Deguine O, Fraysse B. Very far-advanced otosclerosis: stapedotomy or cochlear implantation. *Acta Oto-Laryngologica* 2007;127:574-578.

[13] Siebenmann F. Multiple Spongiosierung der Labyrinthkapsel als Sectionsbefund bei einem Fall von progressiver Schwerhorigkeit [Multiple spongiosis of the labyrinth capsule as a section finding in a case of progressive heavy hearing]. *Z Ohrenheilk* 1899;34:356-374.

[14] Bretlau P, Causse J, Jorgensen MB, et al. Histiocytic activity in the otosclerotic bone. *Arch Klin Exp Ohren Nasen Kehlkopfheilkd* 1971;198:301-316.

[15] Chevance LG, Bretlau P, Jorgensen MB, et al: Otosclerosis: An electron microscopic and cytochemical study. *Acta Otolaryngol* [Suppl] (Stockholm) 1970;272:1-27.

[16] Ruedi L. Histopathologic confirmation of labyrinthine otosclerosis. *Laryngoscope* 1965;75:1582-1609.

[17] Linthicum Jr FH, Filipo R, Brody S. Sensorineural hearing loss due to cochlear otospongiosis: theoretical considerations of etiology. *Ann Otol Rhinol Laryngol* 1975;84:544-551.

[18] Linthicum Jr FH. Histopathology of otosclerosis. *Otolaryngol Clin North Am* 1993;26:335-352.

[19] Linthicum Jr FH, Filipo R, Brody S. Sensorineural hearing loss due to cochlear otospongiosis: theoretic considerations of etiology. *Ann Otol Rhinol Laryngol* 1975;84:544-551.

[20] Cureoglu S, Baylan MY, Paparella MM. Cochlear otosclerosis. *Curr Opin Otolaryngol Head Neck Surg* 2010;18:357-362.

[21] Doherty JK, Linthicum FH. Spiral ligament and stria vascularis. *Otol Neurotol* 2004;25:457-464.

[22] Valvassori GE. Imaging of otosclerosis. *Otolaryngol Clin North Am* 1993;26:359-371.

[23] Palacios E, Valvassori G. Cochlear otosclerosis. *Ear Nose Throat J* 2000;XX:494.

[24] Marx SV, Langman AW. Cochlear otosclerosis. *Am J Otol* 1997;18:404.

[25] Polak M, Ulubil SA, Hodges AV, et al. Revision cochlear implantation for facial nerve stimulation in otosclerosis. *Arch Otolaryngol Head Neck Surg* 2006;132:398-404.

[26] Rotteveel LJ, Proops DW, Ramsden RT, Saeed SR, van Olphen AF, Mylanus EA. Cochlear implantation in 53 patients with otosclerosis: demographics, computed tomographic scanning, surgery, and complications. *Otol Neurotol* 2004;25:943-952.

[27] Shin YJ, Fraysse B, Deguine O, et al. Sensorineural hearing loss and otosclerosis: a clinical and radiological survey of 437 cases. *Acta Otolaryngol* 2001;121:200-204.

[28] Lee TC, Aviv RI, Chen JM, Nedzelski JM, Fox AJ, Symons SP. CT grading of otosclerosis. *AJNR Am J Neuroradiol* 2009;30:1435-1439.

[29] Ruckenstein MJ, Rafter KO, Montes M, Bigelow DC. Management of far advanced otosclerosis in the era of cochlear implantation. *Otol Neurotol* 2001;22:471-474.

[30] Goh JPN, Chan LL, Tan TY. MRI of cochlear otosclerosis. *Br J Radiol* 2002:75;502-505.

[31] Toung JS, Zwolan T, Spooner TR, et al. Late failure of cochlear implantation resulting from advanced cochlear otosclerosis: surgical and programming challenges. *Otol Neurotol* 2004;25:723-726.

[32] Semaan MT, Gehani NC, Tummala N, et al. Cochlear implantation outcomes in patients with far advanced otosclerosis. *Am J Otolaryngol* 2012;33:608-614.

[33] Berrettini S, Ravecca F, Volterrani D, et al. Imaging evaluation in otosclerosis: single photon emission computed tomography and computed tomography. *Ann Otol Rhinol Laryngol* 2010;119:215-224.

[34] Lombardo F, De Cori S, Aghakhanyan G, Montanaro D, De Marchi D, Frijia F, Fortunato S, Forli F, Chiappino D, Berrettini S, Canapicchi R. 3D-Flair sequence at 3T in cochlear otosclerosis. *Eur Radiol* 2016 Oct;26(10):3744-3751.

[35] Marshall AH, Fanning N, Symons S, et al. Cochlear implantation in cochlear otosclerosis. *Laryngoscope* 2005;115:1728-1733.

[36] Kabbara B, Gauche C, Calmels MN, et al. Decisive criteria between stapedotomy and cochlear implantation in patients with far advanced otosclerosis. *Otol Neurotol* 2015;36:73-78.

[37] Sheehy JL. Far-advanced otosclerosis. Diagnostic criteria and results of treatment: report of 67 cases. *Arch Otolaryngol Head Neck Surg* 1964;80:244-248.

[38] Berrettini S, Burdo S, Forli F, et al. Far advanced otosclerosis: stapes surgery or cochlear implantation? *J Otolaryngol* 2004;33:165-171.

[39] Eshraghi AA, Nazarian R, Telischi FF, et al. The cochlear implant: historical aspects and future prospects. *Anat Rec* (Hoboken) 2012;295:1967-1980.

[40] Häusler R, Stieger C, Bernhard H, et al. A novel implantable hearing system with direct acoustic cochlear stimulation. *Audiol Neurootol* 2008;13:247-256.

[41] House WF, Glorig A. Criteria for otosclerosis surgery and further experiences with round window surgery. *Laryngoscope* 1960;70:616-630.

[42] van Loon MC, Merkus P, Smit CF, et al. Stapedotomy in cochlear implant candidates with far advanced otosclerosis: a systematic review of the literature and meta-analysis. *Otol Neurotol* 2014;35:1707-1714.

[43] Frattali MA, Sataloff RT. Far-advanced otosclerosis. *Ann Otol Rhinol Laryngol* 1993;102:433-437.

[44] Marchioni D, Soloperto D, Bianconi L, et al. Endoscopic approach for cochlear implantation in advanced otosclerosis: a case report. *Auris Nasus Larynx* 2016;43:584-590.

[45] Linthicum Jr FH, Galey FR. Histologic evaluation of temporal bones with cochlear implants. *Ann Otol Rhinol Laryngol* 1983;92:610-613.

[46] Fayad J, Moloy P, Linthicum Jr FH. Cochlear otosclerosis: does bone formation affect cochlear implant surgery? *Am J Otol* 1990;11:196-200.

[47] Nadol JB Jr, Young YS, Glynn RJ. Survival of spiral ganglion cells in profound sensorineural hearing loss: implications for cochlear implantation. *Ann Otol Rhinol Laryngol* 1989;98:411-416.

[48] Eisenberg LS, Luxford WM, Becker TS, et al. Electrical stimulation of the auditory system in children deafened by meningitis. *Otolaryngol Head Neck Surg* 1984;92:700-705.

[49] Quaranta N, Bartoli R, Lopriore A, et al. Cochlear implantation in otosclerosis. *Otol Neurotol* 2005;26:983-987 [Erratum in: *Otol Neurotol* 2005; 26(6):1264].

[50] Sainz M, Garcia-Valdecasas J, Ballesteros JM. Complications and pitfalls of cochlear implantation in otosclerosis: a 6-year follow-up cohort study. *Otol Neurotol* 2009;30:1044-1048.

[51] Matterson AG, O'Leary S, Pinder D, et al. Otosclerosis: selection of ear for cochlear implantation. *Otol Neurotol* 2007;28:438-446.

[52] Lenarz T, Lesinski-Schiedat A, Weber BP, et al. The nucleus double array cochlear implant: a new concept for the obliterated cochlea. *Otol Neurotol* 2001;22:24-32.

[53] Balkany T, Gantz BJ, Steenerson RL, Cohen NL. Systematic approach to electrode insertion in the ossified cochlea. *Otolaryngol Head Neck Surg* 1996;114:4-11.

[54] Ramsden R, Bance M, Giles E, Mawman D. Cochlear implantation in otosclerosis: a unique positioning and programming problem. *J Laryngol Otol* 1997;111:262-265.

[55] Muckle RP, Levine SC. Facial nerve stimulation produced by cochlear implants in patients with otosclerosis. *Am J Otol* 1994;15:394-398.

[56] Weber BP, Lenarz T, Battmer R-D, et al. Otosclerosis and facial nerve stimulation. *Ann Otol Rhinol Laryngol Suppl* 1995;166:445-447.

[57] Bigelow D, Kay DJ, Rafter KO, Montes M, Knox GW, Yousem DM. Facial nerve stimulation from cochlear implants. *Am J Otol* 1998;19:163-169.

[58] Flook EP, Broomfield SJ, Saeed S, et al. Cochlear implantation in far advanced otosclerosis: a surgical, audiological and quality of life review of 35 cases in a single unit. *J Int Adv Otol* 2010;7:35-40.

[59] Seyyedi M, Herrmann BS, Eddington DK, et al. The pathologic basis of facial nerve stimulation in otosclerosis and multi-channel cochlear implantation. *Otol Neurotol* 2013;34:1603-1609.

[60] Rayner MG, King T, Djalilian HR, et al. Resolution of facial stimulation in otosclerotic cochlear implants. *Otolaryngol Head Neck Surg* 2003;129:475-480.

[61] Kelsall DC, Shallop JK, Brammeier TG, Prenger EC. Facial nerve stimulation after nucleus 22-channel cochlear implantation. *Am J Otol* 1997;18:336-341.

[62] Gold SR, Miller V, Kamerer DB, et al. Fluoride treatment for facial nerve stimulation caused by cochlear implants in otosclerosis. *Otolaryngol Head Neck Surg* 1998;119:521-523.

[63] Fernandez-Vega S, Quaranta N, Bartoli R, et al. Management of facial nerve stimulation in otosclerosis by revision cochlear implantation. *Audiol Med* 2008;6:155-160.

[64] Ramsden R, Rotteveel L, Proops D, et al. Cochlear implantation in otosclerotic deafness. *Adv Otorhinolaryngol* 2007;65:328-334.

[65] Kludt E, Bu¨chner A, Schwab B, et al. Indication of direct acoustical cochlea stimulation in comparison to cochlear implants. *Hear Res* 2016;340:185-190.

[66] Bernhard H, Stieger C, Perriard Y: New implantable hearing device based on a micro-actuator that is directly coupled to the inner ear fluid. *Conf Proc IEEE Eng Med Biol Soc* 2006;1:3162-3165.

[67] Lenarz T, Verhaert N, Desloovere C, et al. A comparative study on speech in noise understanding with a direct acoustic cochlear implant in subjects with severe to profound mixed hearing loss. *Audiol Neurootol* 2014;19:164-174.

[68] Busch S, Kruck S, Spickers D, et al. First clinical experiences with a direct acousticcochlear stimulator in comparison to preoperative fitted conventional hearing aids. *Otol Neurotol* 2013;34:1711-1718.

[69] Bosman AJ, Smoorenburg GF. Intelligibility of Dutch CVC syllables and sentences for listeners with normal hearing and with three types of hearing impairment. *Audiology* 1995;34:260-284.

[70] Drennan WR, Rubinstein JT. Music perception in cochlear implant users and its relationship with psychophysical capabilities. *J Rehabil Res Dev* 2008;45:779-789.

[71] Thomas, E., Martines, F., Bianco, A., Messina, G., Giustino, V., Zangla, D., Iovane, A., Palma, A. (2018) *Decreased postural control in people with moderate hearing loss Medicine* (United States), 97 (14), DOI: 10.1097/MD.0000000000010244.

[72] Thomas, E., Bianco, A., Messina, G., Mucia, M., Rizzo, S., Salvago, P., Sireci, F., Palma, A., Martines, F. The influence of sounds in postural control (2017) *Hearing Loss: Etiology, Management and Societal Implications*, pp. 1-11.

[73] Glasscock ME, Storper IS, Haynes DS, Bohrer PS. Stapedectomy in profound cochlear loss. *Laryngoscope* 1996;106:831-833.

[74] Quesnel AM, Seton M, Merchant SN, et al. Third-generation bisphosphonates for treatment of sensorineural hearing loss in otosclerosis. *Otol Neurotol* 2012; 33:1308-1314.

[75] Brookler KH, Gilston N. Re: Third-generation bisphosphonates for treatment of sensorineural hearing loss in otosclerosis, *Otology & Neurotology* 33:1308Y1314, 2012. *Otol Neurotol* 2013;34:778-779.

Chapter 9

SUDDEN SENSORINEURAL HEARING LOSS

*Valerio Giustino[1], Francesco Lorusso[2], MD,
Serena Rizzo[3], MD, Pietro Salvago[4], MD
and Francesco Martines[4,5], MD, PhD*

[1]Sport and Exercise Sciences Research Unit,
University of Palermo, Palermo, Italy
[2]A.O.U.P. Paolo Giaccone, Palermo, Italy
[3]University of Palermo, Di. Chir.On.S. Department,
Physical medicine and rehabilitation, Palermo, Italy
[4]University of Palermo, Bio. Ne. C. Department,
Audiology Section, Palermo, Italy
[5]Istituto Euromediterraneo di Scienza e Tecnologia – IEMEST, Palermo, Italy

ABSTRACT

Sudden sensorineural hearing loss (SSNHL), is an important otological disorder that affects up to 5-20 in 100,000 people. It is characterized by a rapid loss of the hearing, usually unilateral, with a sensorineural hearing loss greater than 30 dB over three consecutive frequencies, in less than 72 hours and can be associated with tinnitus and vertigo. It is a real sensorineural emergency that can become a permanent handicap if not adequately treated.

Because of patients recovering rapidly or seeking no medical attention, the true figure might be higher, even if delaying SHL diagnosis and treatment may decrease the effectiveness of treatment. Sudden Hearing Loss can occur at any age but usually affects between 50 and 60 years old and the youngest patients affected are among 20-30 years old. There are not significantly differences in the prevalence between men and women[1-3]. Several pathophysiological mechanisms have been proposed to explain SHL (infective, vascular, and immune disease), but only 10 to 15 percent of the people have an identifiable cause; the majority of cases in fact remain 'idiopathic'[4].

Because no specific cause is identified, the treatments are heterogeneous and can be considered empiric; on one hand therapies' aim is to correct the primary risk factors (smoke, diabetes, hypertension, previous viral or bacterial infections), on the other hand the purpose is to act on the main etiopathogenetic hypotheses (viral infection, immunologic, vascular compromise).

Keywords: sudden hearing loss, sensorineural hearing loss

ETIOLOGY

The etiology of Sudden Hearing Loss (SHL) includes viral/infectious, autoimmune, labyrinthine membrane rupture/trauma, vascular, neurological, and neoplastic causes [5, 6]. Within these broader categories, there are a host of subtypes associated with SHL. An abridged list of recognized causes of SHL is shown in table 1 [7-10].

DIAGNOSTIC EVALUATION

Hearing impairment workup comprehends history, audiometry, tympanometry, including stapedial reflex testing, as well as auditory evoked potentials.

A typical history, per se, often makes for a straightforward diagnosis. In particular, clinicians should focus on the accompanying circumstances, symptom onset and temporal progression, as well as corroborating audiovestibular features (i.e., tinnitus, vertigo/dizziness, aural fullness) [11-13]. Clinically, tinnitus and vertigo affect approximately 77% and 33% of cases, respectively [14-16]. Moreover, the history should include inquiry into prior otologic surgery, exposure to ototoxic agents, viral infections and systemic disorders, such as hypercoagulable states, diabetes and autoimmunity [17-19]. A pure-tone audiometry exam that assesses conventional generated tone frequencies (i.e., 125, 250, 500, 1000, 2000, 4000 and 8000 Hz) is a mainstay of the workup in every patient presenting with SHL, as recommended by the "International Organization for Standardization" (ISO). Furthermore, the clinical utility of the audiogram, together with its morphological features, is not limited to the diagnosis, but rather provides clinician the elements of prognostic value as well (Figure 1).

As for the tympanogram and stapedial reflexes, the utility of these assessments mainly lies in the topographic diagnosis of hearing loss. Finally, via objective estimations of electrophysiological hearing thresholds, the hearing impairment workup avails itself of recordings of auditory evoked potentials, which aid in assessing the integrity of discrete constituents of the acoustic-facial bundle and neural circuitry.

Table 1. Causes of SHL

Infectious	Meningococcal men
	Herpesvirus (simplex, zoster, varicella, cytomegalovirus)
	Mumps
	Human immunodeficiency virus
	Lassa fever
	Mycoplasma
	Cryptococcal meningitis
	Toxoplasmosis
	Syphilis
	Rubeola
	Rubella
	Human spumaretrovirus
Autoimmune	Autoimmune inner ear disease (AIED)
	Ulcerative colitis
	Relapsing polychondritis
	Lupus erythematosus
	Polyarteritis nodosa
	Cogan's syndrome
	Wegener's granulomatosis
Traumatic	Perilymph fistula
	Inner ear decompression sickness
	Temporal bone fracture
	Inner ear concussion
	Otologic surgery (stapedectomy)
	Surgical complication of nonotologic surgery
Vascular	Vascular disease/alteration of microcirculation
	Vascular disease associated with mitochondriopathy
	Vertebrobasilar insufficiency
	Red blood cell deformability
	Sickle cell disease
	Cardiopulmonary bypass
Neurologic	Multiple sclerosis
	Focal pontine ischemia
	Migraine
Neoplastic	Acoustic neuroma
	Leukemia
	Myeloma
	Metastasis to internal auditory canal
	Meningeal carcinomatosis
	Contralateral deafness after acoustic neuroma surgery

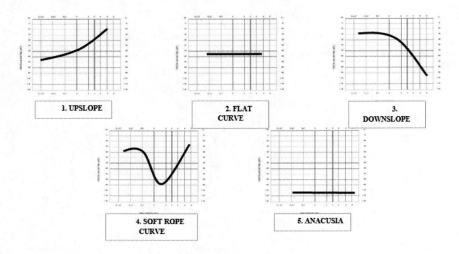

Figure 1. Most common types of curve.

PATHOPHYSIOLOGY OF SUDDEN HEARING LOSS

Although a specific cause may be identified in no more than approximately 10% of cases, most available evidence appears to support inflammation and/or hypoxia as the underlying condition(s) leading to cell injury or dysfunction. Accordingly, three main theories have been advanced to interpret idiopathic Sudden Hearing Loss, all of whose hypotheses regarding the pathophysiological mechanisms converge on the common pathway of inflammation and/or hypoxia: vascular, viral and autoimmune theories.

VASCULAR THEORY

Since the inner ear is supplied by terminal blood vessels, the organ is particularly vulnerable to reduced blood flow and/or hypoxic stress. Moreover, the resulting clinical picture closely matches the physiology of the affected area. Unsurprisingly, circulation within the cochleo-vestibular system can be compromised by conditions such as: increases in blood/plasma viscosity; sludging of blood; vasospasm and/or release of vasoactive substances; embolism or thrombosis.

VIRAL THEORY

In 1957, van Dishoeck first advanced a viral theory to elucidate the onset of Sudden Hearing Loss, positing three alternative mechanisms [20] (Figure 2):

1. direct viral invasion of the inner ear or cochlear nerve via the bloodstream, cerebrospinal fluid, or middle ear;
2. reactivation of a latent virus presents in the inner ear: neurotropic viruses subclinically infect cochlear neurons, become latent and subsequently are reactivated manifesting as acute cochleitis or neuritis, which lead to sudden deafness;
3. viral antigens stimulating an immune response during a systemic infection induce cross-reacting antibodies (i.e., antigenic mimicry) to antigens of the inner ear.

AUTOIMMUNE THEORY

The first report of an autoimmune inner ear disease (AIED), dates back to McCabe (1979) [21]. The autoimmune theory of Sudden Hearing Loss postulates the existence of autoantibodies or activated T-cells that directly target constituents of the inner ear. Antigens occurring on a variety of host molecules, such as type-II collagen, β-actin, cochlin, β-tectorin, cochlear proteins (P30 and P80), cardiolipids, phospholipids, serotonin and gangliosides have been singled out as the putative targets. As of yet, however, the most compelling case concerns a protein called choline transporter-like protein 2 (CTL2).

Finally, the higher frequency of specific HLA alleles in patients that respond well to corticosteroid therapy has been observed, lending further support to the autoimmune theory [22-26].

(A): Reduced blood flow to the cochlear artery affects the medium and apical parts of the cochlea, resulting in audiometric deficit limited to medium - and low frequency tones.

(B): Reduced blood flow at the level of the vestibular-cochlear artery affects the basal part of the cochlea, resulting in audiometric deficit of high-frequency tones associated with vertigo.

(C): Reduced blood flow in vestibular artery manifests clinically as significant vertigo due to injury of the three semicircular canals.

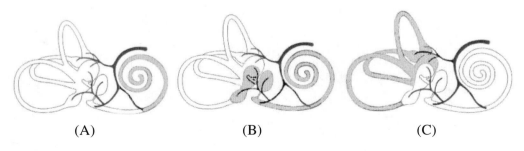

(A)   (B)   (C)

Figure 2. Occlusion of the cochlear (A), vestibular-cochlear (B) and vestibular arteries (C). (From: http://www.orl.uniroma2.it/ischemia.htm).

Table 2. Therapeutic modalities of SHL

Anti-inflammatory/immunologic agents
Steroids
Prostaglandin
Cyclophosphamide
Methotrexate

Diuretics
Hydochlorothiazide/triamterene
Furosemide

Antiviral agents
Acyclovir
Valacyclovir

Vasodilators
Carbogen
Papaverine
Buphenine
Naftidrofuryl
Thymoxamine
Prostacyclin
Nicotinic acid
Pentoxifylline

Volume expanders/hemodilutors
Hydroxyethyl starch
Low-molecular-weight dextran

Defibrinogenators
Batroxobin

Calcium antagonists
Nifedipine

Other agents and procedures
Amidotrizoate
Acupunture
Iron
Vitamins
Procaine

TREATMENT

As mentioned above, treatment of SHL is a controversial matter and the idiopathic category has been treated by a wide range of approaches. Within the various treatments proposed, glucocorticoids remain the agents most relied on, although via different routes of administration: either oral or intratympanic steroids or their combinations [27, 28]. Nonetheless, table 2 includes a list of therapeutic modalities which have been adopted, some of which are currently in use for the treatment of SHL.

PROGNOSIS

Statistical data from case series indicate that 25% of cases evolve with full recovery of hearing, 50% have only partial recovery, while the remaining 25% of patients experience permanent hearing impairment [29-31]. In a study of 270 patients in Sicily, included in one review, the following five prognostic factors were identified:

a) *Type of Therapy*: combined intratympanic and systemic steroids produced more favorable results;
b) *Type of Curve*: an upward curve increased the margins for improvement;
c) *Hypertension*: a hypertensive state reduced the likelihood of recovery;
d) *Vertigo*: severe vertigo correlated with significantly worse outcomes than no vertigo;
e) *OAE*: presence of OAEs had positive prognostic significance [32].

CONCLUSION

Sudden sensorineural hearing loss is an issue of primary concern to otolaryngology, given its clinical relevance and potential for disabling outcomes. Arguably, hearing loss negatively impacts quality of life, social and work-related relationships, often representing not only a communication barrier, but also a disconnect from their surroundings for those affected, with the inherent risk of emotional isolation [33]. Despite the advances made, many aspects regarding etiology, pathogenesis, diagnosis and therapy remain elusive and/or controversial. The recent increase in incidence, reported in the literature, probably due to a host of new and widespread pathological noxae, along with the emergence of new therapeutic protocols, render the discussion regarding these issues quite timely. Finally, there is consensus among authors that Sudden Hearing Loss should not go untreated, because many treatments provide at least some margin of benefit and functional recovery, thus improving the patient's quality of life [34-36].

REFERENCES

[1] Gignoux, M., Martin, H., Cajgfinger, H., (1973) Les surdites brusques [The sudden surgeons]. *J. Med. Lyon*, 44/1043, 1701 - 1718.
[2] Tran Ba Huy, P., Bastian, D., Ohresser, M. (1980) Anatomie de l'oreille interne [Anatomy of the inner ear]. *Encycl. Med. Chir. Paris*, ORL, 20020 A 10.
[3] De Kleyn, A., (1994) Sudden complete or partial loss of function of the octavus-system in apprerently normal persons. *Acta Otolaryngol. (Stockh)*, 32: 407 - 429.
[4] Martines, F., Bentivegna, D., Maira, E., Marasà, S., Ferrara, S. (2012) Cavernous haemangioma of the external auditory canal: Clinical case and review of the literature. *Acta Otorhinolaryngol. Ital.*, 32(1): 54 - 57.
[5] Martines, F., Salvago, P., Bartolotta, C., Cocuzza, S., Fabiano, C., Ferrara, S., La Mattina, E., Mucia, M., Sammarco, P., Sireci, F., Martines, E. (2015) A genotype–phenotype correlation in Sicilian patients with GJB2 biallelic mutations. *Eur. Arch. Otorhinolaryngol.*, 272(8): 1857 - 1865.
[6] Gagliardo, C., Martines, F., Bencivinni, F., Latona, G., Lo Casto, A., Midiri, M. (2013) Intratumoral Haemorrhage Causing an Unusual Clinical Presentation of a Vestibular Schwannoma. *Neuruladiology Journal*, 26: 30 - 34.
[7] Martines, F., Ballacchino, A., Sireci, F., Mucia, M., La Mattina, E., Rizzo, S. (2016) Audiologic profile of OSAS and simple snoring patients: the effect of chronic nocturnal intermittent hypoxia on auditory function. *European Archives of Oto-Rhino-Laryngology*, 273: 1419 - 1424.
[8] Martines, F., Messina, G., Patti, A., Battaglia, G., Bellafiore, M., Messina, A., Rizzo, S., Salvago, P., Sireci, F., Traina, M., Iovane, A. (2015) Effects of tinnitus on postural control and stabilization: A pilot study. *Acta Medica Mediterranea*, 31: 907 - 912.
[9] Ferrara, S., Salvago, P., Mucia, M., Ferrara, P., Sireci, F., Martines, F. (2014) Follow-up after pediatric myringoplasty: Outcome at 5 years. *Otorinolaringologia*, 64: 141 - 146.
[10] Cannizzaro, E., Cannizzaro, C., Plescia, F., Martines, F., Sole, L., Pira, E., Lo Coco, D. (2014) Exposure to ototoxic agents and hearing loss: A review of current knowledge. *Hearing, Balance and Communication*, 12: 166 - 175.
[11] Rizzo, S., Bentivegna, D., Thomas, E., La Mattina, E., Mucia, M., Salvago, P., Sireci, F., Martines, F. (2016) Sudden sensorineural hearing loss, an invisible male: State of art. *Hearing loss: etiology, management and societal implications*, 75 - 86.

[12] Salvago, P., Rizzo, S., Bianco, A., Martines, F. (2017) Sudden sensorineural hearing loss: is there a relationship between routine haematological parameters and audiogram shapes? *International Journal of Audiology*, 56(3): 148 - 153.

[13] Ballacchino, A., Salvago, P., Cannizzaro, E., Costanzo, R., Di Marzo, M., Ferrara, S., La Mattina, E., Messina, G., Mucia, M., Mulè, A., Plescia, F., Sireci, F., Rizzo, S., Martines, F. (2015) Association between sleep-disordered breathing and hearing disorders: Clinical observation in Sicilian patients. *Acta Medica Mediterranea*, 31(3): 607 - 614.

[14] Kiris, M., Cankaya, H., Icli, M., Kutluhan, A. Retrospective analysis of our cases with sudden hearing loss. *J. Otolaryngol.*, 2003; 32: 384 - 7.

[15] Martines, F., Dispenza, F., Gagliardo, C., Martines, E., Bentivegna, D. (2011) Sudden sensorineural hearing loss as prodromal symptom of anterior inferior cerebellar artery infarction. *ORL,* 2011; 73: 137 - 140.

[16] Plescia, F., Cannizzaro, C., Brancato, A., Sireci, F., Salvago, P., Martines, F. (2016) Emerging pharmacological treatments of tinnitus. *Tinnitus: Epidemiology, Causes and Emerging Therapeutic Treatments.* Nova Science Publishers, Inc.; 43 - 64.

[17] Wilson, W. R., Laird, N., Moo-Young, G., Soeldner, J. S., Kavesh, D. A., MacMeel, J. W. (1982) The relationship of idiopathic sudden hearing loss to diabetes mellitus. *Laryngoscope*, 92: 155 - 60.

[18] Campbell, K. C., Klemens, J. J., (2000) Sudden hearing loss and autoimmune inner ear disease. *J. Am. Acad. Audiol.*, 11: 361 - 7.

[19] Martines, F., Maira, E., Ferrara, S. (2011) Age-related hearing impairment (ARHI): A common sensory deficit in the elderly. *Acta Medica Mediterranea*, 27 (1), 47 - 52.

[20] Van Dishoeck, H., Bierman, T. (1957) Sudden perceptive deafness and viral infection (report of the first one hundred patients). *Ann. Otol. Rhinol. Laryngol.*, 66: 963 - 980.

[21] McCabe, Brian F. (1991) Autoimmune inner ear disease: results and therapy. *Adv. Otorhinolaryngol.*, 46:78 - 81.

[22] Boulassel, M. R., Deggouj, N., Tomasi, J. P., Gersdorff, M. (2001) Inner ear autoantibodies and their targets in patients with autoimmune inner ear diseases. *Acta Otolaryngol.*, 121: 28 - 34.

[23] Solares, C. A., Edling, A. E., Johnson, J. M., Baek, M. J., Hirose, K., Hughes, G. B., Tuohy, V. K. (2004) Murine autoimmune hearing loss mediated by CD4+ T cells specific for inner ear peptides. *J. Clin. Invest.*, 113: 1210 - 1217.

[24] Nair, T. S., Kozma, K. E., Hoefling, N. L., Kommareddi, P. K., Ueda, Y., Gong, T. W., Lomax, M. I., Lansford, C. D., Telian, S. A., Satar, B., Arts, H. A., EI-Kashlan, H. K., Berryhill, W. E., Raphael, Y., Carey, T. E. (2004) Identification and characterization of choline transporter-like protein 2, an inner ear glycoprotein of

[25] 68 and 72 kDa that is the target of antibody induced hearing loss. *J. Neurosci.*, 24: 1772 - 1779.
[25] Adams, L. E. (2002) Clinical implications of inflammatory cytokines in the cochlea: a technical note. *Otol. Neurotol.*, 23:316 - 322.
[26] Disher, M. J., Ramakrishnan, A., Nair, T. S., Miller, J. M., Telian, S. A., Arts, H. A., Sataloff, R. T., Altschuler, R. A., Raphael, Y., Carey, T. E. (1997) Human autoantibodies and monoclonal antibody KHRI-3 bind to a phylogenetically conserved inner ear supporting cell antigen. *Ann. NY Acad. Sci.*, 830: 253 - 265.
[27] Wilson, Willimam, R., Byl., Frederick, M. and Laird, Nan. (1980) The efficacy of steroids in the treatment of idiopathic sudden hearing loss. *Archives of Otolaryngology*; 106:772 - 776 (Dec.).
[28] Dispenza, F., De Stefano, A., Costantino, C., Marchese, D., Riggio, F. (2013) Sudden Sensorineural Hearing Loss: results of intratympanic steroids as salvage treatment. *Am. J. Otolaryngol.*, 34:296 – 300.
[29] Lazarini, P. R., Camargo, A. C. (2006) Idiopathic sudden sensorineural hearing loss: etiopathogenic aspects. *Braz. J. Otorhinolaryngol.*, 72:554 - 61.
[30] O'Malley, M. R., Haynes, D. S. (2008) Sudden hearing loss. *Otolaryngol. Clin. North Am.*, 41:633 - 49.
[31] Rauch, S. D. *(2008)* Idiopathic sudden sensorineural hearing loss. *N. Engl. J. Med.*, 359: 833 - 40.
[32] Schweinfurth, J. M. and others. (1997) Clinical applications of otoacoustic emissions in sudden hearing loss. *Laryngoscope*, 107: 1457 - 1463.
[33] Thomas, E., Martines, F., Bianco, A., Messina, G., Giustino, V., Zangla, D., Iovane, A., Palma, A. (2018) Decreased postural control in people with moderate hearing loss. *Medicine* (Baltimore), 97(14): e0244.
[34] Dispenza, F., Amodio, E., De Stefano, A., Gallina, S., Marchese, D., Mathur, N., Riggio, F. (2011) Treatment of sudden sensorineural hearing loss with transtympanic injection of steroids as single therapy: a randomized clinical study. *Eur. Arch. Otorhinolaryngol.*, 268:1273 - 1278.
[35] Dispenza, F., Cappello, F., Kulamarva, G., De Stefano, A. (2013) The discovery of the stapes. *Acta Otorhinolaryngol. Ital.,* 33(5): 357 - 359.
[36] Dispenza, F., Mazzucco, W., Bianchini, S., Mazzola, S., Bennici, E. (2015) Management of labyrinthine fistula in chronic otitis with cholesteatoma: case series. *EuroMediterranean Biomedical Journal,* 10(21): 255 - 261.

Chapter 10

CAUSE, PATHOGENESIS, CLINICAL MANIFESTATIONS AND TREATMENT OF MENIERE'S DISEASE AND ENDOLYMPHATIC HYDROPS

Sergio Ferrara[2], MD and Francesco Dispenza[1,2], MD, PhD
[1]Istituto Euromediterraneo di Scienza e Tecnologia – IEMEST, Palermo, Italy
[2]U.O.C. Otorinolaringoiatria Azienda Ospedaliera
Universitaria Policlinico P. Giaccone, Palermo, Italy

ABSTRACT

Meniere's disease (MD) is characterized by the triad of fluctuating hearing loss, episodic vertigo and tinnitus, and by endolymphatic hydrops found on postmortem examinations. Since the description of endolymphatic hydrops by Hallpike and Cairns all the physiopathology of Meniere's symptoms have been based on assumption that the pathologic lesion was the cause of the symptoms. Paparella came out term and concept towards understanding of a disease was, "pathogenesis," which applies to all otological diseases, in general and in particular within this context of MD, which allows us to better understand this disease. After Schuknecht proposed the theory of membranous rupture causing the mixing up of endo and perilymph leading to the appearance of Meniere's symptoms. Lawrence proved this theory with research on experimental animals. In 1995 the AAO-HNS criteria defines "Possible MD, Probable MD, Definite MD and Certain MD. In 1995 the Committee of Barany Society proposed a classification that is similar to the AAO-HNS criteria, it includes only two categories: definite MD and probable MD. A variety of medical and surgical treatments have been developed to treat or control the symptoms. The treatment can be divided into non-destructive and destructive procedures.

Keywords: meniere disease, hearing loss, deafness, inner ear, endolymphatic hydrops

INTRODUCTION

Endolymphatic hydrops is the increase of fluids in the inner ear. The morphological substrate of Meniere's disease, becomes histomorphologically evident by excavation of the Reissner's membrane in the paraffin sections of the cochlea. Although, Paparella described the cause (multifactorial inheritance, genetic) and pathogenesis (endolymphatic absorption) of Meniere's disease and its symptoms (mechanical and chemical); there are diseases that, according to Paparella, can predispose patients to endolymphatic hydrops and Meniere's disease. These diseases include: advanced otosclerosis with otosclerosis obstructing the vestibular aqueduct, chronic inactive otitis media and mastoiditis, syphilis, delayed MD symptoms, endolymphatic hydrops from childhood measles or mumps and sometimes sudden deafness. The latter responded well to medical and surgical therapy. Pathophysiology of symptoms of MD (vertigo, deafness, pressure, tinnitus, loudness intolerance) can be assessed through animal studies; observations of patients clinically and in sequential histopathological studies in patients with MD. Besides hydrops of pars inferior, there are hydrops of the pars superior, as well, with utricle enlargement. This would have allowed for potassium rich endolymph to bathe the basal surface of hair cells as well as the eighth cranial nerve endings. Repeated exposure to toxic potassium levels could cause vertigo episodes and a decline in hearing. There is currently no gold standard treatment for MD and endolymphatic hydrops. Non-destructive methods aim to reduce the symptoms of MD through dietary restrictions as well as through the use of betamethasone, citicoline, cinnarizine and diuretics. Isosorbide, is also used for MD to improve the endolymphatic hydrops. As with the cases of destructive procedures, surgical decompression of the endolymphatic sac, surgical or chemical labyrinthectomy and vestibular nerve section are applied in intractable cases. Recently, in research literature about MD, improvement in vertigo and hearing in patients with MD were described after application of positive pressure to the middle ear using the Meniett device.

CAUSE OF MENIERE'S DISEASE

In the mid- nineteenth century, the classical triad of episodic disabling vertigo (Thomas et al. 2018), fluctuating sensorineural hearing loss (Salvago et al. 2017, Martines, Maira, and Ferrara 2011), tinnitus (Sireci et al. 2012, Salvago et al. 2012, Neri et al. 2009), and a feeling of aural pressure was known as "apoplectic cerebral congestion" and was felt to be a brain disorder. Meniere demonstrated that this phenomenon was due to a labyrinthine dysfunction rather than a brain disease. After Guild discussed the longitudinal flow of endolymph, leading to the knowledge that the endolymphatic sac is the site of the outflow of endolymph in guinea pigs (Guild 1927). Numerous histopathological studies have clearly described, the importance of endolymphatic hydrops and Meniere's disease. Hydrops has been demonstrated to involve both the scala media and the otolithic organs of the inner ear. Hydrops has rarely been associated in only the vestibular portion, but it has been seen to involve only the cochlear portion (Dispenza, Cappello, et al. 2013). Traditionally, Meniere's symptom-complex has divided into two categories: the so-called Meniere's syndrome for which a known cause exists, and Meniere's disease, in which the process appears to be idiopathic (Paparella 1984). Subsequently, Paparella proposed a new simpler classification: a Meniere's disease extrinsic and a Meniere's disease intrinsic. The first is caused by etiological agents that have been shown, through histopathological correlations, to lead to hydrops and the symptomatology of Meniere's disease. These include etiological agents such as syphilis (Pulec 1972), trauma (Paparella and Mancini 1983), otosclerosis (Yoon, Paparella, and Schachern 1990), chronic otitis media (Martines et al. 2016, Ballacchino et al. 2015), allergy, tumors, leukemia and autoimmune disorders. The second category to consider is the intrinsic factors leading to Meniere's disease. Intrinsic factors are associated with multifactorial inheritance (Paparella 1985), as a cause can include extrinsic contributing factors as well as underlying intrinsic factors such as genetic predispositions and developmental anomalies (Martines et al. 2015, Fung et al. 2002). Of these the most important is genetic. Recently it is been observed the phenotypic and molecular changes in the organ of Corti auditory sensory epithelia and an increase in the number of hair cells and supporting cells, which suggested proliferation of those cells after knockdown of protein Hes 1 (hairy and enhancer of split) and protein COUP-TF1 (COUP Transcription Factor 1) using shRNA (short hairpin RNA) in the organ of Corti organotypic culture of three-day postnatal mice (Tang, Alger, and Pereira 2006). Multiple anomalies were found during endolymphatic sac surgery. These findings were seen in many mastoidectomies for chronic mastoiditis. The findings included hypopneumatization of the mastoid, a sigmoid sinus that is not lateral, but medial and anterior, hypo-development of the aditus and supra pyramidal recess and most importantly Trautmann's triangle, that plate of bone separating the sigmoid sinus from the posterior semi-circular canal which also separates the mastoid from the posterior cranial fossa. Trautmann's triangle may be oriented in a more vertical than horizontal orientation, but most importantly Trautmann's triangle is often reduced in size and can be absent in too many cases. In these patients the sigmoid sinus abuts against the bony wall of the solid angle containing the posterior semi-circular canal. In these cases it can be difficult to gain access to the dura containing the endolymphatic sac beneath the solid angle. Meniere's disease is defined by AAO-HNS as "an idiopathic disease involving the inner ear, that is characterized by vertigo, hearing loss and tinnitus. Meniere's disease has become accepted as the name used to describe these symptoms when they are presumed to be due to hydrops.

PATHOGENESIS OF MENIERE'S SYNDROME

Meniere's syndrome will be described in a number of proposed pathogenic mechanism. These include obstruction of the endolymphatic duct or dysfunction of the endolymphatic sac, overproduction (or up-regulation) of endolymphatic volume, infections, either bacterial or viral, immune-mediated etiologies, genetic causation or predisposition, and vascular disorders.

Endolymphatic hydrops of the membranous labyrinth was described in the pathogenesis of Meniere's syndrome by experiment of Kimura e Schuknecht (Kimura 1982) by surgical obstruction of the endolymphatic duct in the guinea pig. Surgical dissection or cauterization of the sac may cause endolymphatic hydrops in the guinea pig. Histological examination in several human temporal bones showed the presence of peri saccular fibrosis in the endolymphatic duct or sac in patients with Meniere's disease compared to normal (Ikeda and Sando 1984). Hypoplasia of the vestibular aqueduct as a cause of Meniere's syndrome has been suggested by an histological study of the human temporal bone and a difference in the radiographic appearance of the posterior fossa dural plate and the position of the lateral venous sinus. Also, small anatomical size, non-visualization of the duct using RMN and possible obstruction of the vestibular aqueduct by a diverticulum of the jugular bulb, have been described in some patients with Meniere's syndrome. Common to all of these observations is that the size of the duct or its capacity for radiographic visualization is correlated in some way with the function of the sac and fluid homeostasis of the inner ear. Although obstruction of the endolynphatic duct has been seen in a few human temporal bone specimens with endolymphatic hydrops and concomitant otosclerosis, frank obstruction of the endolymphatic space has been seen in a minority of temporal bones from patients who in life had Meniere's syndrome. The obstruction of some part of the endolymphatic compartment in patients with Meniere's syndrome may be the result, rather than the cause, of endolymphatic hydrops and due to displacement and distortion of limiting membranes of the inner ear (Sando and Ikeda 1984) (Masutani et al. 1991).

As an alternative to defective resorption of the endolymph, it has been suggested that the up-regulation, or overproduction, of endolymph could be another cause for the increased volume of the endolymphatic space found in temporal bones from patients with Meniere's syndrome. Plasma vasopressin levels and plasma antidiuretic hormone (P-ADH) have been demonstrated, by Takumida M. et al, to be elevated in patients with a clinical diagnosis of Meniere's syndrome. Keithley et al. could not demonstrate a significant increase in Na^+-K^+ ATPase in the stria vascularis from patients with Meniere's syndrome, compared to normal patients (Keithley, Horowitz, and Ruckenstein 1995). In fact, degenerative changes in the lateral cochlear wall in human Meniere's syndrome, would imply decreased activity in at least some enzymatic systems in endolymphatic hydrops. Sterkers et al. have described two osmotic gradients in the cochlea, one between the perilymphatic and endolymphatic spaces, and another within the endolymphatic space from apex to base. They concluded that interference with either gradient may cause endolymphatic hydrops. Juhn et al. have described the possible role of intrinsic metabolites of arachidonic acid in the fluid homeostasis of the inner ear and the interaction of external factors as drugs, stress hormones, and noise, with intrinsic perilymphatic prostaglandin levels and osmolarity.

Both bacterial and viral pathogens have been proposed as etiological agents in Meniere's syndrome. The classical example of bacterial causation of endolymphatic hydrops is syphilis, involving the endolymphatic duct, which includes generalized mononuclear leukocytic inflammatory response and endarteritis, that may also be involved in the pathogenesis of hydrops. In addition endolymphatic hydrops may also be caused by acute or chronic otitis media secondary to passage of bacterial toxins into the inner ear via the round window membrane. A delayed endolymphatic hydrops provides indirect evidence for viral causation of Meniere's syndrome. Endolymphatic hydrops seems to occur months or years following a previous damage to the inner ear, which in some cases may have been viral.

There are a number of known immune-mediated systemic diseases, which also cause inner ear symptoms and endolymphatic hydrops such as Cogan's syndrome and polyarteritis nodosa. In a number of studies evidence of immune hyperactivity has been demonstrated in patients with Meniere's syndrome. Circulating immune complexes have been demonstrated in the serum of some patients with Meniere's syndrome. More recently, a number of articles have demonstrated that 30% of patients with Meniere's syndrome have been reported to have circulating antibodies that reacted with a 58-kilodalton (kDa) antigen generated from animal inner ear protein. Similarly, circulating serum antibodies to a 68-kDa protein were found in some patients with Meniere's syndrome and in some patients with delayed endolymphatic hydrops (Rauch et al. 1995). Hydrops has been demonstrated following a Type 3 allergic reaction, and immunization against Type II collagen. It is clear that a number of disorders known to be immune-mediated may produce hearing loss and also endolymphatic hydrops (Fattori et al. 1994).

It also suggested that disorders of the microcirculation of the inner ear, including the venous drainage, may be significant in the pathogenesis of Meniere's syndrome. In the classical model of Meniere's syndrome, it has been suggested that endolymphatic hydrops may not be entirely due to physical obstruction of the endolymphatic duct, but may be partially mediated by interference with microcirculation of the endolymphatic sac of the vein at the vestibular aqueduct. It is demonstrated that endolymphatic hydrops in disorders of the microcirculation of the inner ear is immune-mediated in which a significant perivascular inflammatory response is common.

Genetic predisposition to development of endolymphatic hydrops is based on immune-regulatory mechanisms. There is an increased prevalence of the haplotype HLA B8/DR3 in patients with Meniere's syndrome.

Inner ear damage may leads to detachment of the otoliths causing Tumarkin's crisis with drop attack caused by a paroxysmal positional vertigo, which may be treated by maneuvers in the non-active phase (Dispenza, Kulamarva, and De Stefano 2012, Dispenza et al. 2011).

TREATMENT OF MENIERE'S DISEASE AND ENDOLYMPHATIC HYDROPS

The treatment of Meniere's disease remains one of most controversial areas in the field of otolaryngology. The most significant obstacle to define treatment is a lack of understanding of its underlying etiology and a variety of therapeutic options have been studied with conflicting results. Once an attack is established, vestibular suppressant and antiemetic medication have been used to control the vertigo, in association with electrolyte adjustment and rehydration. Treatment can be divided into non-destructive and destructive procedures. Non-destructive methods aim to reduce the symptoms of Meniere disease through dietary restrictions and lifestyle (voluptuary habits, greasy and allergic foods) as well as through the use of diuretics, steroids, drugs modulating the cholinergic system (scopolamine, atropine), or the histaminergic system (dimenhydrate, promethazine), or GABA system (benzodiazepine). On the other hand there are medications acting on voltage-gated ionic channels like the calcium channel blockers (nimodipine, flunarizine, cinnarizine). Betahistine is currently used in European countries for the management of Meniere disease. Recently, experimental and clinical studies on antisecretory system as a clinical innovation in Meniere's disease have been published. As for destructive procedures, surgical decompression of the endolymphatic sac, surgical or chemical labyrinthectomy and vestibular nerve section are applied for intractable cases. Meniett device is used to reduce vertigo and hearing in patients with Meniere disease after application of positive pressure to the middle ear.

A diet low in salt (<2 g) has been the mainstay of therapy. Sodium retention may result from endogenous hormonal responses to stress. No evidence indicates that sodium restriction alters the progression of the hearing loss, but it seems to help control symptoms significantly in many patients. Next, we suggest that patients avoid consuming caffeine, tobacco, alcohol, chocolate and allergens. Those patients who consume these seem to suffer more episodic dizziness and aural pressure.

We routinely use hydrochlorothiazide/triamterene, starting at a low dose (one 25-mg tablet per day for one week, after one 25 mg tablet every other day for two weeks, after one 25 mg tablet twice a week for two weeks) to control metabolic symptoms and reduce the sodium load on the inner ear. With this therapy, there is a need to supplement loss of liquids with potassium. Blood pressure can be measured before treatments and a week after; if it is low to begin with, we may not use diuretic therapy, and it may stop therapy if pressure drops later. It is also described the use of osmotic diuretics (mannitol, glycerol) administered intravenously. The rationale for their use is based on the supposition that these drugs can alter the fluid balance of inner ear, leading to a depletion of endolymph and a correction of hydrops (Stahle 1984).

Oral corticosteroid use is not advisable in patients with classic Meniere disease, but might it be advisable in patients with bilateral Meniere's symptom complex. Treatment with high doses oral of prednisone (1mg/Kg/day for five days and then taper it slowly over a further ten days). If patients' response is significant, we may reinstate the therapy, prolonging the use of the steroid until we reach a stable audiogram and symptomatology. The use of oral or intratympanic (dexamethasone) corticosteroids has also been proposed both to reduce the acuity of the crisis and to promote audio-vestibular recovery (Hargunani et al. 2006, Dispenza, De Stefano, et al. 2013).

In the past many patients used a patch for preventing motion sickness as well as a treatment for chronic low- grade dizziness, but manufacturing problems have made this drug unavailable. A tablet of 0,6 mg of atropine sublingually is an effective method of stopping an attack of vertigo. The atropine is absorbed through the oral mucosa and causes a parasympathomimetic blockade. A subcutaneous injection of atropine 0,4 mg is useful in an emergency room setting to help arrest an active attack.

Histaminergic system drugs are often prescribed for patients with dizziness or vertigo. The anti-emetic action is associated with a sedative effect, which many patients find intrudes on their ability to function during day-to-day. Antihistamines and phenothiazines, strong vestibular suppressants, can be used as anti-emetics in the control of vertigo; patients with Meniere's disease are often plagued with nausea and vomiting, as well as dizziness. Potentially habit- forming drugs must be used with care so as not to create dependency. They must be used only for a few days only because of their side effects (sedation, drowsiness) that delay the spontaneous vestibular compensation and slow down the recovery process. Benzodiazepines act on the cerebellar GABAergic system that inhibits vestibular nuclei response and on glycine receptors of the vestibule-spinal reflex that regulate the postural tone. Among this class, diazepam, clonazepam and lorazepam are used the most (Padoan et al. 1990).

Calcium channel blockers show vestibular suppressant activity because of their anticholinergic and antihistamine properties. They may act on the calcium channel of the vestibular dark cells modifying the ionic concentration in the endolymph. Side effects are tremors, drowsiness, weight gain and depression. Available in this category are flunarizine, cinnarizine, nimodipine and verapamil; these latter have been proposed in treating vertigo of vestibular peripheral origin and Meniere's disease particularly.

All the molecules described, separately or in combination, constitute a possible treatment during a crisis of Meniere's disease. The method of administration depends on the development of vegetative symptoms and the availability in the formulation of each molecule. It could be oral, intramuscularly, intravenously or rectally. It is important to remember that, because of the action inhibiting the vestibular compensation of most of these drugs, their use should be limited to the acute phase and stopped as soon as possible (Martines et al. 2012).

Betahistine favors vestibular compensation and it may play an important role in helping patients to recover more quickly after each episode. Betahistine, an analogue of histamine with strong inverse agonist action on the H3 histamine receptors, is currently used in European countries for the management of Meniere's disease. It significantly reduces the incidence and severity of vertigo when compared to cinnarizine, flunarizine or Ginko biloba. Betahistine efficacy can be explained by mechanisms targeting the histamine receptors at three different levels: the vascular tree, the central nervous system, and the peripheral vestibular system. In patients with Meniere's disease, betahistine reduced the intensity and frequency of vertigo significantly. However, the therapeutic effect of betahistine is dose- and duration dependent. High doses of betahistine (at least 48 mg/day) and long-term betahistine treatment (six to nine months) seem two necessary requirements for the prophylactic treatment of Meniere's disease and the improvement of vestibular compensation. According to the new theory of the Meniere attack as an ischemia/reperfusion disorder of inner ear sensory tissue, betahistine could therefore regulate and normalize the reduced perfusion pressure in the inner ear of patients with endolymphatic hydrops (Lacour 2013).

The anti-secretory factor (AF) is a 41 Kd protein secreted in plasma and other tissue fluids in mammals. This protein provides protection against diarrheal diseases and intestinal inflammation. It has been postulated that AF may act as a modulator of water and ions by regulating chloride homeostasis through membranes, and an interaction with aquaporins has been claimed. The endogenous plasma level of anti-secretory factor is increased by enterotoxins and surprisingly also by certain food constituents. Specially Processed Cereals (SPC) is an AF-inducing medical food, developed by the Swedish R&D company, as well as an AF-rich egg yolk powder, Salovum. SPC-Flakes® are especially processed cereal optimized to increase endogenous AF plasma levels. A 14-28 days-long period of intake of SPC-Flakes® is necessary to obtain a significant AF plasma concentration, commonly followed by a positive clinical outcome. Because of the effects on hypersecretion in the gastro-intestinal tract, it was hypothesized that anti-secretory treatment with SPC could be valuable in other instances where fluid imbalance is thought to play a role, such as Meniere's disease. In an open pilot study, in some patients, the attacks of rotatory vertigo were reduced and hearing was normalized. Studies in rats using immunohistochemistry methods demonstrated that AF was localized to the cochlea and the vestibule of the inner ear, which led the authors to propose that AF could be a new regulator of endolymph. Recently, various authors have reported a significant reduction of vertigo in patients with Meniere' disease treated with SPC-Flakes® ranging between 50% and 60%. Significantly other authors have correlated the reduction of episodes of vertigo with an increase of AF plasma levels in patients with Meniere's disease performing the therapy. Today, the antisecretory factor protein is recognized as a fundamental regulator of fluid balance in mammals (Leong, Narayan, and Lesser 2013).

When intractable incapacitating vertigo cannot be controlled by other means, surgical intervention must be considered. In this situation it is desirable to recommend a procedure that offers a high likelihood of vertigo control with maximum hearing preservation.

We can divide intractable vertigo into conservative (endolymphatic sac surgeries, saculotomy, crioterapy, fistulization of the labyrinth) and destructive (vestibular neurectomies and labyrintectomies). The first type, conservative surgery for Meniere's disease had been used relatively infrequently, and reports by otologists were often not enthusiastic about the procedure's value.

Paparella published very good results of a technique with decompression and drainage. He emphasized that the experimental demonstration of the endolymphatic sac's role has not been conclusive, however, it appears that the sac does have a significant function in endolymphatic homeostasis. When endolymphatic homeostasis is disturbed and hydrops occurs, the sac appears a conceptually excellent site for decompression of the endolymphatic space. The sac is relatively distant from the cochlear and vestibular organs. There is also some evidence that the direction of the flow within the endolymphatic duct is away from these organs toward the sac. The surgical technique is essentially the same as any other trans-mastoid endolymphatic sac procedure, with the exposure of the endolymphatic sac below the lateral sinus. It is important to try to expose as much of the endolymphatic sac as possible. A probe is used to locate the endolymphatic duct to measure the amount of endolymphatic sac hidden by the posterior semicircular canal. The lateral edge of the endolymphatic sac is gently excised and lifted off the underlying dura. A probe can be placed between the endolymphatic sac and the dura. Next, the endolymphatic sac is transected inferiorly using a small knife. The endolymphatic sac can then be lifted off the dura and dissected superiorly, so the only attachment remains at the duct. The duct is then grasped with angled cupped forceps and avulsed to try to remove as much of the intraosseous portion as possible.

Chemical labyrinthectomy consists of instilling into the middle ear streptomycin or gentamicin with the intention to reduce or abolish vestibular activity in the afflicted ear whilst preserving hearing. Gentamicin is less cochleotoxic than streptomycin when instilled directly into the middle ear. The absorption of drugs into the inner ear is via the round window or the anular ligament of the oval window. The treatment protocols using intratympanic gentamicin can be divided into fixed dose protocols and titration protocols. Fixed dose protocols aim to administer a fixed dose of gentamicin over a predetermined interval. The treatment is discontinued earlier only if the patient develops symptoms or signs of ototoxicity. Titration protocols aim to administer gentamicin until the patient demonstrates evidence of ototoxicity. Our protocol consists of instilling gentamicin 40 mg/cc through a single weekly injection technique. The solution is introduced into the middle ear with an epidural needle into the anterior-inferior quadrant of the eardrum until the middle ear is full. A bone conduction audiogram and clinical assessment is performed daily before the next administration. Low dose, varying interval, protocols offer the attraction of a reduced incidence of hearing loss (De Stefano et al. 2007). However, they require a significant time investment and may require multiple treatments for the control of vertigo. Intratympanic gentamicin is an effective treatment modality for the control of vertigo in severe unilateral Meniere's disease. It offers an alternative to the traditional surgical procedures of vestibular neurectomy and labyrinthectomy. Complete or substantial control of vertigo is noted in 90% of patients. Vestibular neurectomy is considered when medical management fails. In the retrolabyrinthine approach to the vestibular nerve combined with the retrolabyrinthine-retrosigmoid approach to the vestibular nerve, the facial nerve is routinely monitored. In the retrolabyrinthine approach an anteriorly based postauricolar flap is elevated with the periosteum and postauricular muscles in a single layer. A mastoidectomy is performed and bone is removed over and behind the sigmoid sinus. The endolymphatic sac and the surrounding dura are widely exposed. The vertical portion of the facial nerve, the posterior wall of the external auditory canal, and the posterior semicircular canal are identified and preserved. The sigmoid sinus is collapsed and retracted posteriorly using a retractor. The dura anterior to the sigmoid sinus is incised, creating an anteriorly based flap around the endolymphatic sac. A 1,5-2 cm wide Penrose drain is placed over the cerebellum, which is gently retracted as the arachnoid is opened with an arachnoid dissector instrument to allow the cerebrospinal fluid to escape. The vestibular nerve section is then performed under high-power magnification. The dura is closed using interrupted 4-0 silk sutures. Temporalis fascia is placed over the dura, the mastoid cavity is then filled with adipose tissue and the wound closed in layers. However a watertight closure is generally not possible and the 10% incidence of cerebrospinal fluid leakage has led to an evolution in technique of the retrosigmoid-internal auditory canal approach (RSG-IAC) and finally of the combined retrolabyrinthine-retrosigmoid approach (RRVN).

The RSG-IAC approach was developed in an attempt to improve results of the vestibular neurectomy near the labyrinth, where the fibers are more clearly delineated and decrease the incidence of cerebrospinal fluid leakage. Within the internal auditory canal, the cleavage plane between the cochlear and vestibular fibers is more developed near the labyrinth and thus a more complete and selective vestibular nerve section can be performed. A posterior fossa craniotomy is performed behind the sigmoid sinus. After the cerebrospinal fluid is released from the cerebellopontine cistern the cerebellum falls away. The jugular dural fold and the VIIIth cranial nerve are identified. The posterior wall of the external auditory canal is drilled with a diamond burr to the singular canal. Next, the dura in the internal auditory canal is incised. The superior vestibular nerve and the singular nerve, the branch of the inferior vestibular nerve to the posterior semicircular superior canal (SSC), are sectioned at this point. The branch of the inferior vestibular nerve to the saccule is preserved since the saccule has no known vestibular function in man and sectioning it would place the hearing at risk. With this procedure, no abdominal fat is needed to fill the defect since this approach does not require a mastoidectomy. Also, the dura can be closed in a watertight fashion. The retrosigmoid approach solved the cerebrospinal fluid leakage problem, however, because of the frequent incidence of severe headaches, this approach was discontinued in1987. The headaches were felt to be related drilling the bone over the internal auditory canal, causing a bone dust arachnoiditis.

The combined RRVN approach represents a further evolution in posterior fossa approaches to vestibular neurectomy. A limited mastoidectomy is performed, opening a few mastoid air cells. The bone over the sigmoid sinus is removed from the transverse sinus to the jugular bulb of about 3 cm. The dura posterior to the sigmoid sinus is exposed for 1,5-2 cm. A dural incision is made 3 mm behind and parallel to the sigmoid sinus. The sigmoid is retracted forward using three stay sutures placed along the dural cuff. This affords visualization of the posterior wall of the temporal bone, the jugular dural fold, and allows wide exposure of the cerebellopontine angle without retraction of the cerebellum. After the cerebellopontine angle cistern is opened and cerebrospinal fluid released, the vestibular nerve is identified and sectioned. On occasion when a cleavage plane cannot be visualized, the internal auditory canal can be opened and the nerve sectioned, as outlined under the RSG-IAC approach. The internal auditory canal is no longer opened for vestibular nerve section. In cases with a poor cleavage plane, the superior half of the VIIIth nerve is sectioned near the brain stem. Once the procedure is completed, the exposed mastoid air cells are sealed with bone wax and the dura is closed in a watertight fashion with interrupted silk sutures. Abdominal fat is used to fill in the bony defect for cosmetic purposes and to reinforce the dural closure. The skin is closed with staples without a drain. This approach was developed in an effort to streamline the procedure further by shortening the operating time, making a watertight closure of the dura possible, and allowing exposure for drilling the internal auditory canal when necessary.

Pressure treatment is regarded as one of the therapeutical options to offer to disable Meniere's disease, when the patients are not responding to any medical treatment. The Meniett device is a portable instrument that allows a patient to self-administer treatments at home, whenever required. The Meniett device has become, at some centers, a conservative procedure without risk of additional damage to the inner ear, such as when applying intra-tympanic gentamicin. This therapy started to be always proposed to those Meniere's patients already selected for vestibular neurectomy surgery. The protocol consisted in insertion of a short-term trans-tympanic ventilation tube and in one-month treatment that started the same day. Each patient was instructed to use the device five times per day, for three minutes per session. During the month of treatment, each patient was asked to fill in a diary, noting any symptom related to Meniere's disease (Gates et al. 2006).

A simple surgical intervention is performed, under local anesthesia, inserting a short-term trans- tympanic ventilation tube, with the aim of reducing intralabyrithine pressure and decreasing the potential high pressure of the middle ear. Some patients report an improvement or a disappearance of vertigo (Park, Chen, and Westhofen 2009, Dispenza et al. 2015).

CONCLUSION

Meniere's disease raises great interest for many reasons:

- It is necessary to make a precise clinical analysis to decide the diagnosis;
- Specific examinations are available to confirm the diagnosis;
- The therapeutic medical or surgical support is various and variable;
- Clinical and research pathways are multiple.

Beyond the clinical expressions, Meniere's disease imposes a better understanding of mechanisms involving homeostasis of the inner ear and its troubles. The diversity of clinical expression, in particular the variability of the intensity and symptoms, justifies individual care to establish appropriate treatment.

REFERENCES

Ballacchino, A, P Salvago, E Cannizzaro, R Costanzo, M Di Marzo, S Ferrara, E La Mattina, G Messina, M Mucia, A Mulè, F Plescia, F Sireci, S Rizzo, and F Martines. 2015. "Association between sleep-disordered breathing and hearing disorders: Clinical observation in Sicilian patients." *Acta Medica Mediterranea* 31:607-614.

De Stefano, A, F Dispenza, G De Donato, A Caruso, A Taibah, and M Sanna. 2007. "Intratympanic gentamicin: a 1-day protocol treatment for unilateral Meniere's disease." *Am J Otolaryngol* 28 (5):289-93.

Dispenza, F, F Cappello, G Kulamarva, and A De Stefano. 2013. "The discovery of the stapes." *Acta Otolaryngol Ital* 33 (5):357-359.

Dispenza, F, A De Stefano, C Costantino, D Rando, M Giglione, R Stagno, and E Bennici. 2015. "Canal switch and re-entry phenomenon in benign paroxysmal positional vertigo: difference between immediate and delayed occurrence." *Acta Otolaryngol Ital* 35:116-120.

Dispenza, F, G Kulamarva, and A De Stefano. 2012. "Comparison of repositioning maneuvers for benign paroxysmal positional vertigo of posterior semicircular canal: advantages of hybrid maneuver." *Am J Otolaryngol* 33:528-532.

Dispenza, F, A De Stefano, C Costantino, D Marchese, and F Riggio. 2013. "Sudden Sensorineural Hearing Loss: Results of intratympanic steroids as salvage treatment." *Am J Otolaryngol* 34 (4):296-300.

Dispenza, F, A De Stefano, N Mathur, A Croce, and S Gallina. 2011. "Benign paroxysmal positional vertigo following whiplash injury: a myth or a reality?" *Am J Otolaryngol* 32:376-380. doi: doi:10.1016/j.amjoto.2010.07.009.

Fattori, B, P Ghilardi, A Casani, P Migliorini, and L Riente. 1994. "Meniere's disease: Role of antibodies against basement membrane antigens." *Laryngoscope* 104:1290-1294.

Fung, K, Y Xie, S F Hall, D P Lillicrap, and S A M Taylor. 2002. "Genetic basis of familial Meniere's disease." *J Otolaryngol* 31:1-4.

Gates, G A, A Verrall, J D Green Jr, D L Tucci, and S A Telian. 2006. "Meniett clinical trial: Long-term follow-up." *Arch Otolaryngol Head Neck Surg* 132:1311-1316.

Guild, S, 1927. "The circulation of endolymph." *Am J Anat*:39-57.

Hargunani, C A, J B Kempton, J M De Gagne, and D R Trune. 2006. "Intratympanic injection of dexamethasone: Time course of inner ear distribution and conversion to its active form." *Otol Neurotol* 27:564-569.

Ikeda, M, and I Sando. 1984. "Endolymphatic duct and sac in patients with meniere's disease: A temporal bone histopathological." *Ann Otol Rhinol Laryngol* 93:540-546.

Keithley, E M, S Horowitz, and M J Ruckenstein. 1995. "Na,K-atpase in the cochlear lateral wall of human temporal bones with endolymphatic hydrops." *Ann Otol Rhinol Laryngol* 104:858-863.

Kimura, R S, 1982. "Animal models of endolymphatic hydrops." *Am J Otolaryngol* 3:447-451.

Lacour, M, 2013. "Betahistine treatment in managing vertigo and improving vestibular compensation: Clarification." *J Vest Res* 23:139-151.

Leong, S C, S Narayan, and T H Lesser. 2013. "Antisecretory factor-inducing therapy improves patient-reported functional levels in Meniere's disease." *Ann Otol Rhinol Laryngol* 122:619-624.

Martines, F, M Agrifoglio, D Bentivegna, M Mucia, P Salvago, F Sireci, and A Ballacchino. 2012. "Treatment of tinnitus and dizziness associated vertebrobasilar insufficiency with a fixed combination of cinnarizine and dimenhydrinate." *Acta Medica Mediterranea* 28:291-296.

Martines, F, E Maira, and S Ferrara. 2011. "Age-related hearing impairment (arhi): A common sensory deficit in the elderly." *Acta Medica Mediterranea* 27:47-52.

Martines, F, A Ballacchino, F Sireci, M Mucia, E La Mattina, S Rizzo, and P Salvago. 2016. "Audiologic profile of OSAS and simple snoring patients: the effect of chronic nocturnal intermittent hypoxia on auditory function." *European Archives of Oto-Rhino-Laryngology* 273 (6):1419-1424. doi: 10.1007/s00405-015-3714-6.

Martines, F, P Salvago, C Bartolotta, S Cocuzza, C Fabiano, S Ferrara, E La Mattina, M Mucia, P Sammarco, F Sireci, and E Martines. 2015. "A genotype–phenotype correlation in Sicilian patients with GJB2 biallelic mutations." *European Archives of Oto-Rhino-Laryngology* 272 (8):1857-1865. doi: 10.1007/s00405-014-2970-1.

Masutani, H, H Takahashi, I Sando, and H Sato. 1991. "Vestibular Aqueduct in Meniere's Disease and Non-Meniere's Disease With Endolymphatic Hydrops: A Computer Aided Volumetric Study." *Auris Nasus Larynx* 18:351-357.

Neri, G, A De Stefano, C. Baffa, G Kulamarva, P Di Giovanni, G Petrucci, A Poliandri, F Dispenza, L Citraro, and A Croce. 2009. "Treatment of central and sensorineural tinnitus with orally administred Melatonin and Sulodexide: personal experience from a randomized controlled study." *Acta Otolaryngol Ital* 29:86-91.

Padoan, S, K Korttila, M Magnusson, I Pyykkö, and L Schalén. 1990. "Reduction of gain and time constant of vestibulo-ocular reflex in man induced by diazepam and thiopental." *J Vest Res* 1:97-104.

Paparella, M M, 1984. "Pathogenesis of Meniere's disease and Meniere's syndrome." *Acta Otolaryngol* 98 (suppl. 406):10-25.

Paparella, M M, 1985. "The cause (multifactorial inheritance) and pathogenesis (endolymphatic malabsorption) of meniere's disease and its symptoms (mechanical and chemical)." *Acta Otolaryngol* 99:445-451.

Paparella, M M, and F Mancini. 1983. "Trauma and meniere's syndrome." *Laryngoscope* 93:1004-1012.

Park, J J H, Y S Chen, and M Westhofen. 2009. "Meniere's disease and middle ear pressure - Vestibular function after transtympanic tube placement." *Acta Otolaryngol* 129:1408-1413.

Pulec, J L, 1972. "Symposium on meniere's disease: I. Meniere's disease: Results of a two and one-halfyear study of etiology, natural history and results of treatment." *Laryngoscope* 82:1703-1715.

Rauch, S D, J E San Martin, R A Moscicki, and L J Bloch. 1995. "Serum antibodies against heat shock protein 70 in Meniere's disease." *Am J Otol* 16:648-652.

Salvago, P, A Ballacchino, M Agrifoglio, S Ferrara, M Mucia, and F Sireci. 2012. "Tinnitus patients: Etiologic, audiologic and psychological profile." *Acta Medica Mediterranea* 28:171-175.

Salvago, P, S Rizzo, A Bianco, and F Martines. 2017. "Sudden sensorineural hearing loss: is there a relationship between routine haematological parameters and audiogram shapes?" *Int J Audiol* 56:148-153.

Sando, I, and M Ikeda. 1984. "The vestibular aqueduct in patients with meniere's disease: A temporal bone histopathological investigation." *Acta Otolaryngol* 97:558-570.

Sireci, F, A Ballacchino, M Agrifoglio, S Ferrara, M Mucia, and P Salvago. 2012. "Psychopathologic diseases in patients with tinnitus: A case-control of an outpatient cohort. Acta Medica Mediterranea 2012; 28 (2):167-170." *Acta Medica Mediterranea* 28:167-170.

Stahle, J, 1984. "Medical treatment of fluctuant hearing loss in Meniere's disease." *Am J Otol* 5:529-533.

Tang, L S, H M Alger, and F A Pereira. 2006. "COUP-TFI controls Notch regulation of hair cell and support cell differentiation." *Development* 133:3683-3693.

Thomas, E, F Martines, A Bianco, G Messina, V Giustino, D Zangla, A Iovane, and A Palma. 2018. "Decreased postural control in people with moderate hearing loss." *Medicine* (United States) 97:e0244. doi: 10.1097/MD.0000000000010244.

Yoon, T H, M M Paparella, and P A Schachern. 1990. "Otosclerosis involving the vestibular aqueduct and Meniere's disease." *Otolaryngol Head Neck Surg* 103:107-112.

Chapter 11

AUTOIMMUNE INNER EAR DISEASE

*Francesco Dispenza[1,2], MD, PhD, Alessia Ceraso[2], MD,
Antonina Mistretta[2], MD, Gabriele Ebbreo[2], MD,
Francesco Barbara[3], MD and Alessia Maria Battaglia[2], MD*

[1]Istituto Euromediterraneo di Scienza e Tecnologia, IEMEST, Palermo, Italy
[2]U.O.C. Otorinolaringoiatria Azienda Ospedaliera Universitaria
Policlinico P. Giaccone, Palermo, Italy
[3]Otolayngology Unit, Department of Basic Medical Science,
Neuroscience and Sensory Organs, University of Bari Aldo Moro, Bari, Italy

ABSTRACT

Nowadays, autoimmune deafness does not appear to be as a well-defined nosological entity, although the ability of the inner ear to react to genetic, environmental and autoimmune phenomena has been demonstrated. The scientific evidence shows sensorineural deafness, usually bilateral, rapidly progressive and debilitating, which mostly affects women (from 30 to 50 years) and is associated with vestibular symptoms and 30% of autoimmune diseases. The clinical diagnosis, without specific laboratory tests, is made most of the time, as exclusion.

Generally, autoimmune deafness is rapidly progressive and is characterized by a reduction of more than 30 db on three adjacent frequencies. It appears over a period of weeks or a few months. The best diagnostic test, in general, is the improvement of hearing observed after treatment with corticosteroids or immunosuppressants.

Regarding the onset of autoimmune deafness, it is possible to identify different factors: genetic hypothesis with particular HLA suggesting genetic susceptibility to pathology and environmental hypotheses, namely exogenous (viral, toxic) factors that ease its onset. Otoscopy is usually within limits, audiometry doesn't show particular features and it is possible to observe curves with falling plateaus on acute sounds. The differential diagnosis is important with diseases such as carcinosis, ear tumors, ototoxicity, syphilis, and Ménière's disease. In absence of specific tests, what is typically provided is: a) dosage of inflammation markers (ESR and PCR); b) search for antibodies that can be found in autoimmune diseases (ANCA, ANA Cryoglobulins, Anti-endomysial antibodies, Anti-core, Anti-Mitochondria, Anti-muscle smooth, etc.); c) viral serology; d) tests to explore humoral and cellular immunity.

Therefore, therapy involves not only the use of corticosteroids (oral or transtympanic) or immunosuppressants, but also of plasmapheresis, gamma globulin and, finally, the installation of a cochlear implant.

Keywords: autoimmune, hearing loss, deafness, immunology, ear

INTRODUCTION

Already in 1958, Lehnhardt studied recursive bilateral cases of deafness, attributing them to the presence of autoantibodies. The immune system is complex and formed by a series of balances that allow to recognize our body the self from non-self. If one of these mechanisms that guarantee equilibrium should fail, an autoimmune pathology occurs.

The Autoimmune Inner Ear Disease (AIED) was first described by McCabe in 1979 as Bilateral Sensorineural Hearing Loss (SNHL) that progressed over weeks to months and was responsive to immunosuppressive agents; hence he proposed an autoimmune mechanism. Since that time, a large body of evidence in support of the immune hypothesis has been proposed; however, the underlying pathophysiology remains unknown and is likely to be varied. Elucidating the underlying immune mechanism is important, because immune-mediated hearing loss is one of the few causes of SNHL that is reversible.

Inner ear, also called labyrinth of the ear, is a part of the ear that contains organs of the senses of hearing and equilibrium. The bony labyrinth, a cavity in the temporal bone, is divided into three sections: the vestibule, the semicircular canals, and the cochlea. (Dispenza, Cappello, et al. 2013). Within the bony labyrinth is a membranous labyrinth, which is also divided into three parts: the semicircular ducts; two saclike structures, the saccule and utricle, located in the vestibule; and the cochlear duct, which is the only part of the inner ear involved in hearing. The cochlear duct forms a shelf across the cochlea dividing it into two sections, the scala vestibuli and the scala tympani. The bony labyrinth contains the otic capsule, which is denser than the surrounding temporal bone. The entire inner ear is bathed in a cushioning fluid, called the endolymph when it lies within the membranous labyrinth and the perilymph when it separates the bony and membranous labyrinths (Martines et al. 2015, Rizzo et al. 2016, Salvago et al. 2017).

AUTOIMMUNE INNER EAR DISEASE PATHOLOGY

It is complex to have a precise definition of the pathology known as autoimmune deafness, since most of the time the diagnosis is made by exclusion or given by the response to the treatment with corticosteroids.

According to the literature data, autoimmune deafness refers to a rapidly progressive bilateral and asymmetric sensorineural deafness, with associated vestibular signs and a slight prevalence for women in their middle age (factor in common with all the other autoimmune diseases) and with a systemic disease associated with a percentage that is around 25% of cases.

AIED manifests clinically as SNHL that progress over weeks. Most commonly affects women between the ages of 20 and 50 years. The inner ear is not an immune-privileged site, and the endolymphatic sac is critical for the immune response.

Sudden autoimmune deafness seems to be very rare, and the self-priming residing in the presence of autoimmune agents would destroy or directly affect the inner ear.

Causes of the pathology can be: environmental factors and genetic factors.

Environmental Factors

These are infectious agents (for example, parts of viruses or other infectious agents) that, according to a mechanism of molecular mimicry, would be recognized as non-self structures of the human organism.

Genetic Factors

In the years 2001-2005, 88 patients were recruited and subjected to routine serological tests and also tests for the determination of antibodies hsp70. Patients were divided into three groups: patients with Autoimmune Sensorineural Hearing Loss (ASNHL), patients with idiopathic ASNHL associated with Cogan Syndrome and patients with ASNHL associated with Systemic Autoimmune Disease (SAD). The study confirmed the value of the anti-hsp70 test in the diagnosis of autoimmune deafness, promoting it as a marker capable of identifying an autoimmune origin of hearing loss (Boulassel et al. 2001, Bovo, Aimoni, and Martini 2006).

MicroRNAs (miRNAs) regulate the differentiation and development of inner ear cells. Mutations in miRNAs lead to deafness in humans and mice. Among inner ear pathologies, inflammation may lead to structural and neuronal defects and eventually to hearing loss and vestibular dysfunction. While the genetic factors of these pathways have not been defined, autoimmunity participates in these processes. Is reported that inflammatory stimuli in the inner ear induce activation of the innate immune system via miR-224 and pentraxin 3 (Ptx3). miR-224 is a transcriptional target of nuclear factor κB, a key mediator of innate immunity. Ptx3 is a regulator of the immune response. It is released in response to inflammation and regulated by nuclear factor κB. Is shown that miR-224 and Ptx3 are expressed in the inner ear and is demonstrated that miR-224 targets Ptx3. As a model for the innate immune response, lipopolysaccharide is injected into the scala tympani of mouse inner ears. This resulted in changes in the levels of miR-224 and Ptx3, in addition to activation of the complement system, as measured by immune cell infiltration and activated C3. This suggests that while miR-224 regulates Ptx3 under normal conditions, upon inflammation, both are recruited to offer a front line of defense in acting as responders to inflammation in the inner ear. miR-224 diminishes the innate immune response by downregulating Ptx3 expression, while Ptx3 stimulates the innate immune response (Rudnicki et al. 2014).

Yet a role for development is suggested by intriguing overlaps in particular organs targeted in autoimmune diseases, in this case type 1 diabetes and Primary Sjogren's Syndrome (PSS). Patients with diabetes type 1 have high rates of concomitant PSS, and both conditions are associated with hearing loss and tongue abnormalities. All of these co-occurrences are found in organs tracing their lineage to the developmental transcription factor Hox11, which is expressed in embryonic cells destined for the pancreas, salivary glands, tongue, cranial nerves and cochlea (Lonyai et al. 2008).

Diagnosis

Making a diagnosis of ASNHL is not simple; it is necessary to have an accurate knowledge of the patient in terms of medical history, collection of instrumental examinations, laboratory tests and radiological examinations useful to diagnose any underlying multi-organ pathology.

An interesting retrospective study in which 19 cases of patients with bilateral ASNHL were presented, with clinical features, laboratory tests, instrumental examinations, audiometric and radiological examinations with relative prognosis for each case described. Among these 19 cases, 78.9% of patients presented non-otological diseases with multisystem and multi-organ disorders, with diseases of the central nervous system such as viral or bacterial meningitis, 5 patients on the other hand had pathologies of the concomitant immune system, with characteristic deafness progressive and simultaneous bilateral autoimmune type. It is therefore necessary, first of all, to identify the etiology of the underlying disease by admitting its treatment to treat and try to resolve the associated deafness (Gao et al. 2015).

Currently, there is any reliable test in order to detect immunocompetent cells or direct and specific circulating antibodies against certain labyrinth structures.

The sensitivity and the specificity of the various tests proposed in the literature must be interpreted with caution, since in the absence of standard comparators, there are numerous methodological distortions that can lead astray and therefore towards incorrectly correct diagnoses.

The implementation of the complementary budget, particularly the laboratory one, is a function of the anamnesis where previous personal and family history, traumas of long standing, recent viral syndrome, recent vaccination or intake of an ototoxic drug, must be sought. The otoscopic and vestibular examination with subjective audiometry (audiometry) and objective measures (auditory evoked potentials, otoemissions) and instrumental vestibular tests, will then be completed (Hervier et al. 2010, Dispenza and De Stefano 2012).

Cogan's Syndrome

Cogan's syndrome (**CS**) is a rare chronic autoimmune disease, characterized by interstitial keratitis and sensorineural hearing loss. It may also be accompanied by systemic vasculitis (large vessel vasculitis, aortitis, medium-sized vessel vasculitis) (St Clair and McCallum 1999). The etiology of CS is still unknown; environmental exposure to toxic substances or pollutants, viral infections, cigarette smoking might be some triggers for the disease (Gluth et al. 2006). The pathogenesis is now supposed to be based on circulating autoantibodies and endothelial antigens that are found in the inner ear in CS patients, but are not found in the sera of patients with other autoimmune diseases. Lunardi et al. identified "the Cogan peptide" as an amino acid sequence related to six autoantigens; CD148 (a transmembrane protein expressed in the inner ear) and connexine 26 (a gap junction protein highly expressed in the inner ear) are two of these six autoantigens that have been studied. They might be two inner ear targets for autoantibodies (Lunardi, Bason, and Leandri 2002).

Crohn's disease, ulcerative colitis, sarcoidosis, hypothyroidism, and interstitial nephritis and other autoimmune diseases may present in association with CS. That supports the hypothesis that CS is an autoimmune disease too (Grasland et al. 2004).

Usually, CS initially presents with vestibule-auditory pathologies. The most common presenting symptom is sudden bilateral sensory hearing loss. Inner ear manifestations of CS are Ménière's-like attacks consisting of vertigo, hearing loss, tinnitus, ataxia, nausea, and vomiting. Vestibular and auditory dysfunctions develop quickly, and recurrent episodes of inner ear disease result frequently in deafness. Once the hearing loss is deep, vertigo and other vestibular symptoms usually disappear.

According to Oshrat et al. mandatory criteria for CS diagnosis are: sensorineural hearing loss, inflammatory ocular disease (classically interstitial keratitis), alternative causes of inflammation or infection ruled out.

Prevalent additional criteria are vertigo and tinnitus, ataxia and dizziness, fever, weight loss, fatigue, lymphadenopathy, and headache. Possible additional criteria are vasculitis and elevation of systemic inflammatory markers.

There are basically three therapeutic approaches. Topical steroid to treat mild ocular disease without other symptoms. Prednisone (1 mg/kg/day) is prescribed when inner ear, ocular and systemic symptoms are present; this treatment should produce a short period of intense immunosuppression. If improvement occurs doses can be tapered down after 2 to 4 weeks. In cases of relapse, corticosteroid dose should be increased again.1 Therapeutic doses are chosen according to clinical response, in order to reduce the steroid dosage below 10 mg/day. Additional immunosuppressive drugs are methotrexate, azathioprine, cyclophosphamide, cyclosporine (D'Aguanno et al. 2018).

A biologic therapy using infliximab (anti-TNF-α) could be considered after treatment with steroids if:

1) Lack of response to steroids within 2–3 weeks;
2) Inability to reduce the steroid dosage below 10 mg/day;
3) The use of steroids is contraindicated in light of the patient's medical status (e.g., diabetes, hypertension, or if there are significant sides effects).

The use of infliximab as first-line therapy could be started in selected patients:

1) Patients with severe ocular involvement, which jeopardizes the patient's eyesight (scarring and elevated intraocular pressure);
2) Rapid hearing loss (hearing level approaching 50 Hz);
3) When both ears are simultaneously affected;
4) Evidence of systemic involvement: large vessels vasculitis, involvement of the heart, kidneys, and nervous system;
5) The patient's general condition precludes the use of high-dose steroids (severe heart failure, uncontrolled diabetes, or hypertension).

Vogt-Koyanagi-Harada Syndrome

Vogt-Koyanagi-Harada (VKH) syndrome is an idiopathic, multisystem autoimmune disorder characterized by bilateral granulomatous uveitis with neurologic, auditory or dermatologic symptoms.

Otologic complaints are sensorineural hearing loss, tinnitus and/or vertigo that typically coincide with the onset of ocular pathology (Ondrey et al. 2006).

The diagnosis of VKH disease is based on both ocular and extraocular symptoms and signs. The current diagnostic criteria only include tinnitus, not hearing loss, as an auditory finding (Read et al. 2001).

Nevertheless, according to Morita et al., 89.4% of the subjects affected by VKH included in their study were found to be suffering from hearing loss on the basis of audiometric findings, while only 34.1% complained of tinnitus. This might be explained by the mild degree of hearing loss that can be noticed easily with audiometry but doesn't match with subjective hearing loss. That's why they suggest to do auditory examinations to every VKH patient, in order to evaluate any degree of hearing loss, whether or not the loss is clinically relevant (Morita et al. 2014).

The diagnosis is clinical; the eye exam is fundamental, looking for iridocyclitis and posterior uveitis.

The cochleo-vestibular involvement appears in 33 to 75% of cases. Evolution in deafness is usually progressive; rarely can it be sudden. The severity of this impairment is variable. The prognosis is improved by early diagnosis and treatment, and adequate management based on prolonged corticosteroid therapy with or without immunosuppressors.

Susac's Syndrome

Susac's syndrome (SS) classically presents with the clinical triad of sensorineural hearing loss, retinal artery occlusion and encephalopathy plus the neuroimaging triad of white matter lesions, deep gray matter lesions, and leptomeningeal disease. It's a rare disease. Initial SS is characterised by incomplete clinical or neuroimaging triads; this makes it difficult to be diagnosed.

It is now thought that it is an immune-mediated endotheliopathy that affects the microvasculature of the brain, retina, and inner ear. The incidence of SS is higher in females than in males (3:1), in fact there is a female predominance in autoimmunity diseases. Antiendothelial cell antibodies (AECAs) mediate the endothelial cell injury with consequent deposition of thrombotic material in the lumen of the small vessel (Magro et al. 2011).

Patients with SS must be treated quickly and aggressively. Medical treatments start with a pulse of highly dosed methylprednisolone (1000 mg/day for 5 days), tapering it in the following weeks, according to the patient condition. It is usually provided also an antithrombotic and anticoagulation treatment (García-Carrasco et al. 2011).

In the worst cases, addition of mycophenolate mofetil or rituximab is required, followed by cyclophosphamide when disease is refractory to other medications.

Rheumatoid Arthritis

Rheumatoid Arthritis (RA) is a chronic autoimmune inflammatory disorder that can affect joints. In some people, the condition also can damage a wide variety of body systems, including the skin, eyes, lungs, ear, heart and blood vessels. The initial site of disease is the synovial membrane, where swelling and congestion lead to infiltration by immune cells. Three phases of progression of RA are an initiation phase (due to non-specific inflammation), an amplification phase (due to T cell activation), and chronic inflammatory phase, with tissue injury resulting from the cytokines, IL–1, TNF-alpha and IL–6. Patients with RA had a high prevalence of sensorineural hearing loss for high and very high frequencies.

RA is thought to induce conductive hearing loss and/or sensorineural hearing loss. Ahmadzadeh et al. evaluated the function of the middle ear and cochlea, and the related factors in patients with RA; they detected higher bone conduction thresholds in some frequencies of RA patients, but not clinically significant. Otherwise they confirmed that sensorineural hearing loss is significantly more prevalent in refractory rheumatoid arthritis patients. This study revealed that sensorineural hearing loss is frequently due to medical treatment with azathioprine, cyclosporine and etanercept (Ahmadzadeh et al. 2017).

Primary Sjögren Syndrome

Primary Sjögren Syndrome (pSS) is a chronic autoimmune disease characterized by lymphocyte infiltration of both the salivary and lacrimal glands; its main symptoms are dry eyes and a dry mouth. Otologic symptoms may be an early indicator of pSS, but they are also a less-common feature of other autoimmune disorders (Tucci, Quatraro, and Silvestris 2005). Ziavra et al. founded SNHL in 22.5% (9/40) of pSS patients (Ziavra et al. 2000).

The most common hearing impairment has cochlear origin; it often involves high frequencies. Autoantibodies of both cardiolipin and M3 muscarinic receptors in the sera are suspected to play a pathogenetic role in the progressive hearing loss of pSS patients(Tucci, Quatraro, and Silvestris 2005).

The mechanism that leads to sensorineural damage might be vasculitis, neuritis, or an ototoxic effect of the drugs used to treat pSS (Tumiati, Casoli, and Parmeggiani 1997).

Polyarteritis Nodosa

Polyarteritis nodosa (PAN), also known as panarteritis nodosa, periarteritis nodosa, Kussmaul disease, or Kussmaul-Maier disease, is a systemic necrotizing inflammation of blood vessels (vasculitis) affecting small- or medium-sized muscular arteries, that typically involves the arteries of the kidneys, of lungs and other internal organs.

According to Wolf et al. the hearing loss that occurs in PAN is due largely to middle ear effusion but usually appears as a mixed type. Pure perceptive hearing loss is rare. A profound, rapidly deteriorating perceptive hearing loss could be the onset and only one symptom of PAN (Wolf et al. 1987).

Gussen detected that the cochlea as well as the vestibular system exhibited ischemic necrosis of the soft tissue structures with extensive fibrosis and bone formation; that is supposed to be one of the pathogenic mechanism of hearing impairment (Gussen 1977).

Systemic Lupus Erythematosus

Systemic Lupus Erythematosus (SLE) is an autoimmune disease with multiorgan involvement and an incidence of 12.5–39.0 per 100,000 people in the general population (Di Stadio and Ralli 2017). The pathophysiology of SLE is based on the production of autoantibodies that react with self-nuclear and cytoplasmic antigens, creating an immunologic attack on body organs, resulting in tissue inflammation and multiorgan damage (McCarty et al. 1995).

Di Stadio et al. performed a systematic literature review about hearing loss in patients affected by SLE. They assessed that SLE can damage tissues and organs through three different mechanisms: antibody/antigen direct reactions, cytotoxic action, and immune complex deposition(Di Stadio and Ralli 2017).

These mechanisms together create hearing impairment: immune complex deposition plays a central role in the development of inner ear vasculitis and is associated with atrophy of the stria vascularis. Progressive reduction of the vessel caliber increases the resistance in the circulatory system, eventually increasing the blood pressure. Oxygen deficit damages inner ear cells.

According to Di Stadio et al., corticosteroids should be considered as the first treatment option to restore hearing in patients with sudden hearing loss and prevent worsening of progressive hearing loss. If steroid therapy is unsuccessful cyclophosphamide should be used. Monoclonal antibodies should be used in patients with proven resistance to other treatments. Plasmapheresis and anticoagulant treatments could be a good preventive therapy for sudden sensorineural hearing loss (Di Stadio and Ralli 2017).

SPECIFIC TESTS OF THE INNER EAR

The Specific tests of the inner ear can be classified as follow: lymphoblastic transformation test concerning cellular immunity (TTL), western blot (humoral immunity) and indirect immunofluorescence test.

Lymphoblastic Transformation Test Concerning Cellular Immunity

The test consists in incubating the lymphocytes of patients stimulated with antigens belonging to the inner ear (human). To collect the material needed to perform the test, the antigens must be extracted by surgery conducted by translabyrintyne route. During these experiments conducted on a small number of patients, given the complexity of finding the biological material to perform the study, an increase in gamma interferon by T cells placed in the presence of antigens coming from the inner ear, was noted (Lorenz, Solares, and Williams 2002).

Western Blot

The test aims to identify specific circulating autoantibodies with respect to different antigens present in the human labyrinth, following their migration on a support according to their size and weight.

On this basis several candidate antigens were studied as targets in autoimmune deafness (Suslu, Yilmaz, and Gursel 2009):

- Type II collagen;
- Po-myelin;
- Beta-actin;
- Beta-tubulin;
- Different proteins with a molecular weight of 30, 32, 33, 34, 35, 58, 68, 220 Kda

Also some autoantibodies directed against non-specific inner ear proteins were initially attentions, such as the antibodies directed against the 68 proteins found in western blot up to 60% of cases of isolated developmental sensorineural hearing loss, but also in extra pathologies labyrinthine.

This protein was subsequently identified in the heat shock protein 70, an intracellular protein released in the event of thermal stress. For other authors it would be the CTL2 protein, fundamental in the role of degeneration of the Corti's cells. However, the distribution of CTL2 would not only be limited to Corti's cells, but its molecular similarity to cyclic, suspects an important function also in the transport of molecules from the intracellular environment to the extra cellular environment of the inner ear. This specific protein of the inner ear, however, seems an interesting track even if, to date, a diagnostic test has not yet been developed to actively and easily tests this protein in the diagnosis of autoimmune deafness.

Indirect Immunofluorescence Test

The principle is based on the visualization, starting from human or animal temporal bone sections, of human antibodies that are fixed and taken first from the patient's serum, which confirms that the serum contains specific proteins of the inner ear or non-specific (Yeom et al. 2003).

However, it is possible to simply evaluate that laboratory tests have neither the sensitivity nor the specificity sufficient to confirm that this is an autoimmune deafness and are nevertheless very expensive.

OTHER USEFUL TESTS FOR DIAGNOSIS

An examination of the fundus oculi is essential to understand the presence of the signs of raisins or episcleritis, always in the context of the systemic autoimmune disease.

A Magnetic Resonance Imaging (MRI) of the posterior cranial fossa and the inner ear would be useful in order to found a retrocochlear pathology in the case of asymmetric sensorineural deafness (Piccirillo et al. 2011, De Stefano, Kulamarva, and Dispenza 2012). A CT of petrous bone also plays an important role in the diagnosis in order to found morphological abnormalities of the labyrinth in children (Dispenza et al. 2015).

The diagnosis is based on history, on physical examination, on laboratory and instrumental tests that lead to a general and global classification (Hervier et al. 2010, De Stefano et al. 2011, Dispenza, Gargano, et al. 2011).

THERAPY

Therapies can be classified as follows: corticosteroids, immunosuppressive, plasmapheresis, gammaglobuline, intratympanic injections, cochlear implants, and new frontiers of research.

Corticosteroids

Validated treatment that demonstrates efficacy in autoimmune deafness. This treatment turns out to be the first therapeutic choice even before the diagnostic phase; in fact it is done before having carried out all the investigations of the case. The recommended dose for adults is 1-2 mg/kg per day of methylprednisone for 4 weeks.

The oral delivery route is recommended due intravenous cortisone boluses are considered off-label with regard to the occurrence of sudden or autoimmune deafness. More the treatment is quickly, the greater the degree of improvement of the symptoms obtained.

The actual duration of steroid treatment seems rather uncertain. Periods of continuation of corticosteroid therapy are recommended for 1-2 months, depending on the response (Harris and Ryan 1984). If there is not response within 4 weeks, then the steroid therapy is recommended to interrupt over a period of seven days in descending order, again to avoid altering the hypothalamic-pituitary axis.

In patients who respond, the hypothesis of continuing with 20-30 mg/day for several weeks can be evaluated. In children up to 14 years of age, must be taken into account all the adverse effects that could occur with the introduction of corticosteroid therapy during growth and evaluate any risks and benefits.

Immunosuppressive

Immunosuppressants drugs may be an alternative treatment to the use of corticosteroids. It can be evaluated:

- in those patients who cannot assume steroid therapy;
- in those patients in whom, side effects due to excessive use of strictures, such as myelosuppression or hemorrhagic cystitis, have already occurred;
- in those patients in whom, having obtained a good result with corticosteroids, they want to maintain and strengthen the therapy and the success of the therapy through the use of this class of drugs.

Specifically, the drugs used are methotrexate and cyclophosphamide. Methotrexate is prescribed at a dose of 7.5 mg/week as a single dose, given in combination with folio acid 1 mg/day to minimize the risk of stomatitis.

It is important to monitor the side effects of methotrexate, which include anemia, thrombocytopenia, hepatotoxicity and lung problems.

The side effects of cyclophosphamide instead include bone marrow suppression, infertility, hemorrhagic cystitis, increased risk of prostate cancer and lymphoma. Another drug that is used as an immunosuppressant is colchycin, an alkaloid that prevents microtubule polymerization by blocking them in metaphase, used in anti-inflammatory gout therapy. In animals, its validity in the modification of fluids within the labyrinth seems to be related. The recommended dose is 1 mg/day, although at the moment none of these drugs was approved by the Food and Drug Administration (FDA) for the treatment of autoimmune sensorineural deafness.

Plasmapheresis

The blood is purified from all the immunoglobulins with a mechanism very similar to that of dialysis. This therapy is invasive, expensive and unapproved in the treatment of sudden autoimmune deafness.

Gammaglobuline

The intravenous route of administration appears to lead to results similar to plasmapheresis, with greater ease of delivery and fewer side effects. The immunoglobulins would seem to interact with a series of complement factors, such as cytokines, mediators of immunity and cellular fractions, in order to attenuate the autoimmune response in autoimmune deafness.

Intratympanic Injections

The local injection of drugs such as corticosteroids locally, would seem to avoid the series of side effects that lead to suspension of therapy. Even this method of delivery presents different disadvantages, e.g., given its proximity to the round window and the Eustachian tube, it could lead to a residual perforation of the tympanic membrane, but also a series of advantages including an ease delivery of therapy that can be repeated over time e also with simultaneity between right ear and left ear(De Stefano, Kulamarva, and Dispenza 2010, Dispenza, De Stefano, et al. 2013, Dispenza, Amodio, et al. 2011).

Cochlear Implants

To be evaluated very carefully and after having tried medical therapy according to the various steps. The indication clearly is never given in urgency but assessed over time and varies from case to case.

Table 1. Autoimmune investigation: main complementary 1st-intention examinations

EMS-platelets, PCR, blood ionogram, creatinine, liver tests
CPK, LDH, serum protease electrophoresis, 24-hour proteinuria
Antinuclear factors, native anti-DNA, anti-ENA
Latex-Waaler Rose, circulating anticoagulant, anticardiolipin, C3, C4, CH50
Ophthalmologic examination (including fundus of the eye and research of a sicca syndrome) Capillaroscopy
Biopsy of accessory salivary glands
X-ray of hands

EMS: blood count; PCR: C reactive protein; CPK: creatine phosphokinase; LDH: lactate dehydrogenase; DNA: deoxyribonucleic acid; ENA: extractable nuclear antigen.

Table 2. Autoimmune investigation: main complementary 2nd-intention examinations

Outside specialized laboratories
HLA typing
Search for an increase in the HSP-70
Ac anticollagene II
Ac antimelin P0
Specialized laboratories
Ac directed against proteins present in large quantities in the cochlea, but not only:
- Ac anti-betatubulin
- Ac anti-lamanina
- Ac anti-Raf 1 protein
Ac directed against proteins present only in the cochlea:
- Ac anti-betatectorine
- Ac anti-coclina

HLA: human leucocyte antigen; Ac: antibodies.

Table 3. Systemic autoimmune diseases associated with autoimmune inner ear disease

Vogt_Koyanagi_Harada Syndrome
Cogan Syndrome
Susac Syndrome
Antiphospholipid syndrome
Rheumatoid Arthritis
Systemic vasculitis
Panarteritis nodosa
Granulomatosis with polyangiitis
Goodpasture Syndrome
Behcet disease
Sarcoidosis
Sjogren Syndrome
Hashimoto thyroiditis
Relapsing polychondritis
Myasthenia gravis
Polymyositis_dermatomyositis
Crohn's disease
Ulcerative colitis
Guillain-Barré syndrome
Multiple sclerosis

CONCLUSION

ASNHL is a rare kind of sensorineural deafness, difficult to detect and to diagnose correctly. In those patients who suffer from a well-known systemic autoimmune disease, diagnosis is easier and it is supported sometimes by a regression after corticosteroid or immunosuppressive therapies. In patients without a systemic autoimmune disease, the diagnosis is often given when other possible causes are excluded. A medical team made by ENTs, audiologists, rheumatologists, and ophthalmologists is required to manage as well as possible the patient with a suspect of ASNHL.

In order to increase results especially in those patients who can't be delivered with corticosteroid, immunosuppressor and other drugs, local therapies have to be improved. When therapies aren't working, the cochlear implant can be alternatively chosen as a good solution.

REFERENCES

Ahmadzadeh, A, M Daraei, M Jalessi, A A Peyvandi, E Amini, L A Ranjbar, and A Daneshi. 2017. "Hearing status in patients with rheumatoid arthritis." *J Laryngol Otol* 13:895-899.

Boulassel, M R, N Deggouj, J P Tomasi, and M Gersdorff. 2001. "Inner ear autoantibodies and their targets in patients with autoimmune inner ear diseases." *Acta Otolaryngol* 121:28-34.

Bovo, R, C Aimoni, and A Martini. 2006. "Immune-mediated inner ear disease." *Acta Otolaryngol* 126:1021.

D'Aguanno, V., M. Ralli, M. de Vincentiis, and A. Greco. 2018. "Optimal management of Cogan's syndrome: A multidisciplinary approach." *Journal of Multidisciplinary Healthcare* 11:1-11. doi: 10.2147/JMDH.S150940.

De Stefano, A., F. Dispenza, L. Citraro, A. G. Petrucci, P. Di Giovanni, G. Kulamarva, N. Mathur, and A. Croce. 2011. "Are postural restrictions necessary for management of posterior canal benign paroxysmal positional vertigo?" *Ann Otol Rhinol Laryngol* 120 (7):460-4.

De Stefano, A., G Kulamarva, and F Dispenza. 2010. "Intratympanic management for autoimmune inner ear disease." *Otorinolaringologia* 60 (3):155-163.

De Stefano, A., G. Kulamarva, and F. Dispenza. 2012. "Malignant paroxysmal positional vertigo." *Auris Nasus Larynx* 39:378-382.

Di Stadio, A, and M Ralli. 2017. "Systemic Lupus Erythematosus and hearing disorders: Literature review and meta-analysis of clinical and temporal bone findings." *J Int Med Res* 45:1470-1480.

Dispenza, F, F Cappello, G Kulamarva, and A De Stefano. 2013. "The discovery of the stapes." *Acta Otorhinolaryngol Ital* 33 (5):357-359.

Dispenza, F, and A De Stefano. 2012. "Vertigo in childhood: a methodological approach." *Bratisl Med J* 113:256-259.

Dispenza, F., E. Amodio, A. De Stefano, S. Gallina, D. Marchese, N. Mathur, and F. Riggio. 2011. "Treatment of sudden sensorineural hearing loss with transtympanic injection of steroids as single therapy: a randomized clinical study." *Eur Arch Otorhinolaryngol* 268 (9):1273-8.

Dispenza, F., A. De Stefano, C. Costantino, D. Marchese, and F. Riggio. 2013. "Sudden Sensorineural Hearing Loss: Results of intratympanic steroids as salvage treatment." *Am J Otolaryngol* 34 (4):296-300.

Dispenza, F., R. Gargano, N. Mathur, C. Saraniti, and S. Gallina. 2011. "Analysis of visually guided eye movements in subjects after whiplash injury." *Auris Nasus Larynx* 38:185-189.

Dispenza, F., W. Mazzucco, S. Bianchini, S. Mazzola, and E. Bennici. 2015. "Management of labyrinthine fistula in chronic otitis with cholesteatoma: Case series." *EuroMediterranean Biomedical Journal* 10 (21):255-261. doi: 10.3269/1970-5492.2015.10.21.

Gao, X, L Liu, Y Huang, H Lu, J Ouyang, and Y Wang. 2015. "Etiologies and clinical features of 19 cases with bilateral acute sensorineural hearing loss." *Zhonghua Er Bi Yan Hou Tou Jing Wai Ke Za Zhi* 50:3-7.

García-Carrasco, M, C Jiménez-Hernández, M Jiménez-Hernández, S Voorduin-Ramos, C Mendoza-Pinto, G Ramos-Alvarez, A Montiel-Jarquin, J Rojas-Rodríguez, and R Cervera. 2011. "Susac's syndrome: an update." *Autoimmun Rev* 10:548-552.

Gluth, M B, K H Baratz, E L Matteson, and C L Driscoll. 2006. "Cogan syndrome: a retrospective review of 60 patients throughout a half century." *Mayo Clin Proc* 81:483-488.

Grasland, A, J Pouchot, E Hachulla, O Blétry, T Papo, and P Vinceneux. 2004. "Typical and atypical Cogan's syndrome: 32 cases and review of the literature." *Rheumatology* 43:1007-1015.

Gussen, P. 1977. "Polyarteritis nodosa and deafness. A human temporal bone study." *Arch Otorhinolaryngol* 217:263-271.

Harris, J P, and A F Ryan. 1984. "Immunobiology of the inner ear." *Am J Otolaryngol* 5:418-425.

Hervier, B, P Bordure, M Audrain, C Calais, A Masseau, and M Hamidou. 2010. "Systematic screening for nonspecific autoantibodies in idiopathic sensorineural hearing loss: no association with steroid response." *Otol Neurotol* 31:687-690.

Lonyai, A, S Kodama, D Burger, and D L Faustman. 2008. "The promise of Hox11+ stem cells of the spleen for treating autoimmune diseases." *Immunol Cell Biol* 86:301-309.

Lorenz, R R, C A Solares, and P Williams. 2002. "Interferon-gamma production to inner ear antigens by T cells from patients with autoimmune sensorineural hearing loss." *J Neuroimmunol* 130:173-178.

Lunardi, C, C Bason, and M Leandri. 2002. "Autoantibodies to inner ear and endothelial antigens in Cogan's syndrome." *Lancet* 360:915-921.

Magro, C M, J C Poe, M Lubow, and J O Susac. 2011. "Susac syndrome: an organ-specific autoimmune endotheliopathy syndrome associated with anti-endothelial cell antibodies. 2011;136:903–12." *Am J Clin Pathol* 136:903-912.

Martines, F., P. Salvago, C. Bartolotta, S. Cocuzza, C. Fabiano, S. Ferrara, E. La Mattina, M. Mucia, P. Sammarco, F. Sireci, and E. Martines. 2015. "A genotype–phenotype correlation in Sicilian patients with GJB2 biallelic mutations." *European Archives of Oto-Rhino-Laryngology* 272 (8):1857-1865. doi: 10.1007/s00405-014-2970-1.

McCarty, D J, S Manzi, T A Jr Medsger, R Ramsey-Goldman, R E LaPorte, and C K Kwoh. 1995. "Incidence of systemic lupus erythematosus. Race and gender differences." *Arthritis Rheum* 38:1260-1270.

Morita, S, Y Nakamaru, N Obara, M Masuya, and S Fukuda. 2014. "Characteristics and Prognosis of Hearing Loss Associated with Vogt-Koyanagi-Harada Disease." *Audiol Neurotol* 19:49-56.

Ondrey, F G, E Moldestad, M A Mastroianni, A Pikus, D Sklare, E Vernon, R Nusenblatt, and J Smith. 2006. "Sensorineural hearing loss in Vogt-KoyanagiHarada syndrome." *Laryngoscope* 116:1873-1876.

Piccirillo, E., A. De Stefano, F. Dispenza, G. Kulamarva, G. De Donato, and M. Sanna. 2011. "Intermediate nerve schwannoma: a rare tumour." *B-Ent* 7 (3):219-23.

Read, R W, G N Holland, N A Rao, K F Tabbara, S Ohno, L Arellanes-Garcia, P Pivetti-Pezzi, H H Tessler, and M Usui. 2001. "Revised diagnostic criteria for Vogt-Koyanagi-Harada disease: report of an international committee on nomenclature." *Am J Ophthalmol* 131:647-652.

Rizzo, S., Bentivegna, D., Thomas, E., La Mattina, E., Mucia, M., Salvago, P., Sireci, F., Martines, F. (2016) Sudden sensorineural hearing loss, an invisible male: State of art. *Hearing loss: etiology, management and societal implications*, 75-86.

Rudnicki, A, S Shivatzki, L A Beyer, Y Takada, Y Raphael, and K B Avraham. 2014. "MicroRNA-224 regulates Pentraxin 3, a component of the humoral arm of innate immunity, in inner ear inflammation." *Hum Mol Genet* 23:3138-3146.

Salvago, P., S. Rizzo, A. Bianco, and F. Martines. 2017. "Sudden sensorineural hearing loss: is there a relationship between routine haematological parameters and audiogram shapes?" *International Journal of Audiology* 56 (3):148-153. doi: 10.1080/14992027.2016.1236418.

St Clair, E W, and R M McCallum. 1999. "Cogan's syndrome." *Curr Opin Rheumatol* 11:47–52.

Suslu, N, T Yilmaz, and B Gursel. 2009. "Utility of immunologic parameters in the evaluation of Meniere's disease." *Acta Otolaryngol* 129:1160-1165.

Tucci, M, C Quatraro, and F Silvestris. 2005. "Sjögren's syndrome: an autoimmune disorder with otolaryngological involvement." *Acta Otolaryngol Ital* 25:139-144.

Tumiati, B, P Casoli, and A Parmeggiani. 1997. "Hearing loss in the Sjögren syndrome. *Ann Intern Med.* 1997 Mar 15; 126:450-3." *Ann Intern Med* 126:450-453.

Wolf, M, J Kronenberg, S Engelberg, and G Leventon. 1987. "Rapidly progressive hearing loss as a symptom of polyarteritis nodosa." *Am J Otolaryngol* 8:105-108.

Yeom, K, J Gray, T S Nair, H A Arts, and S A Telian. 2003. "Antibodies to HSP-70 in normal donors and autoimmune hearing loss patients." *Laryngoscope* 113:1770-1776.

Ziavra, N, E N Politi, I Kastanioudakis, A Skevas, and A A Drosos. 2000. "Hearing loss in Sjögren's syndrome patients. A comparative study." *Clin Exp Rheumatol* 18:725-728.

In: Sensorineural Hearing Loss
Editors: F. Dispenza and F. Martines
ISBN: 978-1-53615-048-3
© 2019 Nova Science Publishers, Inc.

Chapter 12

OCCUPATIONAL HEARING LOSS

*Giampietro Ricci, MD[1], Egisto Molini[1], Mario Faralli[1], Lucia Calzolaro[2] and Luca D'Ascanio[3],**

[1]Department of Biological and Surgical Sciences, ENT Section,
University of Perugia, Perugia, Italy
[2]Department of Otolaryngology, Civil Hospital Città di Castello, Italy
[3]Department of Otolaryngology - Head & Neck Surgery,
Carlo Poma Civil Hospital – ASST Mantova, Italy

ABSTRACT

Occupational hearing loss is a condition that results from exposure to noise (noise induced hearing loss, NIHL) or to non-noise agents in a work environment. NIHL is usually caused by continuous or intermittent noise exposure which usually develops slowly over several years. Hearing loss from non-noise agents results from exposure to organic solvents, metals, and carbon monoxide. Occupational hearing loss is a prominent global topic affecting individuals, families, businesses and communities, since it is one of the major causes of adult-onset hearing loss at different ages all over the world. Furthermore, occupational noise may have harmful effects eventually independent or associated to hearing loss. Non auditory effects of noise exposure and hearing loss are: physical effects (tinnitus, increased cardiovascular disease risk, fatigue and sleeplessness, increased accident and injury risk, impaired communication), psychological and social effects (annoyance, depression, memory loss, impaired decision making, reduced quality of life, lower confidence and self-esteem, social isolation, relational difficulties) and economic effects (employment and income disruption, increased work absenteeism, increased employee turnover, reduced productivity and performance). Occupational NIHL is typically bilateral, with a classical "notch" at the high frequencies (3000, 4000, or 6000 Hz) and recovery at 8000 Hz, in contrast to presbycusis, indicating a hearing impairment in the middle of the frequency range of human voice. The notch becomes

---

*Corresponding Author's Email: giampietro.ricci@unipg.it.

deeper and wider and affects adjacent frequencies in case of continued noise exposure, with a consequent increased impact on speech communications. Making a diagnosis of occupational NIHL is an important step in preventing further hearing loss in the affected worker and identifying the potential for NIHL in co-workers. Complete hearing loss prevention programs are needed to effectively reduce the global burden of occupational hearing loss.

Keywords: occupational hearing loss, noise induced hearing loss

INTRODUCTION

Sound is energy in the form of pressure waves that vary rapidly as they move through the air and other media. Sound waves enter the cochlea where they stimulate hair cells (HCs). Such cells convert the vibratory sound energy into electrical impulses that travel via the auditory nerve to the brain, where they are interpreted. In case of HCs destruction, a permanent hearing loss will develop. Sound frequency (pitch) is the number of pressure variations per second and is measured in hertz (Hz). The magnitude or intensity of a sound (loudness) is measured by the sound pressure level in units of decibels (dB). The decibel is used to describe both noise exposure and hearing loss. While sound magnitude is measured as sound pressure level (dB SPL), hearing threshold is measured as hearing level (dB HL).

Averaged thresholds at specific tested frequencies are referred as pure tone average (PTA). The typical pure tone audiometric test includes frequencies at 0.25, 0.5, 1, 2, 4, and 8 kHz, which include the speech frequency range of 0.3 – 4 kHz. Many epidemiological and population-based studies on occupational noise induced hearing loss focus on PTAs that include 0.5, 1, 2, and 4 kHz frequencies.

The perceived loudness of sounds varies with sound frequency as well as with dB level. To account for this, a spectral sensitivity factor (A-filter) is used to weight sound pressure levels to de-emphasise lower and higher frequencies and emphasise the mid-range frequencies to which the human ear is most sensitive (i.e., around the 1–6 kHz range). These A-weighted sound pressure levels are expressed in units of dB(A) [1-3].

Long-term exposure to noise levels beyond 80 dB(A) carries an increased risk of hearing loss, which increases with noise level. Exposure to loud noise is the most common preventable cause of hearing loss and impairment (a weighted average hearing loss at 1, 2, 3, and 4 kHz greater than 25 dB) [4].

Occupational noise hearing loss in workers at different ages accounts for 7% to 21% (mean 16%) of the forms of adult-onset hearing impairment all around the world [5]. Besides hearing loss, occupational noise is associated with tinnitus, cardiovascular disease, depression, increased risk of accidents, and decreased productivity. Occupational hearing loss is a permanent sensorineural hearing loss due to acoustic overstimulation that has the potential for damaging cochlear cells (noise induced hearing loss, NIHL). Occupational NIHL is caused by continuous or intermittent noise exposure and usually develops slowly over several years. However, occupational hearing loss can also result from exposure to non-noise agents, such as chemicals (organic solvents, metals, carbon monoxide) and pharmaceuticals (ototoxins). In case of contemporary causes (i.e., noise and ototoxic chemicals), the effects on hearing loss are usually additive [6]. Many chemicals, either alone or in association with noise, may damage hearing organs and nerves after inhalation or dermal exposure. Potential ototoxic chemicals in the occupational environment are fuels, carbon monoxide, lead and derivatives, toluene, xylene, stoddard solvent, mercury and derivatives, organophosphate pesticides, chemical warfare nerve agents, perchloro-ethylene, n-hexane, ethyl benzene, trichloroethylene, manganese, styrene monomer, cyanide, organic tin, arsenic, carbon disulfide, paraquat [7].

PATHOPHYSIOLOGY OF OCCUPATIONAL HEARING LOSS

The mechanisms of cochlear damage are mechanical: the exaggerated movements of the basilar membrane cause an increase in oxidative metabolism with a consequent production of free radicals, glutamatergic excitotoxicity, ionic and ischemic disorders responsible for delayed HCs death in the inner ear by necrosis and apoptosis. Increased levels of reactive oxygen species (ROS: molecules or ions formed by the incomplete single-electron reduction of oxygen, superoxide, peroxides, hydroxyl radicals, and hypochlorous acid) and reactive nitrogen species (RNS: nitric oxide-derived compounds that include nitroxyl anion, nitrosonium cation, higher oxides of nitrogen, S-nitrosothiols, and dinitrosyl iron complexes) play a significant role in noise-induced hair cell death [8-10].

Oxidative stress is an imbalance between the production of reactive oxygen species (ROS) and antioxidant defences, potentially resulting in oxidative damage [11]. ROS cause damage by chemically reacting with DNA, proteins, cytosolic molecules, cell surface receptors, and membrane lipids [12] and have been detected in cochlear tissue just after noise exposure [13] just before any morphological sign of damage [14]. The initial mechanical HCs damage occurs in conjunction with transient intense ROS formation; HCs loss progresses over time and stabilizes two or more weeks after the insult when the late formation of free radicals of ROS/RNS causes a delayed HCs loss spreading from the basal turn to the apex [15]. ROS cause the activation of cellular defence pathways such as autophagy [16], a protective process that delivers damaged cellular components to lysosomes for degradation [17]. Such procedure attenuates noise-induced hearing loss (NIHL) by reducing the consequences of oxidative stress [18]. ROS can also cause the production of pro-inflammatory cytokines [19] and tumour necrosis factor [20] which can produce cochlear damage [21]. Calcium homeostasis plays a significant role in regulating ROS release from mitochondria into the cytoplasm [22]. Aminoglycoside antibiotics drastically alter calcium homeostasis by increasing cytoplasmic ROS in HCs; free calcium triggers mitogen-activated protein kinase (MAPK) responsible of HCs damage [23].

Glutamate excitotoxicity is defined as cell death produced by the toxic actions of the essential amino-acid glutamate. Neuronal excitotoxicity is the injury and death of neurons arising from prolonged exposure to glutamate and the associated excessive calcium overload in HCs responsible for the activation of enzymes that degrade proteins, membranes and nucleic acids [24]. High-level noise exposure causes the release of a large amount of glutamate within inner hair cells (IHCs) that overstimulate NMDA receptors, thus producing high intracellular synapses calcium levels. Excessive postsynaptic ion influx into the auditory nerve terminals at the IHCs synapse results in dendritic swelling and vacuolization [25].

In addition, an increased potassium concentration, due to high-level noise exposure, may be toxic for HCs [26] since it increases intracellular calcium concentration which activates a series of enzymes that degrade proteins, membranes and nucleic acids [27].

High-level noise exposure causes cochlear vasoconstriction and reduced inner ear blood flow as well, by means of prostaglandins [28]. Noise-induced ischemia and subsequent re-perfusion further potentiate the generation of ROS [29].

Following intense noise exposure activation of ROS, RNS and MAPK stress pathways, cochlear HCs can undergo apoptosis and/or necroptosis [30-35].

Apoptosis results in the orderly disassembly of cells into membrane-packaged fragments that can be eliminated by phagocytes in a non-inflammatory process. Apoptosis appears extremely rapidly after noise stresses and has been shown to be the primary cell death pathway in the first day following noise exposure [31,32,36]. Necroptosis permeabilizes intra- and extracellular membranes, releasing cellular and organelle contents into the extracellular medium, where they induce inflammation.

Noise exposure has been shown to up-regulate cochlear production of cytokines [20,37] and chemotactic chemokines that attract inflammatory cells to the cochlea [38]. Another potential source of inflammatory mediators is the release of intracellular components into the extracellular environment. Such release develops in case of necrosis or necroptosis, both of which have been implicated in noise-induced cochlear damage [39].

The accumulation of ROS in cells is opposed by the action of native antioxidant enzyme systems, and HCs are no exception to this process. Glutathione, superoxide dismutase (SOD), catalase (CAT), glutathione peroxidase, glutathione reductase and coenzyme Q10 have all been detected in cochlear tissues [40-42]. These natural defences have to be overcome by ROS before cell damage develops. The antioxidant glutathione in the organ of Corti is distributed in a high-to-low gradient from the apex to the base [43].

This distribution may explain the familiar pattern of HCs damage due to several causes, with initial appearance in the base and progressive extension towards the apex.

CLINICAL AND AUDIOMETRIC CHARACTERISTICS OF NIHL

Occupational NIHL is always sensorineural, typically bilateral. Its first sign is a "notching" of the audiogram on high frequencies (3000, 4000, or 6000 Hz) with recovery at 8000 Hz [44]. This notch typically develops on one of these frequencies and affects adjacent frequencies with continued noise exposure. The exact location of the notch depends on multiple factors including the frequency of the damaging noise and size of the ear canal. In early NIHL, the average hearing thresholds at the lower frequencies (500, 1000, and 2000 Hz) are better than the average thresholds at 3000, 4000, and 6000 Hz, and the hearing level at 8000 Hz is usually better than the deepest part of the notch. Noise exposure alone usually does not produce a loss greater than 75 dB at high frequencies and greater than 40 dB at lower frequencies. Hearing loss due to noise exposure increases most rapidly during the first 10 to 15 years of exposure, while the pattern of hearing loss decelerates later on: previously noise-exposed ears are less sensitive to future noise exposure. Furthermore, it is unlikely that NIHL progresses if noise exposure is discontinued.

The presence of a temporary threshold shift (TTS: the temporary loss of hearing, which largely disappears 16–48 hours after exposure to loud noise) with or without tinnitus is a risk indicator that permanent threshold shift (PTS) will occur if hazardous noise exposure continues. Except for ototraumatic accident, workers always develop TTS before sustaining PTS [45].

When evaluating cases of asymmetric loss, a referral to rule out a retrocochlear lesion, such as an acoustic neuroma, is required before attributing the loss to noise. The addition of very intense and frequent impulse/impact noise to steady-state noise can be more harmful than steady-state noise of the same A-weighted energy exposure. There are a number of other causes of sensorineural hearing loss besides occupational noise. These include non-occupational noise exposure (recreational noise), exposure to ototoxic compounds including drugs [46,47], mutations in deafness genes [48-51], infections such as labyrinthitis or prenatal cytomegalovirus [52-56], aging [57,58], head injury, therapeutic radiation exposure, neurologic disorders, cerebral vascular disorders, immune disorders, bone diseases (Paget disease), central nervous system neoplasms, and Ménière disease [59].

NIHL is irreversible. Detection and intervention are critical to prevent this condition to develop. A significant threshold shift (STS) of 10-dB from the baseline in PTA at 2000, 3000, and 4000 Hz is an important early indicator of permanent hearing loss [60]. TTS is an important early and reversible indicator that potential cochlea HCs damage can progress to a STS. Tinnitus is another early warning symptom for NIHL [61-64]. One of the main components of the hearing conservation programme is the annual pure tone audiogram (PTA), designed to detect workers with NIHL early and to submit them to subsequent interventions that might arrest hearing lossprogression. The use of PTA at 2, 3 and 4 kHz has shown the highest sensitivity and specificity amongst the other pure tone averages [65].

Otoacoustic Emissions (OAEs) are an important technological advance in audiological assessment.OAEs are sounds produced by the cochlea, specifically the outer hair cells (OHCs), and measured in the outer ear canal. Transient Otoacoustic Emissions (TEOAEs)are evoked responses from stimulating the cochlea with a transient signal such as a click or tone burst acoustic signal. TEOAEs are a wide frequency response in 500 to 5000 Hz range.Distortion Products (DPOAEs) are evoked response OAEs from stimulating the cochlea with two simultaneously presented pure tones of different frequency. This type of OAE can be recorded in individuals with a more severe hearing loss, at higher frequencies with more frequency specificity. DPOAEs are obtainable in the frequency range of 500 to 8000 Hz. They typically do not occur in hearing losses greater than 30 dB.The production of OAEs by the OHCs of the cochlea is due to the cochlear active processes. In case of OHCs damage producing a mild hearing loss, OAEs are not present.

OAE testing is twice as sensitive as audiometry to detect a change in hearing threshold level and could improve monitoring for noise-induced hearing loss in the workplace [66]. Furthermore, OAEs indicate noise-induced changes in the inner ear undetected by audiometric tests [67].More studies are needed to show whether OAE testing can replace standard audiometry or whether the two techniques have complementary roles.

NON AUDITORY EFFECTS OF NOISE EXPOSURE

Occupational and environmental noise exposure may have important non-auditory effects, eventually independent or associated to hearing loss. Such effects can be manifold, bothersome and, sometimes, serious.

Among them, tinnitus is one of the most frequent and annoying. It can have low intensity or can be extremely severe, thus causing distress, depression and sleep discomfort [68,69].

Environmental or occupational exposure to noise can have effects on the cardiovascular system, causing tachycardia and high systolic and diastolic blood pressure, in addition to other risk factors such as blood lipid concentration, blood viscosity and blood glucose concentration [70-74].Chang et al. (2013) [75], found that high noise exposure (≥85 dBA) increased systolic pressure by 3.2 mm Hg and diastolic pressure by

2.5 mm Hg. Such conditions can increase the risk of severe events such as myocardial infarction and stroke (Basner et al., 2014). Potential mechanisms are emotional stress reactions with release of catecholamines and glucocorticoids (indirect pathway) and non-conscious physiological stress from interactions between the central auditory system and other regions of the CNS (direct pathway) [76-78].

In 2009, WHO published the Night Noise Guidelines for Europe, an expert consensus that mapped four noise exposure groups to negative health outcomes ranging from no biological effects to increased risk of cardiovascular disease (below 30 $dB_{aeq,night,outside}$; 30-40 dB; 40-55 dB; above 55 $dB_{aeq,night,outside}$: in this group the situation is considered increasingly dangerous for public health [76].

Exposure to loud noise has been linked to adverse psychological and social effects. It can cause anxiety, depression, annoyance, sleeplessness [79]. Particularly, sleep disturbances are thought to be one the most deleterious non-auditory effect of environmental noise exposure, since a sufficient undisturbed sleep is considered necessary for a good quality of life [80]. The effects of environmental noise exposure depend not only on the acoustical properties of the sound [76] but also on the momentary sleep stage [81] and individual noise susceptibility [82]. Elderly people, children, shift-workers and people with a pre-existing sleep disorder are thought to be the major risk groups for noise induced sleep disturbance [76-78].

Other authors reported negative effects of chronic noise exposure on memory (IEH, 1996) [83], decision-making ability [84] and after-work irritability [85]. Many studies demonstrated environmental noise exposure has a negative effect on children's learning outcomes and cognitive performance [86]. Postulated mechanisms for these effects are communication difficulties, impaired attention, increased arousal, learned helplessness, frustration, noise annoyance and consequences of sleep-disorders [76].

Recently, Sorensen et al. (2014) [87] have shown a relation between exposure to traffic noise and post-menopausal breast cancer, while some other authors have demonstrated the association between noise exposure and obesity [88,89].

Many of these conditions seem to be associated with a higher frequency of workplace [90,91]. In conclusion, the consequences of chronic noise exposure have a significant social cost, since they are associated with a high frequency of working days loss and reduced productivity [92, 93].

According to the WHO, more than one million healthy life years (disability adjusted life years, DALY) are lost annually in the European Union because of community noise exposure. Noise-induced sleep disturbance is responsible for about 900.000 DALYs, annoyance for 650.000, ischemic heart disease for 65.000 and children's cognitive impairment for 45.000 DALYs [94].

INNER EAR PROTECTION FROM NOISE

Occupational NIHL is permanent. At the moment, no effective treatment to regenerate damaged sensory receptors after noise exposure has been reported, leaving amplification as the only option. However, the risk of NIHL can be greatly minimized if noise is reduced to below 80 dB(A) [95].

The maximum daily occupational noise exposure level at an eight-hour equivalent continuous A-weighted sound pressure level is 85 dB(A). The preferred solution to excessive noise exposure is to completely eliminate the source of loud noise. When this is not possible or practical, the legal requirement is to minimise exposure through a hierarchy of controls: substitute the noise source with quieter machinery or processes, isolate the noise source from workers, apply engineering solutions and install noise guards or enclosures, apply administrative solutions, provide signs and quiet areas for breaks, and when none of the above are reasonably practicable, provide personal hearing protectors (e.g., ear muffs and plugs).

The high rate of occupational NIHL casts doubts upon the effectiveness of prevention programs or people's compliance to them. The average hearing loss prevention programs show the poor effectiveness of non-pharmaceutical interventions for preventing occupational noise exposure and occupational NIHL and do not reduce the risk of hearing loss to below a level at least equivalent to that of workers who are exposed to 85 dB(A) [96].

There are two therapeutic strategies to reduce cochlear damage in NIHL: inhibit pathways that lead to the damage of HCs and enhance processes that enable HCs survival. Antioxidants protect HCs and hearing from noise induced noise [97-100].

The antioxidant N-acetyl cysteine (NAC) in military trainees showed some degree of protection [101] in contrast to other studies, where no protective effect of NAC was found during stapes surgery [102] and on TTS induced by loud music [103].

Reduction of inflammation also has the potential to protect against NIHL: steroid dexamethasone, delivered to the round window membrane, has also been shown to reduce hearing loss after noise [104]. The patients suffering from recently NIHL receiving intratympanic treatment showed significantly more improvement in thresholds than patients receiving systemic steroid alone [105]. Delivery to the inner ear across the round window membrane into the perilymph provides the possibility to utilize a wider variety of potential therapies for inner ear protection from noise.

REFERENCES

[1] Pederson, O.J. (1989). Noise and people. *Noise ContrEngin J, 32*(2), 73–78.

[2]   Roeser, R.J., Buckley, K. A. & Stickney, G.S. (2000). Pure tone tests. In: Roeser, R.J., Valente, M. and Hosford-Dunn, H. (Eds.). *Audiology diagnosis*. New York: Thieme Medical Publishers.

[3]   Gates, G. A. & Hoffman, H.J. (2008). *What the numbers mean: an epidemiological perspective on hearing*. www.nidcd.nih.gov/health/statistics/measuring.htm.

[4]   John, A.B., Kreisman, B. M. & Pallett, S. (2012). Validity of hearing impairment calculation methods for prediction of self-reported hearing handicap. *Noise & Health*, *14*, 13–20.

[5]   *Occupational noise: assessing the burden of disease from work-related hearing impairment at national and local levels*. World Health Organization, Series Number 9, Geneva 2004.

[6]   Tak, S. & Calvert, G.M. (2008). Hearing Difficulty Attributable to Employment by Industry and Occupation: An Analysis of the National Health Interview Survey—United States, 1997 to 2003. *J Occup Environ Med*, *50*(1), 46-56.

[7]   Morata, T.C. (2003). Chemical Exposure as a Risk Factor for Hearing Loss. *J Occup Environ Med*, *45*(7), 676-682.

[8]   Henderson, D., Bielefeld, E.C., Harris, K. C. & Hu, B.H. (2006). The role of oxidative stress in noise-induced hearing loss. *Ear Hear*, *27*(1), 1-19.

[9]   Fubini, B. & Hubbard, A. (2003). Reactive oxygen species (ROS) and reactive nitrogen species (RNS) generation by silica in inflammation and fibrosis. *Free Radic Biol Med*, *34*, 1507–1516.

[10] Martinez, M. C. & Andriantsitohaina, R. (2009).Reactive nitrogen species: molecular mechanisms and potential significance in health and disease. *Antioxid Redox Signal*, *11*(3), 669–702.

[11] Sies, H. (1997). Oxidative stress: oxidants and antioxidants. *Exp Physiol*, *82*, 291–295.

[12] Dröge, W. (2002). Free radicals in the physiological control of cell function. *Physiol Rev*, *82*, 47-95.

[13] Yamane, H., Nakai, Y., Takayama, M., Iguchi, H., Nakagawa, T. & Kojima, A. (1995).Appearance of free radicals in the Guinea pig inner ear after noise-induced acoustic trauma. *Eur Arch Otorhinolaryngol*, *252*(8), 504-508.

[14] Choung, Y.H., Taura, A., Pak, K., Choi, S. J., Masuda, M. & Ryan, A.F.(2009). Generation of highly-reactive oxygen species is closely related to hair cell damage in rat organ of Corti treated with gentamicin. *Neurosci*, *161*(1), 214-226.

[15] Yamashita, D., Jiang, H.Y., Schacht, J. & Miller, J.M. (2004). Delayed production of free radicals following noise exposure. *Brain Res*, *1019*(1-2), 201-209.

[16] Vernon, P. J. & Tang, D. (2013).Eat-me: autophagy, phagocytosis, and reactive oxygen species signaling. *Antioxid Redox Signal*, *18*(6), 677–691.

[17] Wang, C. W. & Klionsky, D.J. (2003). The molecular mechanism of autophagy. *Mol Med*, *9*(3-4), 65–76.

[18] Yuan, H., Wang, X., Hill, K., Chen, J., Lemasters, J., Yang, S. M. & Sha, S.H. (2015). Autophagy Attenuates Noise-Induced Hearing Loss by Reducing Oxidative Stress. *Antioxid Redox Signal.*, *22*(15), 1308–1324.

[19] Wakabayashi, K., Fujioka, M., Kanzaki, S., Okano, H.J., Shibata, S., Yamashita, D., Masuda, M., Mihara, M., Ohsugi, Y., Ogawa, K. & Okano, H. (2010). Blockade of interleukin-6 signaling suppressed cochlear inflammatory response and improved hearing impairment in noise-damaged mice cochlea. *Neurosci Res*, *66*(4), 345-35.

[20] Keithley, E. M., Wang, X. & Barkdull, G.C. (2008).Tumor necrosis factor alpha can induce recruitment of inflammatory cells to the cochlea. *Otol Neurotol*, *29*(6), 854-859.

[21] Tan, W.J., Thorne, P. R. & Vlajkovic, S.M. (2016). Characterization of cochlear inflammation in mice following acute and chronic noise exposure. *Histochem Cell Biol*, *146*(2), 219-230.

[22] Batandier, C., Leverve, X. & Fontaine, E. (2004). Opening of the mitochondrial permeability transition pore induces reactive oxygen species production at the level of the respiratory chain complex I. *J Biol Chem*, *279*(17), 17197-17204.

[23] Maeda, Y., Fukushima, K., Omichi, R., Kariya, S. & Nishizaki, K. (2013). Time courses of changes in phospho- and total- MAP kinases in the cochlea after intense noise exposure. *PLoS One*, *8*(3), e58775.

[24] Berliocchi, L., Bano, D. & Nicotera, P. (2005).Ca2+ signals and death programmes in neurons. *Philos Trans R Soc Lond B Biol Sci*, *360*(1464), 2255–2258.

[25] Pujol, R., Puel, J. L., d'Aldin, C. & Eybalin, M. (1990). Physiopathology of the glutamatergic synapses in the cochlea. *Acta Oto-Laryngol*, *113*, 330–334.

[26] Zenner, H. (1986). K+-induced motility and depolarization of cochlear hair cells. Direct evidence for a new pathophysiological mechanism in Meniere's disease. *Arch Otorhinolaryngol*, *243*(2), 108–111.

[27] Sendowski, I. (2006). Magnesium therapy in acoustic trauma. *Magnes Res*, *19*(4), 244-254.

[28] Miller, J.M., Brown, J. N. & Schacht, J. (2003). 8-iso- prostagladin F(2alpha), a product noise of exposure, reduces inner ear blood flow. *Audiol Neurootol*, *8*(4), 207–221.

[29] Kurabi, A., Keithley, E. M., Housley, G.D., Ryan, A. F. & Wong, A.C. (2017). Cellular mechanisms of noise-induced hearing loss. *Hearing Research*, *349*, 129-137.

[30] Hu, B.H., Guo, W., Wang, P. Y., Henderson, D. & Jiang, S.C. (2000). Intense noise-induced apoptosis in hair cells of Guinea pig cochleae. *ActaOtolaryngol*, *120*(1), 19-24.

[31] Hu, B. H., Henderson, D. & Nicotera, T.M. (2002a). F-actin cleavage in apoptotic outer hair cells in chinchilla cochleas exposed to intense noise. *Hear Res*, *172*, 1-9.

[32] Hu, B. H., Henderson, D. & Nicotera, T.M. (2002b). Involvement of apoptosis in progression of cochlear lesion following exposure to intense noise. *Hear Res*, *166*, 62-71.

[33] Wang, X., Truong, T., Billings, P.B., Harris, J. P. & Keithley, E.M. (2003). Blockage of immune-mediated inner ear damage by etanercept. *Otol Neurotol*, *24*, 52-57.

[34] Nicotera, T., Hu, B. & Henderson, D. (2004). The caspase pathway in noise-induced apoptosis of the chinchilla cochlea. *JARO*, *4*, 466-477.

[35] Yang, W.P., Henderson, D., Hu, B. H. & Nicotera, T.M. (2004). Quantitative analysis of apoptotic and necrotic outer hair cells after exposure to different levels of continuous noise. *Hear Res*, *196*, 69-76.

[36] Hu, B. H., Henderson, D. & Nicotera, T.M. (2006). Extremely rapid induction of outer hair cell apoptosis in the chinchilla cochlea following exposure to impulse noise. *Hear Res*, *211*, 16-25.

[37] Fujioka, M., Kanzaki, S., Okano, H.J., Masuda, M., Ogawa, K. & Okano, H. (2006).Proinflammatory cytokines expression in noise-induced damaged cochlea. *J Neurosci Res*, *83*, 575-583.

[38] Tornabene, S.V., Sato, K., Pham, L., Billings, P. & Keithley, E.M. (2006). Immune cell recruitment following acoustic trauma. *Hear Res*, *222*, 115-124.

[39] Zheng, H. W., Chen, J. & Sha, S.H. (2014). Receptor-interacting protein kinases modulate noise-induced sensory hair cell death. *Cell Death Dis*, *29*(5), 1262.

[40] Jacono, A.A., Hu, B., Kopke, R.D., Henderson, D., Van De Water, T. R. & Steinman, H.M. (1998). Changes in cochlear antioxidant enzyme activity after sound conditioning and noise exposure in the chinchilla. *Hear Res*, *117*, 31-38.

[41] McFadden, S.L., Ding, D., Reaume, A.G., Flood, D. G. & Salvi, R.J. (1999). Age-related cochlear hair cell loss is enhanced in mice lacking copper/zinc superoxide dismutase. *Neurobiol Aging*, *20*, 1-8.

[42] Fetoni, A.R., De Bartolo, P., Eramo, S.L., Rolesi, R., Paciello, F., Bergamini, C., Fato, R., Paludetti, G., Petrosini, L. & Troiani, D. (2013).Noise-induced hearing loss (NIHL) as a target of oxidative stress-mediated damage: cochlear and cortical responses after an increase in antioxidant defense. *J Neurosci*, *33*, 4011-4023.

[43] Sha, S. H., Taylor, R., Forge, A. & Schacht, J. (2001). Differential vulnerability of basal and apical hair cells is based on intrinsic susceptibility to free radicals. *Hear Res*, *155*, 1-8.

[44] McBride, D. I. & Williams, S. (2001). Audiometric notch as a sign of noise induced hearing loss. *Occup Environ Med*, *58*, 46–51.

[45] U.S. Department of Health and Human Services. *Criteria for a Recommended Standard: Occupational Noise Exposure*. Publication No. 98–126, 36-60. Cincinnati, 1998.

[46] Haynes, D. S., Rutka, J., Hawke, M. & Roland, P.S. (2007). Ototoxicity of ototopical drops – an update. *Otolaryngol Clin North Am*, *40*(3), 669-683.

[47] Cannizzaro, E., Cannizzaro, C., Plescia, F., Martines, F., Sole, L., Pira, E. & Lo Coco, D. (2014).Exposure to ototoxic agents and hearing loss: A review of current knowledge. *Hearing, Balance and Communication*, *12*, 166-175.

[48] Vona, B. & Haaf, T. (2016). Genetics of deafness. In: *Monographs in Human Genetics*. Karger, Basel, Switzerland.

[49] Martines, F., Salvago, P., Bartolotta, C., Cocuzza, S., Fabiano, C., Ferrara, S., La Mattina, E., Mucia, M., Sammarco, P., Sireci, F. & Martines, E. (2015).A genotype–phenotype correlation in Sicilian patients with GJB2 biallelic mutations. *Eur Arch Otorhinolaryngol*, *272*(8), 1857-1865.

[50] Bartolotta, C., Salvago, P., Cocuzza, S., Fabiano, C., Sammarco, P. & Martines, F. (2014).Identification of D179H, a novel missense GJB2 mutation in a Western Sicily family. *European Archives of Oto-Rhino-Laryngology*, *271* (6), pp. 1457-1461.

[51] Salvago, P., Martines, E., La Mattina, E., Mucia, M., Sammarco, P., Sireci, F. & Martines, F. (2014). Distribution and phenotype of GJB2 mutations in 102 Sicilian patients with congenital non syndromic sensorineural hearing loss. *International Journal of Audiology*, *53* (8), pp. 558-563.

[52] Furutate, S., Iwasaki, S., Nishio, S. Y., Moteki, H. & Usami, S. (2011).Clinical profile of hearing loss in children with congenital cytomegalovirus (CMV) infection: CMV DNA diagnosis using preserved umbilical cord. *Acta Otolaryngol*, *131*, 976-982.

[53] Ferrara, S., Salvago, P., Mucia, M., Ferrara, P., Sireci, F. & Martines, F. (2014).Follow-up after pediatricmyringoplasty: Outcome at 5 years. *Otorinolaringologia*, *64*, 141-146.

[54] Rizzo, S., Bentivegna, D., Thomas, E., La Mattina, E., Mucia, M., Salvago, P., Sireci, F. & Martines, F. (2016).Sudden sensorineural hearing loss, an invisible male: State of art. *Hearing loss: etiology, management and societal implications*, 75-86.

[55] Salvago, P., Rizzo, S., Bianco, A. & Martines, F. (2017).Sudden sensorineural hearing loss: is there a relationship between routine haematological parameters and audiogram shapes? *International Journal of Audiology*, *56*(3), 148-153.

[56] Dispenza, F., De Stefano, A., Costantino, C., Marchese, D. & Riggio, F. (2013).Sudden Sensorineural Hearing Loss: results of intratympanic steroids as salvage treatment. *Am J Otolaryngol*, *34*, 296-300.

[57] Zhang, Q., Liu, H., McGee, J., Walsh, E. J., Soukup, G. A. & He, D. Z. (2013). Identifying micro RNAs involved in degeneration of the organ of Corti during age-related hearing loss. *PLoS One*, *8*, e62786.

[58] Martines, F., Maira, E. & Ferrara, S. (2011).Age-related hearing impairment (ARHI): A common sensory deficit in the elderly. *Acta Medica Mediterranea, 27* (1), 47-52.

[59] Kirchner, D.B., Evenson, E., Dobie, R.A., Rabinowitz, P., Crawford, J., Kopke, R. & Hudson, T.W. (2012). Occupational Noise-Induced Hearing Loss: ACOEM Task Force on Occupational Hearing Loss. *J Occup Environ Med, 54*(1), 106-108.

[60] Dobie, R.A. (2005). Audiometric threshold shift definitions: simulations and suggestions. *Ear Hear, 26,* 62–77.

[61] Dobie, R.A. (2001). Structure and function of the ear. In: Dobie RA, ed. *Medical-Legal Evaluation of Hearing Loss.* 2nd ed. San Diego.

[62] Plescia, F., Cannizzaro, C., Brancato, A., Sireci, F., Salvago, P. & Martines, F. (2016). Emerging pharmacological treatments of tinnitus. *Tinnitus: Epidemiology, Causes and Emerging Therapeutic Treatments.* Nova Science Publishers, Inc., 43-64.

[63] Cavallaro, A., Martines, F., Cannizzaro, C., Lavanco, G., Brancato, A., Carollo, G., Plescia, F., Salvago, P., Cannizzaro, E., Mucia, M., Rizzo, S., Martini, A. & Plescia, F. (2016).Role of cannabinoids in the treatment of tinnitus. *Acta Medica Mediterranea, 32,* 463-469.

[64] Martines, F., Messina, G., Patti, A., Battaglia, G., Bellafiore, M., Messina, A., Rizzo, S., Salvago, P., Sireci, F., Traina, M. & Iovane, A. (2015). Effects of tinnitus on postural control and stabilization: A pilot study. *Acta Medica Mediterranea, 31,* 907-912.

[65] Razali, A. & Rampal, K.G. (2012). *Validity of various methods of pure tone audiogram averaging in diagnosing hearing impairment in a hearing conservation programme.* Kulliyah of Medicine, IIUM Kuantan Perdana University, Graduate School of Medicine, Kuala Lumpur. GRF One Health Summit, Davos.

[66] Hall, A. J. & Lutman, M.E. (2000). Methods for early identification of noise-induced hearing loss. *Audiol, 38*(5), 277-280.

[67] Lapsley Miller, J.A., Marshall, L., Heller, L. M. & Hughes, L.M. (2006). Low-level otoacoustic emissions may predict susceptibility to noise-induced hearing loss. *J Acoust Soc Am, 120*(1), 280–296.

[68] Axelsson, A. & Prasher, D. (2000). Tinnitus induced by occupational and leisure noise. *Noise and Health, 2*(8), 47–54.

[69] Stormer, C. C. L., Sorlie, T. & Stenklev, N.C. (2017). Tinnitus, Anxiety, Depression and Substance Abuse in Rock Musicians a Norwegian Survey. *Int Tinnitus J, 21*(1), 50-57.

[70] Sbihi, H., Davies, H. W. & Demers, P.A. (2008). Hypertension in noise-exposed sawmill workers: a cohort study. *J Occup Environ Med, 65,* 643–646.

[71] Babisch, W. (2008). Road traffic noise and cardiovascular risk. *Noise and Health, 10*(38), 27–33.

[72] Goyal, S., Gupta, V. & Walia, L. (2010). Effect of noise stress on autonomic function tests. *Noise Health*, *12*(48), 182-186.

[73] Münzel, T., Knorr, M., Schmidt, F., von Bardeleben, S., Gori, T. & Schulz, E. (2016). Airborne disease: a case of a Takotsubocardiomyopathie as a consequence of nighttime aircraft noise exposure. *Eur Heart J*, Oct 1, *37*(37), 2844.

[74] Skogstad, M., Johannessen, H.A., Tynes, T., Mehlum, I.S., Nordby, K. C. & Lie, A. (2016). Systematic review of the cardiovascular effects of occupational noise. *Occup Med* (Lond), Jan, *66*(1), 10-16.

[75] Chang, T.Y., Hwang, B.F., Liu, C.S., Chen, R.Y., Wang, V.S., Bao, B.Y., et al. (2013). Occupational noise exposure and incident hypertension in Men: a prospective cohortstudy. *Am J Epidemiol*, *177*(8), 818-825.

[76] Basner, M., Babisch, W., Davis, A., Brink, M., Clark, C., Janssen, S. & Stansfeld, S. (2014). Auditory and non-auditoryeffects of noise on health. *Lancet*, Apr 12, *383*(9925), 1325-1332.

[77] Ballacchino, A., Salvago, P., Cannizzaro, E., Costanzo, R., Di Marzo, M., Ferrara, S., La Mattina, E., Messina, G., Mucia, M., Mulè, A., Plescia, F., Sireci, F., Rizzo, S. & Martines, F. (2015).Association between sleep-disordered breathing and hearing disorders: Clinical observation in Sicilian patients. *Acta Medica Mediterranea*, *31*(3), 607-614.

[78] Martines, F., Ballacchino, A., Sireci, F., Mucia, M., La Mattina, E. & Rizzo, S. (2016).Audiologic profile of OSAS and simple snoring patients: the effect of chronic nocturnal intermittent hypoxia on auditory function. *European Archives of Oto-Rhino-Laryngology*, *273*, 1419-1424.

[79] Raffaello, M. & Maass, A. (2002). Chronicexposure to noise in industry: the effects on satisfaction, stress, symptoms, and companyattachment. *Environ Behav*, *34*(5), 651–671.

[80] Fritschi, L., Brown, A.L., Kim, R., Schwela, D. H. & Kephalopoulos, S. (2011). *Burden of disease from environmental noise*. Bonn: World Health Organization.

[81] Basner, M., Müller, U. & Griefahn, B. (2010). Practical guidance for riskassessment of traffic noise effects on sleep, *Appl Acoust*, *71*, 518–522.

[82] Dang-Vu, T.T., McKinney, S.M., Buxton, O.M., Solet, J. M. & Ellenbogen, J.M. (2010). Spontaneous brain rhythms predict sleep stability in the face of noise. *Curr Biol*, *20*, 626–627.

[83] IEH (Institute for Environment and Health). (1997). *The non-auditory effects of noise*. University of Leicester.

[84] Siegel, J. M. & Steele, C.M. (1980). Environmental distraction and interpersonal judgments. *Br J Soc Clin Psyc*, *19*(1), 23–32.

[85] Melamed, S. & Bruhis, S. (1996). The effects of chronicindustrial noise exposure on urinary cortisol, fatigue, and irritability: a controlled field experiment. *J Occup Environ Med*, *38*(3), 252-256.

[86] Evans, G. & Hygge, S. (2007). Noise and performance in adults and children. In: Luxon L, Prasher D, editors. *Noise and its effects*. London: Whurr Publishers.

[87] Sørensen, M., Ketzel, M., Overvad, K., TjØnneland, A. & Raaschou-Nielsen, O. (2014). Exposure to road traffic and railway noise and post menopausal breast cancer: A cohort study, *Int J Cancer*, *134*(11), 2691-2698.

[88] Eriksson, C., Hilding, A., Pyko, A., Bluhm, G., Pershagen, G. & Östenson, C.G. (2014). Long-termaircraft noise xposure and body mass index, waistcircumference and type 2 diabetes: a prospective study. *Environ Health Perspect*, *122*(7), 687-694.

[89] Oftedal, B., Krog, N.H., Pyko, A., Eriksson, C., Graff-Iversen, S., Haugen, M., et al. (2015). Road traffic noise and markers of obesity – a population-basedstudy, *Environ Res*, *138C*, 144-153.

[90] Léger, D., Guilleminault, C., Bader, G., Lévy, E. & Paillard, M. (2002). Medical and socio-professional impact of insomnia. *Sleep*, *25*(6), 621–625.

[91] Chau, N., Mur, J.M., Benamghar, L., Siegfried, C., Dangelzer, J.L., Français, M., et al. (2004). Relationships between certain individual characteristics and occupational injuries for various jobs in the construction industry: a case-control study. *Am J Ind Med*, *45*(1), 84–92.

[92] Fried, Y., Melamed, S. & Ben-David, H.A. (2002). The joint effects of noise, job complexity, and gender on employee sickness absence: an exploratory study across 21 organizations—the CORDIS study. *J Occup Organiz Psychol*, *75*(2), 131–44.

[93] Thomas, E., Martines, F., Bianco, A., Messina, G., Giustino, V., Zangla, D., Iovane, A. & Palma, A. (2018). Decreased postural control in people with moderate hearing loss. *Medicine* (Baltimore), *97*(14), e0244.

[94] Belojević, G. & Paunović, K. (2016). Recent advances in research on non-auditory effects of community noise. *Srp Arh Celok Lek*, Jan-Feb, *144*(1-2), 94-98.

[95] International Standard Organisation. ISO (1999). *Acoustics – Determination of occupational noise exposure and estimation of noise-induced hearing impairment*. Geneva: ISO, 2013.

[96] Verbeek, J.H., Kateman, E., Morata, T.C., Dreschler, W. A. & Mischke, C. (2014). Interventions to prevent occupational noise-induced hearing loss: A Cochrane systematic review. *Int J Audiol*, Mar, *53*, Suppl 2, S84-96.

[97] Bielefeld, E.C., Kopke, R.D., Jackson, R.L., Coleman, J. K., Liu, J. & Henderson, D. (2007). Noise protection with N-acetyl-l-cysteine (NAC) using a variety of noise exposures, NAC doses, and routes of administration. *Acta Otolaryngol*, *27*, 914-919.

[98] Fetoni, A.R., Mancuso, C., Eramo, S.L., Ralli, M., Piacentini, R., Barone, E., Paludetti, G. & Troiani, D.(2010). *In vivo* protective effect of ferulic acid against noise-induced hearing loss in the Guinea-pig. *Neurosci*, *169*, 1575-1588.

[99] Fetoni, A. R., Eramo, S., Troiani, D. & Paludetti, G. (2011). Therapeutic window for ferulic acid protection against noise-induced hearing loss in the Guinea pig. *Acta Otolaryngol*, *131*, 419-427.

[100] Le Prell, C.G., Gagnon, P.M., Bennett, D. C. & Ohlemiller, K.K. (2011).Nutrient-enhanced diet reduces noise-induced damage to the inner ear and hearing loss. *Transl Res*, *158*, 38-53.

[101] Lindblad, A. C., Rosenhall, U., Olofsson, A. & Hagerman, B. (2011). The efficacy of Nacetylcysteine to protect the human cochlea from subclinical hearing loss caused by impulse noise: a controlled trial. *Noise Health*, *13*, 392-401.

[102] Bagger-Sjöbäck, D., Strömback, K., Hakizimana, P., Plue, J., Larsson, C., Hultcrantz, M., Papatziamos, G., Smeds, H., Danckwardt-Lillieström, N., Hellström, S., Johansson, A., Tideholm, B. & Fridberger, A. (2015). A randomised, double blind trial of NAC for hearing protection during stapes surgery. *PLoS One*, Mar 12, *10*(3), e0115657.

[103] Kramer, S., Dreisbach, L., Lockwood, J., Baldwin, K., Kopke, R., Scranton, S. & O'Leary, M. (2006). Efficacy of the antioxidant N-acetylcysteine (NAC) in protecting ears exposed to loud music. *J Am Acad Audiol*, *17*, 265-278.

[104] Harrop-Jones, A., Wang, X., Fernandez, R., Dellamary, L., Ryan, A. F., LeBel, C. & Piu, F. (2016). The sustained-exposure dexamethasone formulation OTO-104 offers effective protection against noise-induced hearing loss. *Audiol Neurotol*, *21*, 12-21.

[105] Zhou, Y., Zheng, G., Zheng, H., Zhou, R., Zhu, X. & Zhang, Q. (2013). Primary observation of early transtympanic steroid injection in patients with delayed treatment of noise-induced hearing loss. *Audiol Neurootol*, *18*, 89-94.

Chapter 13

SINGLE SIDE DEAFNESS IN CHILDREN

Antonio della Volpe, Arianna Di Stadio, Antonietta De Lucia, Valentina Ippolito and Vincenzo Pastore
Otology and Cochlear Implant Unit,
Santobono-Posilipon Children's Hospital, Naples-Italy

ABSTRACT

The importance of a good hearing function to preserve memory and cognitive abilities has been shown in the adult population but studies on the pediatric population are currently lacking. To date we have investigated memory and cognition; Memory was studied in children affected from Single Side Deafness (SSD) and treated with Bone Anchored Hearing Implant (BAHI) while the cognition was studied in a sample of children affected from Unilateral Asymmetric Hearing Loss (UAHL) evaluating the effect of Adhesive Anchored Prosthesis (AAP). Both studies aimed evaluating the effects of BAHI or AAP on speech perception, speech processing, and memory in children with SSD or UAHL. We enrolled in the two studies a total of 35 children (25 with SSD and 10 with AUHL) and assessed them prior to BAHI implantation or AAP use. In the case control study (BAHI) children were evaluated at 1-month and 3-month follow-up using tests of perception in silence and perception in phonemic confusion, dictation in silence and noise, working memory and short-term memory function in conditions of silence and noise. We also enrolled end evaluated N = 15 children with normal hearing. In the AUHL study, instead, we evaluated speech perception test, dictation test, working memory and short-term memory function tests prior to the intervention (no Hearing Aid (NoHeAi)), immediately after the intervention (AAPT0), and 1week post-intervention (AAPT1).

Keywords: single side deafness, hearing loss, bilateral hearing

In the BAHI study we found a statistically significant difference in performance between healthy children and children with Single Side Deafness (SSD) before BAHI implantation in the scores of all tests. After 3 months from BAHI implantation, performance of children with SSD was comparable to that of healthy subjects in speech perception, working memory and short-term memory function in silence, while differences persisted in the scores of the dictation (both in silence and noise condition) and working memory function test in noise condition.

The AAP study showed at AdHeT1 statistically significant improvement compared to their pre-intervention baseline (NoHeAi) in speech perception ($p = 0.01$) and dictation ability both in noise ($p = 0.03$) and silence ($p = 0.02$) conditions. Scores of the short-term memory test ($p = 0.01$) and of the working memory test in noise ($p = 0.01$) and silence ($p = 0.01$) conditions were also improved. Similar results were obtained for subjects with mild and severe SSHL. At AdHeT0 subjects showed an improvement in the scores of all tests compared to NoHeAi, but the changes were not statistically significant.

Our data suggests that in children with SSD BAHI improves speech perception and memory; the AAP might be helpful in the treatment of AUHL for the same reason of BAHI in SSD. Speech rehabilitation may be necessary to further improve speech processing both with BAHI that with AAP.

INTRODUCTION

The importance of recovery of bilateral hearing function is a widely accepted concept in the treatment of patients with bilateral deafness[1]; conversely, single side Hearing Loss (SSHL) are rarely treated with hearing aids [2], bone anchored hearing aid [3], or cochlear implants (CI) [4]. In patients with SSHL, both adult and pediatric, a good unilateral hearing function is typically considered acceptable, and the option of using a hearing aid is often underexplored. However, bilateral hearing function is not only important for hearing correctly, but it is also necessary for identifying origin and direction of sound [5], perceiving nuances of music [6], and improving the hearing ability function in noise situations [3, 4]; in children, it is key for developing normal auditory pathways [7]. As it has been shown by recent studies, bilateral hearing improves quality of life, social life, speech perception [8], and memory function [8-11]. While most studies focus on assessing these outcomes in CIs recipients [4, 8, 9], the effects of hearing aids and bone anchored systems are rarely studied [14].

Recently it was demostred on adult population that working memory performances are influenced by hearing function [14-16]. Infact it has been shown that hearing impairments affect working memory function in subjects who are asked to identify spoken sentences with semantic ambiguity [14, 15]. Increased auditory thresholds decrease scores in the Text Reception Threshold test [17, 18] which suggests that hearing impairments also ultimately affect reading performance. Finally, in a recent study, Saunders et al. showed that improvement in hearing via a personal frequency modulation system led to an enhancement of word recognition ability in veterans [19].

The link between hearing impairment and working memory shown by the aforementioned studies is not surprising. In fact, working memory which is part of the short-term memory and whose main role is managing the information temporarily stored in the short-term memory, is composed of four main parts, one of which (phonological loop) is specifically dedicated to storing and manipulating verbal information [20]. The phonological loop works in synergy with the central executive (an attentional control system), the episodic buffer [21], and the visuospatial sketchpad (useful for visual and spatial information) for ensuring a correct higher-level processing of verbal data, such as word recognition, reading, and speech production.

While current literature on the relationship between hearing abilities, memory and speech processing mainly focuses on adults, studies on the pediatric population are lacking. In particular, little is known on how hearing abilities affect memory function in children with Single Side Deafness (SSD). Understanding this relationship in this population is particularly important as both these functions affect learning, and thus potentially academic performances.

HOW TO TEST AUDITORY AND MEMORY

The screening tests for children affected from Single Side Deafness (SSD) includes auditory test and study on memory functions.

During each evaluation session, all subjects undergo tests for evaluating speech perception, memory (working memory and short-term memory), and dictation performances. Speech perception is evaluated by using the Common Evaluation Protocol in Rehabilitative Audiology (CEPRA) [22], where we evaluate Perception in silence (PS) and Perception in Phonemic Confusion (PPC), also evaluated in silence condition.

The PS test allows an integrated evaluation of hearing and brain function (working memory), while the PPC test allows a mere evaluation of the actual hearing ability (sounds perception) [22].

Working memory and short-term memory are evaluated respectively with the non-sense word repetition test and the verbal span test, both from the PROMEA battery of tests [22]. In the non-word repetition task, the assessor read aloud a list of forty non-sense words of different length. The subject was asked to listen and repeat each word. The total test score was calculated as the number of correct words. The verbal span test included six lists of words of different frequency of use, length, and level of similarity. Each list was composed of seven blocks of word sequences and each block identifies a different span level (from 2 to 8). The subject was asked to repeat the sequences read by the assessor maintaining the same words order. The span level corresponded to the highest number of words correctly repeated in at least three sequences out of five. Working memory tests were performed in silence (WMS) and noise (WMN, cocktail party noise) conditions [23, 24]. Short-term memory (SM) tests were performed in silence condition. The dictation tests were taken from DDE-2 test [23], and tested overall speech recognition ability including hearing function, short term memory, working memory, signal integration, and writing skills; they were performed in silence (DS) and noise (DN) conditions. The stimuli included non-sense words. In the tasks the examiner read 24 nonsense words, one by one. The subject was asked to repeat each word aloud and write it down.

STUDIES RESULTS

We completed two different study to investigate the effect of bilateral hearing restoration on working memory function by using bone adhesive prosthesis (AAP) and bone anchorage hearing implant (BAHI); the first was a cross-sectional pilot study in which we analyzed children without and with AAP for evaluating the variance in working memory performance, then in the second one we compared the working memory performance between children with SSD with and without BAHI and a group homogeneous for age and sex of healthy children.

In the first study we observed that all children showed an improvement in speech perception and dictation, short term and working memory function tests when we compared their performance without hearing aids and with AAP. The study analyzed the use of AAP at two different times, when children used AAP for a day only and when they used it for a week at least. In all cases (single day and one week) children improved their performance.

We observed that in single day use of AAP, children improved 15% and 32% their dictation performance, respectively in silence and noise. The working memory scores were better than without hearing aids both in silence (25% of gain) and in noise (40%). The short memory notevolly improved when children used AAP (22% of gain).

After 1 week of constant use of AAP every day, children improved their performances in dictation test of 40.3% when they used AAP, specifically they gained a 31% in silence condition until a 51% of improved performance in noise.

We observed that the working memory scores improved by 33% in silence and 58% in noise when children used AAP; short term in particular improved 17%.

In the second study we compared the performance of children with SSD with a healthy group, without and with BAHI; we studied as the first study, the speech perception, the dictate ability and the working memory.

Children with SSD presented statistically significant difference when compared with the healthy, in all tests when they did not use the BAHI. These differences completely disappeared when children used BAHI and in this way the bilateral hearing function was restored.

The only test in which we did not observe equal performance after use of BAHI was the dictation, in fact even the children with BAHI really improved their performance when compared with themselves with single hearing function, the recovery was not big enough to pair with the healthy children.

DISCUSSION

The overall results of our studies, showed that a bilateral hearing function is fundamental to reach good performance in speech perception, dictate test and working memory function.

In fact, both patients with AAP and the ones with BAHI really ameliorated their personal performance when the prosthesis was applied on the SSD ear, by supporting the idea that also in presence of good function of a single ear the bilateral hearing function have to be always searched, in fact authors have been shown that in pediatric subjects even a mild loss of hearing function can trigger fatigue and ultimately reduce subjects' academic performance [26], as well as reduce intellectual abilities [27].

In our first study patients using AAP showed an overall improvement in speech perception, dictation, and working memory tests; improvements tended to increase with prolonged use (7 days) of the prosthesis.

In the speech perception test, all subjects displayed an improvement with AAP when compared with no use of hearing aids. The improvement in this test was, however, smaller compared to the improvements in the other tests.

The dictation was improved also by analyzing performance after 1-day use of AAP even obviously the major increasing of the performances was observed after 1 week of AAP use.

Memory abilities largely improved with use of AAP, both in terms of working memory and short-term memory. The working memory, a part of short- memory, is the cognitive function involved in manipulating the information temporarily stored in the short-term memory. According to the multi-component model of Baddeley and Hitch [20] working memory can be divided into the following components: 1) phonological loop, which stores and manipulates verbal information; 2) visuospatial sketchpad, useful for visual and spatial information; 3) the central executive, that works as an attentional control system, and at least 4) the episodic buffer. The episodic buffer component stores information from the subsystems in a multimodal code and combines it with information from long-term memory into a unitary episodic representation [21]. The fact that subjects improved in both memory and dictation tests is not surprising, as a short-term and working memory amelioration not only enhances the quantity of storable information, but also facilitates data manipulation and translation from the phonological to the graphemic code.

The biggest gain in working memory function was achieved at after 1 week of use of AAP when the children were tested in the noise and silence conditions. The improvement in silence condition was smaller than the one in noise. After 1 week of AAP use, short term memory function was also greatly improved, and displayed a trend in improvement similar to the one observed for working memory.

These results are on line with the several studies that have shown how the bilateral hearing function is fundamental for maintaining good memory function [27-29], verbal abilities [30, 31, 32], and word recollection performance [33]; all these functions require the ability to identify and recall sounds in the voice frequency band [27].

In our second study, we reinforced the results obtained in the first one, in fact we observed a statistically significant difference between children with SSD without BAHI and healthy controls, in speech perception, dictate test and working memory function.

We chose to measure subjects' performance in speech perception, dictation, and working memory function tests as these skills are known to be related.

When children with SSD used BAHI, they displayed impaired performance compared to healthy subjects only in the dictate and working memory tests in noise, all other scores instead were similar to those recorded from the control group.

The comparison between subjects with SSD using BAHI and healthy controls did not show a statistically significant difference for speech perception both in silence and in noise, indicating that BAHI improves speech perception ability in terms by improving subjects' ability to perceive sound [25, 34].

The dictation abilities of children with SSD using BAHI, although improved when compared to not use of hearing aids, did not reach results statistically significant enough for defining a performance that was the same of the healthy.

We think that this result may be due to a combination of the complexity of the dictation test and the relatively short follow-up we used in this study. Multiple abilities are required to reach high scores in a dictation test, including good hearing function, concentration, short-term memory, and overall confidence of being able to complete the task. Re-acquiring all these skills may take time, possibly longer than the 3 months of our observation period [22].

We investigated working memory both in silence and noise condition to assess the effect of environmental conditions [35]. Children with SSD using BAHI showed performance similar to the healthy for working memory in silence and short memory; the gain that they have had in working memory performance in noise comparing SSD without BAHI and with BAHI, was not big enough to reach the same performance of the healthy. The difference we observed in the working memory in noise scores might be due to the fact that BAHI increases sound perception; as previously shown by other authors [9-14, 19], this increase can cause difficulty in concentration, especially if subjects perceive the noise as meaningful [36].

The key role of bilateral hearing function in preserving good memory function [10, 27, 37-39], verbal abilities [27, 28], and word recollection performance [29] has been shown by a number of studies; all these functions require the ability to identify and recall sounds in the audible frequency band [35]. Our results show that even children who preserved good unilateral hearing function can benefit from the use of BAHI, and that bilateral hearing function positively affects memory function [10, 32, 36, 40]. The bilateral hearing function gained through BAHI allowed SSD children to achieve speech perception abilities comparable to those from healthy subjects in the same age range as well as similar results in terms of short-term memory and working memory function in the noise condition. Performance in the dictation and working memory tests of children with BAHI might be further improved by speech rehabilitation.

CONCLUSION

The results of our studies confirm that bilateral hearing function needs to be achieved always, even in case of quite satisfactory quality of life with a single

The effect of bilateral hearing improves not only the speech perception but also superior brain function.

It is known that in case of deafness there is not a re-organization of brain area, in opposite to that happen in blindness, but we still don't know what happens in SSD

Our results showed that by using AAP of BAHI the performances of children affected by SSD become similar to the heathy ones in the same age range.

In our opinion SSD or asymmetric hearing loss (HL) should be treated with hearing aids, in case of SSD and severe form of HL, BAHI is the more appropriate technology. In case of mild and mild to severe HL the AAP is the best solution, because is a minimally invasive high-performance system.

Anyway, speech rehabilitation after BAHI implantation or AAP application might help fill the gap in performance between subjects with SSD and healthy controls and help the former to achieve full recovery of complex functions such as those required by the dictation and working memory tests in noise condition.

REFERENCES

[1] Martines, F., Maira, E. & Ferrara, S. (2011). Age-related hearing impairment (ARHI): A common sensory deficit in the elderly. *Acta Medica Mediterranea*, *27* (1), 47-52.

[2] James, R. & Dornhoffer, John L. Dornhoffer. (2016). Pediatric unilateral sensorineural hearing loss. *Current Opinion in Otolaryngology & Head and Neck Surgery*, *24*, 6, pages 522-528.

[3] Monini, S., Musy, I., Filippi, C., Atturo, F. & Barbara, M. (2015). Bone conductive implants in single-sided deafness. *Acta Otolaryngol.*, Apr, *135*(4), 381-8.

[4] Arndt, S., Aschendorff, A., Laszig, R., Beck, R., Schild, C., Kroeger, S., Ihorst, G. & Wesarg, T. (2011). Comparison of pseudobinaural hearing to real binaural hearing rehabilitation after cochlear implantation in patients with unilateral deafness and tinnitus. *Otol Neurotol.*, Jan, *32*(1), 39-47.

[5] Seeber, B. U., Baumann, U. & Fastl, H. (2004). Localization ability with bimodal hearing aids and bilateral cochlear implants. *J Acoust Soc Am.*, Sep, *116* (3), 1698-709.

[6] Polonenko, M. J., Giannantonio, S., Papsin, B. C., Marsella, P. & Gordon, K. A. (2017). Music perception improves in children with bilateral cochlear implants or bimodal devices. *J Acoust Soc Am.*, Jun, *141* (6), 4494.

[7] Fallon, J. B., Irvine, D. R. & Shepherd, R. K. (2008). Cochlear implants and 231 brain plasticity. *Hear Res.*, Apr, *238*(1-2), 110-7.

[8] Nahm, E. A., Liberatos, P., Shi, Q., Lai, E. & Kim, A. H. (2017). Quality of Life after Sequential Bilateral Cochlear Implantation. *Otolaryngol Head Neck Surg.*, Feb, *156*(2), 334-340.

[9] van Zon, A., Smulders, Y. E., Stegeman, I., Ramakers, G. G., Kraaijenga, V. J., Koenraads, S. P., Zanten, G. A., Rinia, A. B., Stokroos, R. J., Free, R. H., Frijns, J. H., Huinck, W. J., Mylanus, E. A., Tange, R. A., Smit, A. L., Thomeer, H. G., Topsakal, V. & Grolman, W. (2017). Stable benefits of bilateral over unilateral cochlear implantation after two years: A randomized controlled trial. *Laryngoscope.*, May, *127*(5), 1161-1168.

[10] McCoy, S. L., Tun, P. A., Cox, L. C., Colangelo, M., Stewart, R. A. & Wingfield, A. (2005). Hearing loss and perceptual effort: downstream effects on older adults' memory for speech. *Q J Exp Psychol A.*, Jan, *58*(1), 22-33.

[11] Salvago, P., Rizzo, S., Bianco, A. & Martines, F. (2017). Sudden sensorineural hearing loss: is there a relationship between routine haematological parameters and audiogram shapes? *International Journal of Audiology*, *56* (3), pp. 148-153.

[12] Rizzo, S., Bentivegna, D., Thomas, E., La Mattina, E., Mucia, M., Salvago, P., Sireci, F. & Martines, F. (2016). Sudden sensorineural hearing loss, an invisible

male: State of art. *Hearing loss: etiology, management and societal implications*, 75-86.

[13] Marsella, P., Scorpecci, A., Cartocci, G., Giannantonio, S., Maglione, A. G., Venuti, I., Brizi, A. & Babiloni, F. (2017). EEG activity as an objective measure of cognitive load during effortful listening: A study on pediatric subjects with bilateral, asymmetric sensorineural hearing loss. *International Journal of Pediatric Otorhinolaryngology*, *99*, pp. 1-7.

[14] Zeitooni, M., Mäki-Torkko, E. & Stenfelt, S. (2016). Binaural Hearing Ability With Bilateral Bone Conduction Stimulation in Subjects With Normal Hearing: Implications for Bone Conduction Hearing Aids. *Ear Hear*. Nov/Dec, *37*(6), 690-702.

[15] Koeritzer, M. A., Rogers, C. S., Van Engen, K. J. & Peelle, J. E. (2018). The Impact of Age, Background Noise, Semantic Ambiguity, and Hearing Loss on Recognition Memory for Spoken Sentences. *J Speech Lang Hear Res.*, Feb 15, 1-12. doi: 10.1044/2017_JSLHR-H-17-0077.

[16] Dispenza, F., Cappello, F., Kulamarva, G. & De Stefano, A. (2013). The discovery of the stapes. *Acta Otorhinolaryngol Ital.*, *33*(5), 357-359.

[17] Zekveld, A. A., Pronk, M., Danielsson, H. & Rönnberg, J. (2018). Reading Behind the Lines: The Factors Affecting the Text Reception Threshold in Hearing Aid Users. *J Speech Lang Hear Res.*, Feb 13, 1-14. doi: 10.1044/2017_JSLHR-H-17-0196.

[18] Besser, J., Zekveld, A. A., Kramer, S. E., Rönnberg, J. & Festen, J. M. (2012). New measures of masked text recognition in relation to speech-in-noise perception and their associations with age and cognitive abilities. *J Speech Lang Hear Res.*, Feb, *55*(1), 194-209. doi: 10.1044/1092-4388(2011/11-0008).

[19] Saunders, G. H., Frederick, M. T., Arnold, M. L., Silverman, S. C., Chisolm, T. H. & Myers, P. J. (2018). A Randomized Controlled Trial to Evaluate Approaches to Auditory Rehabilitation for Blast-Exposed Veterans with Normal or Near-Normal Hearing Who Report Hearing Problems in Difficult Listening Situations. *J Am Acad Audiol.*, Jan, *29*(1), 44-62. doi: 10.3766/jaaa.16143.

[20] Baddeley, A. D. (2000). The episodic buffer: A new component of working memory? *Trends in Cognitive Science*, *4*, 417-423.

[21] Baddeley, A. D. & Hitch, G. J. (1974). Working 256 memory. In G. A. Bower (Ed.), *Recent advances in learning and motivation*, (Vol. *8*, pp. 47-89). New York: Academic Press.

[22] Schindler, A., Vernero, I. & Aimar, E. (2009). Fisiologia della percezione uditiva. In: Allenamento della percezione uditiva nei bambini con impianto cocleare. [Physiology of auditory perception. In: Training of auditory perception in children with a cochlear implant] *Metodologie Riabilitative in Logopedia*, vol 16. Springer, Milano.

[23] Hutcherson, R. W., Dirks, D. D. & Morgan, D. E. (1979). Evaluation of the speech perception in noise (SPIN) test. *Otolaryngol Head Neck Surg*, Mar-Apr, *87*(2), 239-45.

[24] Sartori, G., Job, R. & Tressoldi, P. E. (2007). *DDE-2 Batteria per la Valutazione della Dislessia e della Disortografia Evolutiva-2 Giunti O.S.* [*DDE-2 Battery for the Evaluation of Dyslexia and Evolutionary Disorthography-2 Joints O.S.*]

[25] Sheffield, B. M. & Zeng, F. G. (2012). The relative phonetic contributions of a cochlear implant and residual acoustic hearing to bimodal speech perception. *J Acoust Soc Am.*, Jan, *131*(1), 518-30.

[26] Hornsby, B. W., Werfel, K., Camarata, S. & Bess, F. H. (2014). Subjective fatigue in children with hearing loss: some preliminary findings. *Am J Audiol.*, Mar, *23*(1), 129-34. doi: 10.1044/10590889 (2013/13-0017).

[27] Rabbitt, P. (1990). Mild hearing loss can cause apparent memory failures which increase with age and reduce with IQ. *Acta Otolaryngol Suppl.*, *476*, 167-75, discussion 176.

[28] McCoy, S. L., Tun, P. A., Cox, L. C., Colangelo, M., Stewart, R. A. & Wingfield, A. (2005). Hearing loss and perceptual effort: downstream effects on older adults' memory for speech. *Q J Exp Psychol A.* Jan, *58*(1), 22-33.

[29] EeLynn, Ng. & Kerry, Lee. (2010). *Children's task performance under stress and non-stress conditions: A test of the processing efficiency theory Cognition and Emotion*, Vol. 24, Iss. 7.

[30] Rezai, M., Lofti, G. & Wiesi, F. (2012). Comparison of Working Memory in Hearing Loss and Normal Children. *Pajouhan Scientific Journal*, North America, *11*, dec.

[31] Wong, C. G. (2017*). Hearing Loss and Verbal Memory Assessment in Older Adults.* Wayne State University, ProQuest Dissertations Publishing. 10267327.

[32] Ballacchino, A., Salvago, P., Cannizzaro, E., Costanzo, R., Di Marzo, M., Ferrara, S., La Mattina, E., Messina, G., Mucia, M., Mulè, A., Plescia, F., Sireci, F., Rizzo, S. & Martines, F. (2015). Association between sleep-disordered breathing and hearing disorders: Clinical observation in Sicilian patients, *Acta Medica Mediterranea*, *31* (3), pp. 607-614.

[33] Skinner, B. F. (1957). *Verbal Behavior*. Acton, MA: Copley Publishing Group.

[34] Roman, S., Nicollas, R. & Triglia, J. M. (2011). Practice guidelines for bone-anchored hearing aids in children. *Eur Ann Otorhinolaryngol Head Neck Dis.*, Nov, *128* (5), 253-8.

[35] Ng, E. H., Rudner, M., Lunner, T., Pedersen, M. S. & Rönnberg, J. (2013). Effects of noise and working memory capacity on memory processing of speech for hearing-aid users. *Int J Audiol.*, Jul, *52*(7), 433-41.

[36] Lyxell, B. & Rönnberg, J. (1993). The effects of background noise and working memory capacity on speechreading performance. *Scand Audiol.*, *22*(2), 67-70.

[37] Ng, EeLynn. & Kerry, Lee. (2010). Children's task performance under stress and non-stress conditions: A test of the processing efficiency theory. *Cognition and Emotion, 24* (7), 1229-1238.

[38] Dispenza, F., Battaglia, A. M., Salvago, P. & Martines, F. (2018). Determinants of failure in the reconstruction of the tympanic membrane: A case-control study. *Iranian Journal of Otorhinolaryngology, 30* (6), pp. 341-346.

[39] Dispenza, F., De Stefano, A., Costantino, C., Marchese, D. & Riggio, F. (2013). Sudden Sensorineural Hearing Loss: results of intratympanic steroids as salvage treatment. *Am J Otolaryngol, 34*, 296-300.

[40] Dispenza, F., Mazzucco, W., Bianchini, S., Mazzola, S. & Bennici, E. (2015). Management of labyrinthine fistula in chronic otitis with cholesteatoma: case series. *EuroMediterranean Biomedical Journal, 10*(21), 255-261.

Section 3. Treatment of Sensorineural Hearing Loss

Chapter 14

PHARMACOLOGICAL TREATMENT OF SENSORINEURAL HEARING LOSS

Angela Cavallaro[1], Carla Cannizzaro[1], MD,
Francesco Martines[2], MD, Gianluca Lavanco[3],
Pietro Salvago[2], MD, Fabiana Plescia[4], PhD,
Anna Brancato[1], PhD and Fulvio Plescia[1],*, PhD

[1]Department of Sciences for Health Promotion and Mother and Child Care "Giuseppe D'Alessandro," University of Palermo, Palermo, Italy
[2]Bio.Ne.C. Department, University of Palermo, Palermo, Italy
[3]Department of Biomedical and Biotechnological Sciences, University of Catania, Catania, Italy
[4]Dipartimento di Scienze e Tecnologie Biologiche, Chimiche e Farmaceutiche, Sezione di Chimica e Tecnologie Farmaceutiche, Università degli Studi di Palermo, Palermo, Italy

ABSTRACT

Sudden sensorineural hearing loss is a common and alarming symptom of about 360 million people that suffer from hearing impairment worldwide. The sudden sensorineural hearing loss usually arises unilaterally and it is habitually described as greater than 30dB hearing reduction, attributable to lesions of the cochlea, cranial nerve VIII, brainstem and temporal lobe. There are many factor that promote the onset of this lesions such us infections, circulatory diseases, inner ear neoplasia and neurological disorders. This pathology is characterized by primary symptoms such as the impairment of the comprehension of spoken language and the struggling to listen to music. Subsequently,

---

* Corresponding Author's Email: fulvio.plescia@unipa.it.

secondary symptoms arise as well as anxiety, inadequate coping with illness and psychosomatic disturbances that have a negative impact on patients with a significant reduction in the quality of life. Treatment of the sudden sensorineural hearing loss remains one of the most problematic issues for contemporary otorhinolaryngology, because of the wide array of the presumed mechanisms that underpin this disorder. Although the pharmacological treatment remain even now empirical and the management is not standardized in term of medical treatment, duration and route of administration, different agents are used. In the past, pharmacological approaches have included antiviral agents, vitamin, herbal preparations, carbogen inhalations or magnesium, administered on either an inpatient or outpatient procedures. Nowadays, the corticosteroids therapy remains the mainstay strategy, but considering the multifaceted aspects of this disorder, diuretics, anticoagulants, vasodilatators and fibrinolityc agents have also been tried. In this chapter, we will focus mainly on the principal pharmacological approaches of the sudden sensorineural hearing loss that will be described and examined in terms of mechanism of action and effectiveness.

Keywords: sudden sensorineural hearing loss, glucocorticoids, prostaglandine E1

INTRODUCTION

Hearing well is synonymous with living well. A high quality of hearing reflects a fully participation in everything that happens around us, in fact, hearing is the sense that receives sounds which come from outside the human body, transmitting them, through complex mechanisms that originates in the auricle, in the temporal cortex, the area of the brain able to receive and decode sounds.

The correct functioning of the hearing system has a positive effect also at cognitive levels; in fact, there is a direct correlation between hearing loss and ability of the brain to process information and recall memories.

Given the importance of corret functioning of the hearing system, appear clear how troubled and disabililing could be a total or partial perceptual hearing loss.

The Sudden Sensorineural Hearing Loss (SSHL), defined by US National Institute for Deafness and Communication Disorders (NICDC) as an idiopathic loss of hearing of at least 30 dB, nearly always unilateral, is one of the most common human ailments and the most ordinary complaint of patients evaluated by hearing impairment specialists. It occurs at any age making verbal communication and comprehension of spoken language more difficult. Usually patients notice that the hearing loss appears instantaneously in the morning even if others describe that it rapidly developed over a period of hours or days [1].

The onset of the symptoms is subjective, but generally it occurs over less than a 72-hour period and the severity of the harm also varies from patient to patient [2].

SSNHL affect the inner ear and the neural pathways to the auditory cortex. Although the pathology predominantly affects adults, children also can be affected [3].

The diagnosis of deaf patients is difficult and impose a specify analysis of the primary symptoms such as impairment of the localization of sound, the difficulty on comprehension of spoken language in a noisy environment, and the enjoyment of music. These symptoms are frequently associated with secondary symptoms as anxiety, inadequate coping with illness, various types of psychosomatic disturbance, and damage quality of life [4]. Considering the multifaceted aspects of the SSNHL, such as patient age, presence of vertigo and/or tinnitus at onset, exposure to ototoxic agents, degree of hearing loss, audiometric configuration, time between onset of hearing loss, and co-morbidities such as hypertension and diabetes, treatments have traditionally been empirical [5-9].

Corticosteroids, *via* systemic and/or intratympanic administration, have been the most commonly agents used to treat SSNHL, even if a large array of other drugs, such as antivirals, antibiotics, diuretics, vasodilators, osmotic agents, plasma expanders, anticoagulants, mineral supplements, and hyperbaric oxygen or carbon dioxide rich gases, among others, have been used [10].

Although the etiopathology of this disease is still unclear, this chapter aims to understand the pathophysiology and the appropriate drug therapies, by answering four simple questions: *What is Sudden Hearing Loss? What Causes Sudden Hearing Loss? How is Sudden Hearing Loss Diagnosed? How is Sudden Hearing Loss Treated?*

SUDDEN SENSORINEURAL HEARING LOSS: INTO THE MEDICAL HISTORY

SSNHL, described as a medical emergency in search of appropriate diagnostic techniques and treatments, is generally defined as a rapidly developing hearing loss with a threshold reduction of ≥30 dB in at least three contiguous audiometric frequencies [11].

According to the World Health Organization, about 360 million people suffer from hearing impairment worldwide and in the European Union, the number is expected to amount to 434,000 people suffering from deafness and 44,000,000 people suffering from hearing impairment [12, 13].

All ages and both sexes are affected, with peak ages ranging between 30 and 60 years [14, 15]. According to the otolaryngologist guidelines, SSNHL is a suddenly appearing, generally as an unilateral hearing loss of cochlear origin with unknown cause (i.e., idiopathic), expressing different degrees of severity, up to complete deafness (*anacusis*), sometimes additionally with vertigo and/or tinnitus [16].

The SSNHL etiology remains unknown in the most of patients and the causes can be numerous and could be congenital or acquired [Table 1]. Although the list of potential etiologies is lengthy, the more substantial evidence seems to support that SSNHL is most commonly the result of viral infections, vascular disruption, inner ear problems, such as Meniere's disease, neoplastic, traumatic, metabolic, neurologic and cochlear injuries and also autoimmune processes, toxic damage and alcohol use. None of these etiologies has undisputed evidence supporting its role in the cause of SSNHL, therefore, these cases remain idiopathics [17-19].

Regarding its pathophysiological, still unclear, three major categories of hearing loss could be considered to the differential diagnosis: the impeded sound conduction through the external ear, middle ear or both; hearing loss that occurs within the cochlea or the neural pathway to the auditory cortex; and eventually a mixed hearing loss, concomitant with a conductive loss and sensorineural one [20].

Generally, SSNHL has a rapid onset, occurring over a 72-hour period, of a subjective sensation of hearing impairment in one or both ears. It indicates an abnormalities of the cochlea and auditory nerve, with negative impact to the central auditory perception or processing. The most frequently used audiometric criterion is a decrease in hearing and since premorbid audiometry is generally unavailable, hearing loss is defined as related to the opposite ear's thresholds [21].

But *what should we take account of SSNHL?* The majority (96–99%) of sudden hearing loss is unilateral [22, 23]. Causes of bilateral sudden hearing loss are due to autoimmune diseases, syphilis, especially if rapidly progressive, and it occurs commonly in older patients with pre-existing diabetes mellitus and lipid abnormalities. Therefore, it is relevant a full medical history. Detailed otolaryngological experiences indicate that prognosis for recovery is dependent on other factors, including patient age, degree of hearing loss, audiometric configuration, time between onset of hearing loss and treatment, and also presence of vertigo or tinnitus at onset [24, 25].

Table 1. Etiological factors for hearing loss

Infection	Meningitis (bacterial, fungal), labyrinthitis (bacterial, fungal, viral, parasitic, spirochaetal), mumps, measles, chicken pox, syphilis.
Congenital	Large vestibular aqueduct, Mondini dysplasia.
Traumatic	Head injury (with or without fractures), barotrauma (with or without perilymphatic fistula), acoustic trauma, iatrogenic injury.
Neoplastic processes	Vestibular schwannoma and metastases of the meningeal temporal bone, leukemia, multiple myeloma.
Immunological disease	Systemic lupus erythematosus, Cogan syndrome, Wegener's granulomatosis.
Ototoxic agents	Medical product, drugs, tissue toxins
Vascular disease	Hypertensive crisis, hypotonia, AICA (anterior inferior cerebellar artery infarct) infarction.
Neurological diseases	Neurofibromatosis type II, multiple sclerosis, focal ischemia pontine.
Metabolic disorder	Iron metabolic disorder, renal failure/dialysis.

Tinnitus, defined as an abnormal noise perceived in one or both ears or in the head in which a patient has a conscious hearing percept in absence of external sound, is usually reported in patients with SSNHL [26-28]. Given the considerable correlation between tinnitus and sudden hearing loss, studies have been reported that the incidence seems to be 5-30 per 100,000 persons per year [29, 30] and accounts for 1% of all sensorineural hearing loss cases [31].

SSNHL commonly occurs in patients aged between 25 and 60 years old, with a peak in prevalence for patients between 46 and 49 years old with increasing incidence with age and male are equally affected as females [32-34].

Although SSNHL has a greater impact on adults, it also affects children, but it is very rare and its cause is still unclear. It has been reported that 6.6% of patients with SSNHL were under 18 years of age, 3.5% under 14 years, and only 1.2% under 9 years [35]. Due to the rarity of SSNHL in the pediatric population, research regarding etiology, treatment outcomes and prognosis of SSNHL in children is limited.

SYMPTOMS: FROM THE MECHANISTIC DAMAGE TO THE DISTORTED PERCEPTION

Sound waves are conducted via the external ear and the external auditory canal to the tympanic membrane. The mechanical vibrations are transmitted by the ossicles way of the middle ear to the cochlear perilymph and endolymph. Thus, all the disturbances that arise along the sound conduction pathway, have a mechanical nature that terms into a hearing loss [36].

People who get a hearing loss, usually refer a reduction in hearing ability, describing the feeling that have hair in the auricle or a large wool pad into the ear canal.

The subsequent *hypoacusia* has also a perceptive nature, since the inner ear (cochlea, acoustic nerve) cannot transmit, through the central acoustic way, the correct nervous impulse from sound vibrations [37]. This results in a distorted perception of sounds, impairment of the comprehension of spoken language and the struggling to listen to music. In fact, people often compensate to the hearing impairment by turning up the volume of the radio or television set, or (in unilateral hearing impairment) by turning the healthy ear to the sound sources.

In addition to a great insecurity among people affected, toward the environment, it is very common taking advantage from vision to speech recognition with an increasing reliance on lip-reading, in order to prevent the consequent inappropriate answers to misheard questions and an excessively loud speaking voice.

But the simultaneous presence of other symptoms, makes the sudden hearing loss even more disabling. In fact, patients often report disorders such as vertigo, tinnitus and buzzing and just about to the numerous symptoms reported, experts' opinions about causes and therapies are enough controversial [38].

DIAGNOSTIC MEASURES: THE STATE OF THE MULTIPLE EVIDENCES

SSNHL defined as a rapid onset, occurring over a 72-hour period, of a subjective sensation of hearing impairment in one or both ears, has a sensorineural nature and meets audiometric criteria. The most frequently used audiometric criterion is a decrease in hearing of ≥30 decibels (dB), affecting at least 3 consecutive frequencies. Because premorbid audiometry is generally unavailable, hearing loss is defined as related to the opposite ear's thresholds. [39]

Although patients often underestimate a tangible disease, clinical experiences indicate that a range from 32% to 65% of cases of SSNHL may recover spontaneously [40, 41].

Many of the discoverable causes of SSNHL induce permanent hearing loss due to the damage to hair cells or other inner ear structures. Prognosis for recovery depend on a several number of factors, in fact, the evaluation usually lay the groundwork for a careful history on physical examination, beginning to patient age, presence of vertigo or tinnitus at onset, degree of hearing loss and time between onset of hearing loss [5,42]. Moreover, it is essential looking for potential infectious causes such as otitis media, systemic diseases and exposure to known ototoxic medications.

Table 2. Diagnostic measures

Otoacoustic emissions (OAE)
Auditory evoked brainstem potentials (ABR)
Speech audiometry
Stapedius reflex measurement
Functional examination of the cervical spine
Laboratory tests: blood glucose, CRP, procalcitonin, small blood count, differential blood count, creatinine, fibrinogen level.
Serologic testing: borreliosis, syphilis, herpes simplex virus type 1, varicella zoster virus, CMV, HIV.
MRI: exclusion of a tumor of the cerebello pontine angle
CT scan: skull, temporal bone, cervical spine
Electrocochleography: coclear damage, exclusion of hydrops
Auditory steady state responses (ASSR)
Tympanoscopy

Given the decline in hearing, the first step to diagnose the SSNHL, usually requires an audiogram.

Instead, blood studies are usually performed to rule out potential systemic causes (i.e., syphilis, Lyme disease, metabolic, autoimmune and circulatory disorders) [43]. Moreover, in order to investigate the presence of acoustic neuroma, which is reported to be existent up to 15% of patients with sudden hearing loss, Magnetic Resonance Imaging of the brain is frequently recommended [44].

Considering the large amount of etiological causes, the different and usual procedures, required in individual cases, are reported in Table 2.

PHARMACOLOGICAL MANAGEMENT: GLUCOCORTICOIDS MECHANISMS OF ACTION

Numerous agents have been suggested and used to treat of the SSNHL, in concert with alternative approaches (i.e., acoustic, electrical, surgical and radiological strategies). A large number of different drugs have been investigated for the treatment of idiopathic SSNHL including antiinflammatory agents, antimicrobials, calcium antagonists essential minerals, vasodilators, volume expanders, defibrinogenators, diuretics and hyperbaric oxygen [41]. On the basis of the etiology of this disorder, still unclear, there are insufficient evidences supporting the daily application of antiviral, vasodilatory or antioxidant drugs, together with alternative therapeutic methods, which also include vitamins or Ginko Biloba [45, 46].

The most common approach to treatment of SSHL is with glucocorticoids (GC), which are considered, around the world, to be the gold standard of therapy, because it is thought the disorder might be due to an infectious/inflammatory or autoimmune process [4, 47]. GC act on almost all organs, mainly carrying out their effects through a DNA-mediated induction of protein biosynthesis after transformation of an intracellular GC receptor (GCR). In the cytoplasm, the non-active receptor is present in a complex with chaperones. The GC-activated GCR undergoes an initial conformation change, resulting in the dissociation of the chaperone–GCR complex. In this way the GC–GCR complex is activated and can translocate to the nucleus where it dimerizes. As a homodimer, it can bind to the DNA regulatory sequences, called GC response elements (GRE) and found in the promoter regions of glucocorticoid-regulated genes. If the GC–GCR complex binding leads to gene activation, the GRE sequence termed as 'positive' GRE. Negative GRE is also described where GC–GCR leads to gene suppression (direct repression) [48, 49]. GCs action includes their influence (direct or indirect) on the human genome (DNA within the nucleus) transcription and translation, for many genes encoding inflammatory mediators. Its actions become evident within 1 to 2 hours and the cytoplasmatic effects, mostly at very high doses, occur after only a few minutes [50]. Each cell contains 2 classes of GCR, type I (glucocorticoid) and type II (mineralocorticoid), both of which are present in the cochlear and vestibular tissues of mammals [51, 52]. The activation of cytoplasmatic GCR lead to the triggering of transcription processes and also the expression of specific genes, that inhibit the synthesis of inflammatory mediators and cytokines, which are responsible for the anti-inflammatory effects of GC. GC also affect carbohydrate and protein metabolism and change the physicochemical characteristics of cell membranes, promoting their stabilization and reducing the permeability of cations (cytoplasmic effect). Finally, they are able to regulate cellular osmolarity through the binding of type II mineralocorticoid receptors, which activate the enzyme Na,K-ATPase [53]. This enzyme is found at the base of the external and internal hair cells, the tympanic nerve fibers and the spiral ganglion cells of mammals [54, 55]. The activation of Na, K-ATPase by GC could have positive effects on unbalanced intracellular and extracellular osmolarity, electrochemical gradients and neuronal activities, which are disturbed by noise-related cellular, functional cochlear damage and autoimmune inner ear disease [56, 57]. It is interesting that GC, despite their conventional effects at physiological concentrations, have various therapeutic application at higher doses, through different mechanisms: immunosuppressive effects (inhibition of the activation of T lymphocytes), anti-inflammatory (trough blockade of proinflammatory mediators), antiproliferative effect (through suppression of collagen synthesis and fibroblast formation) and immunosuppressive one (through the inhibition of the activation of T lymphocytes) [58]. The use of GC is justified by the fact that steroids are able to reduce inflammation and edema in the inner ear, typical in the idiopathic, SSNHL. Despite the numerous clinical trials, the value of steroids in the treatment of SSNHL remains unclear, but the administration of high-doses of corticosteroids is recommended and primary performed in clinical routine practice [59, 60].

PHARMACOLOGICAL MANAGEMENT: ORAL AND INTRATYMPANIC CORTICOSTEROID THERAPY

Oral/systemic corticosteroid administration is the most frequent primary pharmacological treatment and is widely considered most efficacious for its ability to reduce the inflammation and the edema in the inner ear [10]. Although, there aren't many data to support this recommendation, in fact, different studies showed that oral steroids administration, such as methylprednisolone or dexamethasone, administered over a period of 10 to 12 days, was able to induce a significant higher rates of improvement among patients [61]. The efficacy of systemic corticosteroid treatment seems directly related to the time between the onset of the disease and the start of the pharmacological treatment [62]. Studies taking into account the relationship between the duration of SSNHL before pharmacological therapy and outcomes have reported the greatest recovery of hearing when corticosteroids were given within the first one to two week after symptom onset, and little if any when initiated four weeks or longer after the onset of the symptoms [63-65].

Some clinical studies evaluated the effects of oral corticosteroids *vs* oral placebo for the treatment of SHHL [65]. Wilson et al., [61] showed that dexamethasone (0.75 mg twice daily to 4.5 mg twice daily) or metylprednisolone (4 mg/d to 16 mg three times daily) have the same anti-inflammatory effects. In particular, these clinical research showed that corticosteroids was able to reduce the pure-tone average, measured at four and three months after the onset of SSNHL, thus bringing to a greater rate of recovery in patients treated with steroids than to placebo control group [61]. In contrast with these studies, randomized controlled studies conducted by Nostrati-Zerenoe and Cinamon have failed to demonstrate a beneficial effect of systemic steroids administration [66, 67]. In particular, Cinamon and collegues have find that prednisone (1mg/kg daily) was not able to reduce the pure-tone average scores, speech frequency, high tone hearing levels, and discrimination scores at 6 days and 14 to 90 days (follow-up) after treatment.

These reports together with the side effects induced by corticosteroid administration (mood changes, elevated blood pressure and sugar levels, loss of appetite, weight gain, gastritis, sleep disorders and hyperglycemia) ensure that oral therapy is to be considered carefully, in particular in patients with other chronic diseases such as sleep disorders or diabetes mellitus.

In alternative of oral corticosteroids, some otolaryngologists recommend local corticosteroid therapy for SSNHL. This treatment is based on the local glucocorticoid injection, directly into the ear in order to reduce the risk of systemic side effects, typical of oral administration, allowing glucocorticoids to penetrate directly into the cochlea and achieve a high concentration there even when low doses are used [65-69]. This procedure consists in the administration of methylprednisolone, dexamethasone and prednisolone, drugs able to affect the immune suppression and the ion homeostasis [70], by intratympanic or as eardrops by means of ventilating tube or a 'wick' running from a ventilating tube to the round window membrane in the medial wall of the middle ears. In this way, corticosteroids are available in high concentrations in the target tissue, promoting a reduction of inflammation associated with labyrinthitis, an enhancement in cochlear blood flow and improving striavascularis functions.

During the last years, different researches have taken into account the use of intratympanic steroid as the primary treatment of idiopathic SSNHL. Two multicenter studies, conducted by Battaglia et al., [71, 72], have found that association between intratympanic dexamethasone (12 and 10 mg/ml) and hight-dose oral prednisone resulted in a significant improvement of hearing, respect to the treatment with oral prednisone alone.

Two reports about the efficacy of local corticosteroid therapy showed that the association between 5 mg/ml dexamethasone with i.v steroid are able to induce an improvement of the hearing functions in patients affected by SSNHL [73, 74]. These studies, taking together, demonstrated that a combined therapy was more effective for SSNHL in achieving hearing gain than corticosteroids alone. Furthermore, when administered alone as primary therapy, intratympanic steroids have been shown to be as effective as systemic steroids. An elegant research conducted by Rauche and collegues [75] showed that metylprednisolone (40 mg/ml) was able to improve the pure tone average when compared to oral corticosteroid treatment, rejecting the hypothesis of the inferiority of intratympanic administration with respect oral prednisolone. In conclusion intratympanic injection may be an alternative method, particularly for patients who have high risks of complications, due to the oral therapy, although the evidences supporting this strategy is even more limited.

PHARMACOLOGICAL MANAGEMENT: VASODILATORS AGENTS

The speculation about the pathogenesis of the SSNHL lead to the investigation of several other pharmacological agents to treat this disorder.

The hypothesis about the involvement of microvascular dysfunction in the cochlea as major cause of idiopathic SSNHL, different vasodilators and blood thinners are widely suggested as agents able to increase the caliber and blood flow in vessels, in order to rule out the problem.

A research by Zhuo and colleague [76] pointed out the attention on the role played by the Prostaglandine E1 (PGE1), a prostanoid with vasodilator properties, in the treatment of SSNHL. In this study the author showed that PGE1 might be beneficial, probably due to its ability to increase cardiac output, improving cochlear blood flow [77]. Although this study appeared to be favorable to the use of PGE1, a prospective, double blind, randomized controlled study, showed that either PGE1 or placebo, used in addition to a steroid in each experimental condition, do not have a beneficial effect on the treatment of idiopathic SSNHL [78].

Moreover, in order to enhance the microcirculation, other compounds with cerebral vasodilator activity have been studied. A prospective, single blind, randomized controlled study investigated the efficacy of carbogen, a gaseous mixture of 5% carbon dioxide and 95% oxygen, known for its ability to increasing the partial oxygen pressure of perilinfatic fluids, on idiopathic SSNHL. This study showed that carbogen treatment was able to increase the hearing ability with respect to control group [79].

CONCLUSION

Despite specialists are unanimous about the identification of the typical symptoms of the SSNHL, the research and the evaluation of the main causes that trigger this auditory disability are characterized by contrasting opinions. Nevertheless, different pharmacological treatment are known and have been engaged to ameliorate the idiopathic SSNHL. Treatment regimens have included minerals, essential minerals, antimicrobials, vitamin, antiviral and diuretics agents, in addition to herbal preparations. Although initially promising results are found in different case reports and small trials, surprisingly there is a little persuasive evidence that supports the efficacy of these pharmacological agents in alleviating the simptomatologycal conditions that afflict patients with SSNHL. Among all the different therapies, corticosteroids appear the prominent current standard care to improve or restore hearing.

REFERENCES

[1] O'Connell, B. P., Hunter, J. B., Haynes, D. S. (2016) Current concepts in the management of idiopathic sudden sensor neuronal hearing loss. *Curr Opin Otolaryngol Head Neck Surg,* 24:413–419.

[2] National Institute of Health. Sudden Deafness. Bethesda, Md: National Institutes of Health; 2000. *NIH publication* 00-4757.

[3] Martines, F., Salvago, P., Ferrara, S., Messina, G., Mucia, M., Plescia, F., Sireci, F. (2016) Factors influencing the development of otitis media among Sicilian children affected by upper respiratory tract infections. *Braz J Otorhinolaryngol,* 82(2): 215-222.

[4] Suckfüll, M. (2009) Perspectives on the Pathophysiology and Treatment of Sudden Idiopathic Sensorineural Hearing Loss. *Dtsch Arztebl Int,* 106(41): 669–676.

[5] Conlin, A. E., Parnes, L. S. (2007) Treatment of sudden sensorineural hearing loss, I: a systematic review. *Arch Otolaryngol Head Neck Surg,* 133(6):573–81.

[6] Fetterman, B. L., Saunders, J. E., Luxford, W. M. (1996) Prognosis and treatment of sudden sensorineural hearing loss. *Am J Otol,* 17(4):529–36.

[7] Cannizzaro, E., Cannizzaro, C., Plescia, F., Martines, F., Soleo, L., Pira, E., Lo Coco, D. (2014) Exposure to ototoxic agents and hearing loss: A review of current knowledge. *Hearing, Balance and Communication,* 12(4): 166-175.

[8] Plescia, F., Cannizzaro, E., Brancato, A., Martines, F., Di Naro, A., Mucia, M., Plescia, F., Vita, C., Salvago, P., Mulè, A., Rizzo, S., Sireci, F., Cannizzaro, C. (2015) Acetaldehyde effects in the brain. *Acta Med Med,* 31 (4): 813-817.

[9] Watford, K., Labadie, R. F. (2007) Intratympanic dexamethasone for sudden sensorineural hearing loss after failure of systemic therapy. *Laryngoscope,* 117(1): 3–15.

[10] Wei, B. P. C., Mubiru, S., O'Leary, S. (2006) Steroids for idiopathic sudden sensorineural hearing loss. *Cochrane Database Syst Rev*;(1) Art. No.: CD003998.

[11] Haberkamp, T. J., Tanyeri, H. M. (1999) Management of idiopathic sudden sensorineural hearing loss. *Am J Otol,* 20:587–95.

[12] Olzowy, B., Osterkorn, D., Suckfüll, M. (2005) The incidence of sudden hearing loss is greater than previously assumed. *MMW Fortschr Med,* 147(14):37-8.

[13] Klemm, E., Deutscher, A., Mösges, R. (2009) Aktuelle Stichprobe zur Epidemiologie des idiopathischen Hörsturzes [A present 20. investigation of the epidemiology in idiopathic suddensensorineural hearing loss]. *Laryngo,* 88(8): 524-7.

[14] Megighian, D., Bolzan, M., Barion, U., Nicolai, P. (1986) Epidemological considerations in sudden hearing loss: a study of 183 cases. *Arch Otorhinolaryngol,* 243(4):250–3.

[15] Ballacchino, A., Salvago, P., Cannizzaro, E., Costanzo, R., Di Marzo, M., Ferrara, S., La Mattina, E., Messina, G., Mucia, M., Mulè, A., Plescia, F., Sireci, F., Rizzo, S., Martines, F. (2015) Association between sleep-disordered breathing and hearing disorders: Clinical observation in Sicilian patients. *Acta Med Med,* 31(3): 607-614.

[16] Schick, B., Brors, D., Koch, O., Schäfers, M., Kahle, G. (2011) Magnetic resonance imaging in patients with sudden hearing loss, tinnitus and vertigo. *Otol Neurotol,* 22(6):808-12.

[17] Hughes, G. B., Freedman, M. A., Haberkamp, T. J., Guay, M. (1996) Sudden sensorineural hearing loss. *Otolaryngol Clin North Am,* 29:393–405.

[18] Lazarini, P. R., Camargo, A. C. (2006) Idiopathic sudden sensorineural hearing loss: etiopathogenic aspects. *Rev Bras Otorrinolaringol,* 72(4):554–61.

[19] Rybak, L. P. (1985) Treatable sensorineural hearing loss. *Am J Otol,* 6(6):482–9.

[20] Zahnert, T. (2011) The Differential Diagnosis of Hearing Loss. *Dtsch Arztebl Int,* 108(25): 433–444.

[21] National Institute of Deafness and Communication Disorders. *Sudden deafness.* 2000. http://www.nidcd.nih.gov/health/hear- ing/sudden.htm.

[22] Burton, M., Harvey, R. (2007) Idiopathic sudden sensorineural hearing loss. In *Scott-Brown's Otolaryngology*, Gleeson, M. Chapter 131. Butterworth-Heinemann, Oxford.

[23] Oh, J. H., Park, K., Lee, S. J., Shin, Y. R., Choung, Y. H. (2007) Bilateral versus unilateral sudden sensorineural hearing loss. *Otolaryngol Head Neck Surg,* 136:87–91.

[24] Chiossoine-Kerdel, J. A., Baguley, D. M., Stoddart, R. L., Moffat, D. A. (2000) An investigation of the audiologic handicap associated with unilateral sudden sensorineural hearing loss. *Am J Otol,* 21(5):645-651.

[25] Wie, O. B., Pripp, A. H., Tvete, O. (2010) Unilateral deafness in adults: effects on communication and social interaction. *Ann Otol Rhinol Laryngol,* 119(11):772-781.

[26] Cavallaro, A., Martines, F., Cannizzaro, C., Lavanco, G., Brancato, A., Carollo, G., Plescia, F., Salvago, P., Cannizzaro, E., Mucia, M., Rizzo, S., Martini, A., Plescia, F. (2016) Role of cannabinoids in the treatment of tinnitus. *Acta Med Med,* 32: 463-469.

[27] Plescia, F., Cannizzaro, C., Brancato, A., Sireci, F., Salvago, P., Martines, F. (2016) Emerging pharmacological treatments of tinnitus. *Tinnitus: Epidemiology, Causes and Emerging Therapeutic Treatments,* 43-64.

[28] Bennett, M., Kertesz, T., Yeung, P. (2005) Hyperbaric oxygen therapy for idiopathic sudden sensorineural hearing loss and tinnitus: a systematic review of randomised controlled trials. *J Laryngol Otol,* 119: 791–8.

[29] Nosrati-Zarenoe, R., Arlinger, S., Hultcrantz, E. (2007) Idiopathic sudden sensorineural hearing loss: Results drawn from the Swedish national database. *Acta Oto-Laryngol,* 127:1168-1175.

[30] Wu, C. S., Lin. H. C., Chao. P. Z. (2006) Sudden sensorineural hearing loss: evidence from Taiwan. *Audiol Neuro-Otol,* 11:151-6.

[31] Treviño González, J. L., Soto-Galindo, G. A., Moreno Sales, R., Morales Del Ángel, J. A. (2018) Sudden sensorineural hearing loss in atypical Cogan's syndrome: A case report. *Ann Med Surg,* 30;30:50-53.

[32] Byl, F. M. (1984) Jr Sudden hearing loss: Eeight years' experience and suggested prognostic table. *Laryngoscope,* 94(5 Pt 1):647-661.

[33] Ottaviani, F., Cadoni, G., Marinelli, L., Fetoni, A.R., De Santis, A., Romito, A., Vulpiani, P., Manna, R. (1999) Anti-endothelial autoantibodies in patients with sudden hearing loss. *Laryngoscope,* 109(7):1084–7.

[34] Li, F. J., Wang, D. Y., Wang, H. Y., Wang, L., Yang, F. B., Lan, L., Guan, J., Yin, Z. F., Rosenhall, U., Yu, L., Hellstrom, S., Xue, X. J., Duan, M. L., Wang, Q. J. (2016) Clinical Study on 136 Children with Sudden Sensorineural Hearing Loss. *Chin Med J,* 20;129(8):946-52.

[35] Lai, D., Zhao, F., Jalal, N., Zheng, Y. (2017) Intratympanic glucocorticosteroid therapy for idiopathic sudden hearing loss: Meta-analysis of randomized controlled trials. *Medicine,* 96(50):e8955.

[36] Areias, B., Santos, C., Natal Jorge, R.M., Gentil, F., Parente, M.P. (2016) Finite element modelling of sound transmission from outer to inner ear. *Proc Inst Mech Eng H,* 230(11):999-1007.

[37] Okamoto, H., Fukushima, M., Teismann, H., Lagemann, L., Kitahara, T., Inohara, H., Kakigi, R., Pantev, C. (2014) Constraint-induced sound therapy for sudden sensorineural hearing loss--behavioral and neurophysiological outcomes. *Sci Rep*, 29:4:3927.

[38] Kuhn, M., Heman-Ackah, S. E., Shaikh, J. A., Roehm, P. C. (2011) Sudden sensorineural hearing loss: a review of diagnosis, treatment, and prognosis. *Trends Amplif,* 15(3):91-105.

[39] *National Institute on Deafness and Other Communication Disorders (NIDCD).*

[40] Mattox, D. E., Simmons, F. B. (1997) Natural history of sudden sensorineural hearing loss. *Ann Otol Rhinol Laryngol*, 86(4, pt 1):463-480.

[41] Conlin, A. E., Parnes, L. S. (2007) Treatment of sudden sensorineural hear- ing loss, II: a meta-analysis. *Arch Otolaryngol Head Neck Surg,* 133(6):582-586.

[42] Haynes, D. S., O'Malley, M., Cohen, S., Watford, K., Labadie, R. F. (2007) Intratym- panic dexamethasone for sudden sensorineural hearing loss after failure of systemic therapy. *Laryngoscope,* 117(1):3-15.

[43] Aimoni, C., Bianchini, C., Borin, M., Ciorba, A., Fellin, R., Martini, A., Scanelli, G., Volpato, S. (2010) Diabetes, cardiovascular risk factors and idiopathic sudden sensorineural hearing loss: a case-control study. *Audiol Neurootol,* 15(2):111-5.

[44] Cho, J., Cheon, H., Park, J. H., Lee, H. J., Kim, H. J., Choi, H. G., Koo, J. W., Hong, SK. (2017) Sudden sensorineural hearing loss associated with inner ear lesions detected by magnetic resonance imaging. *PLoS One* 12(10): e0186038.

[45] Plontke, S.K. (2017) Diagnostics and therapy of sudden hearing loss. *GMS Current Topics in Otorhinolaryngology - Head and Neck Surgery,* Vol. 16, ISSN 1865-1011.

[46] Stachler, R. J., Chandrasekhar, S. S., Archer, S. M., Rosenfeld, R. M., Schwartz, S. R., Barrs, D. M., Brown, S. R., Fife, T. D., Ford, P., Ganiats, T. G., Hollingsworth, D.B., Lewandowski, C. A., Montano, J. J., Saunders, J. E., Tucci, D. L., Valente, M., Warren, B. E., Yaremchuk, K. L., Robertson, P. J. (2012) Clinical practice guideline: sudden hearing loss. *Otolaryngol Head Neck Surg,* 146(3 Suppl):S1-35.

[47] Chandrasekhar, S.S. (2003) Update son methods to treat sudden hearing loss. *Oper Tech Otolaryngol Head Neck Surg*, 14:288-292.

[48] Barnes, P. J. (2006) How corticosteroids control inflammation: Quintiles Prize Lecture 2005. *Br J Pharmacol,* 148(3):245-54.

[49] Ito, K., Chung, K. F., Adcock, I. M. (2006) Update on glucocorticoid action and resistance. *J Allergy Clin Immunol,* 117:522–543.

[50] Kaiser, H., Kley, H. K. (1997) *Cortisontherapie.* 10th ed. Stuttgart, Germany: Georg Thieme Verlag, 19-21.

[51] Erichsen, S., Bagger-Sjöbäck, D., Curtis, L., Zuo, J., Rarey, K. E., Hultcrantz, M. (1996) Appearance of glucocorticoid receptors in the inner ear of the mouse during development. *Acta Otolaryngol*, 116:721-725.

[52] Furuta, H., Mori, N., Sato, C., Hoshikawa, H., Sakai, S., Iwakura, S., Doi, K. (1994) Mineralocorticoid type I receptor in the rat cochlea: mRNA identification by polymerase chain reaction (PCR) and in situ hybridization. *Hear Res*, 78(2):175-80.

[53] Pitovski, D. Z., Drescher, M. J., Kerr, T. P., Drescher, D. G. (1993) Aldosterone mediates an increase in [3H]ouabain binding at Na,K-ATPase sites in the mammalian inner ear. *Brain Res*, 601:273-278.

[54] Zuo, J., Curtis, L., Yao Xten Cate, W. J. F., Rarey, K. (1995) Expression of Na,K-ATPase a- and b-isoforms in the neonatal rat cochlea. *Acta Otolaryngol*, 115:497-503.

[55] Erichsen, S., Zuo, J., Curtis, L., Rarey, K., Hultcrantz, M. (1996) Na,K-ATPase a- and b-isoforms in the developing cochlea of the mouse. *Hear Res*; 100:143-149.

[56] Trune, D. R., Wobig, R. J., Kempton. J. B., Hefeneider, S. H. (1999a) Steroid treatment improves cochlear function in the MRL. MpJ-Fas(lpr) autoimmune mouse. *Hear Res*, 137:160-166.

[57] Trune, D. R., Wobig, R. J, Kempton, J. B., Hefeneider, S. H. (1999b) Steroid treatment in young MRL. MpJ-Fas(lpr) autoimmune mice prevents cochlear dysfunction. *Hear Res*, 137:167-173.

[58] Forth, W., Henschler, D., Rummel, W., Förstermann, U., Starke, K. (2001) *Allgemeine und Spezielle Pharmakologie und Toxikologie*. 8. Auflage ed. [*General and Special Pharmacology and Toxicology*. 8th Edition ed.]. Urban & Fischer Verlag München Jena.

[59] Merchant, S. N., Durand, M. L., Adams, J. C. (2008) Sudden deafness: is it viral? *Journal of Oto-rhino-laryngology and its Related Specialities*, 70(1), 52-60.

[60] Wei, B. P., Mubiru, S., O'Leary, S. (2006) Steroids for idiopathic sudden sensorineural hearing loss. *Cochrane Database of Systemic Review*, 1CD003998.

[61] Wilson, W. R., Byl, F. M., Laird, N. (1980) The efficacy of steroids in the treatment of idiopathic sudden hearing loss: a doubleblind clinical study. *Arch Otolaryngol*, 106:772-6.

[62] Mattox, D. E., Simmons, F. B. (1977) Natural history of sudden sensorineural hearing loss. *Ann Otol Rhinol Laryngol*, 86:46380.

[63] Byl, F. M. Jr. (1984) Sudden hearing loss: eight years' experience and suggested prognostic table. *Laryngoscope*, 94:647-61.

[64] Fetterman, B. L., Saunders, J. E., Luxford, W. M. (1996) Prognosis and treatment of sudden sensorineural hearing loss. *Am J Otol*, 17:529-3.

[65] Parnes, L. S., Sun, A. H., Freeman, D. J. (1999) Corticosteroid pharmacokinetics in the inner ear fluids: an animal study followed by clinical application. *Laryngoscope*, 109:1-17.

[66] Cinamon, U., Bendet, E., Kronenberg, J. (2001) Steroids, carbogen or placebo for sudden hearing loss: a prospective double-blind study. *Eur Arch Otorhinolaryngol*, 258:477-480.

[67] Nosrati-Zarenoe, R., Hultcrantz, E. (2012) Corticosteroid treatment of idipathic sudden sensorineural hearing loss: randomized triple-blind placebo-controlled trial. *Otol Neurotol,* 33:523-531.

[68] Plescia, F., Sardo, P., Rizzo, V., Cacace, S., Marino, R. A., Brancato, A., Ferraro, G., Carletti, F., Cannizzaro, C. (2014) Pregnenolone sulphate enhances spatial orientation and object discrimination in adult male rats: evidence from a behavioural and electrophysiological study. *Behav Brain Res* 258:193-201.

[69] Silverstein, H., Choo, D., Rosenberg, S. I., Kuhn, J., Seidman, M., Stein, I. (1996) Intratympanic steroid treatment of inner ear disease and tinnitus (preliminary report). *Ear Nose Throat J*, 75(8):468-71.

[70] Hamid, M., Trune, D. (2008) Issue, indication, and controversies regarding intratympanic steroid perfusion. *Curr Opin Otolaryngol Head Neck Surg,* 16:434-440.

[71] Battaglia, A., Burchette, R., Cueva, R. (2008) Combination therapy (intratympanic dexamethasone + high-dose prednisone taper) for the treatment of idiopathic sudden sensorineural hearing loss. *Otol Neurotol*, 29(4):453-60.

[72] Battaglia, A., Lualhati, A., Lin, H., Burchette, R., Cueva, R. (2014) A prospective, multi-centered study of the treatment of idiopathic sudden sensorineural hearing loss with combination therapy versus high-dose prednisone alone: a 139 patient follow-up. *Otol Neurotol*, 35(6):1091-8.

[73] Jungda, J., Park, J. H., Jang, J. H., Lee, K. Y. (2016) The efficacy of combination therapy for idiopathic sudden sensorineural hearing loss. *Laryngoscope,* 126(8):1871-6.

[74] Lee, J. B., Choi, SJ. (2016) Potential Benefits of Combination Therapy as Primary Treatment for Sudden Sensorineural Hearing Loss. *Otolaryngol Head Neck Surg*, 154(2):328-34.

[75] Rauch, S. D., Halpin, C. F., Antonelli, P. J., Babu, S., Carey, J. P., Gantz, B. J., Goebel, J.A., Hammerschlag, P.E., Harris, J.P., Isaacson, B., Lee, D., Linstrom, C. J., Parnes, L. S., Shi, H., Slattery, W. H., Telian, S. A., Vrabec, J. T., Reda, D. J. (2011) Oral vs intratympanic corticosteroid therapy for idiopathic sudden sensorineural hearing loss: a randomized trial. *JAMA*, 305(20):2071-9.

[76] Zhuo, X. L., Wang, Y., Zhuo, W. L., Zhang, X. Y. (2008) Is the application of prostaglandin E1 effective for the treatment of sudden hearing loss? An evidence-based meta-analysis. *J Int Med Res*, 8;36(3):467-70.

[77] Nishimura, T., Noario, K., Hosoi, H. (2002) Effects of intravenous administration of prostaglandin E1 on cochlear blood flow in guinea pigs. *Eur Arch Othorhinolaryngol*, 259:253-256.

[78] Ogawa, K., Takei, S., Inoue, Y., Kanzaki, J. (2002) Effect of prostaglandin E1 on idiopathic sudden sensorineural hearing loss: a double-blinded clinical study. *Otology and Neurotology,* 23:665–8.

[79] Ni, Y., Zhao, X. (2004) Carbogen combined with drugs in the treatment of sudden deafness. *Lin Chuang Er Bi Yan Hou Ke Za Zhi,* 18 (7):414–5.

Chapter 15

MANAGEMENT OF SENSORINEURAL HEARING LOSS WITH HEARING AIDS

Pasquale Marsella, MD, Alessandro Scorpecci[*], *MD, PhD and Sara Giannantonio, MD, PhD*

Audiology and Otosurgery Unit, Cochlear Implant Referral Center,
"Bambino Gesù" Children's Hospital and Research Institute, Rome, Italy

ABSTRACT

Sensorineural hearing loss (SNHL) is a disease affecting the hair cells of the cochlea. Congenital SNHL is mainly due to genetic mutations, infectious agents and hypoxia, whereas acquired forms are mostly caused by aging (presbycusis), noise exposure and ototoxic drugs, although genetic mutations and infections by neurotropic viral agents are recognized etiologic factors in this category, as well. SHL can also be classified according to laterality into bilateral and unilateral, and according to the degree of hearing loss into mild, moderate, severe and profound.

Modern hearing aids are digital amplifiers receiving sound energy at their microphones, converting it into digital information by means of their processor, and transforming it back into an analogue signal for the receiver. Traditionally they are divided into behind-the-ear and in-the-ear hearing aids, based on the position.

Hearing aids represent an effective treatment of SHL when there is a cochlear reserve, i.e., in cases where residual hair cells are in a sufficient number to be appropriately stimulated. Especially in children affected by prelingual, profound deafness, they can still be used in to get the subject trained to acoustic stimulation before he/she receives cochlear implantation.

Whereas hearing aids are the standard treatment of mild, moderate and severe forms of bilateral SNHL, their indication in patients with unilateral SNHL is much debated.

---

[*] Corresponding Author's Email: alessandro.scorpecci@opbg.net.

Keywords: hearing loss, hearing aids

INTRODUCTION

Hearing loss is the most frequent sensory deficit in human populations, affecting more than 250 million people in the world [1]. Its causes may be congenital, such as for example the 35delG mutation of the connexin 26 gene [2] and intrauterine cytomegalovirus infection, or acquired, such as hearing loss determined by noise exposure [3-8]. Consequences of hearing impairment include inability to interpret speech sounds, often producing a reduced ability to communicate, delay in language acquisition, economic and educational disadvantage, social isolation and stigmatization.

Hearing loss is the most prevalent sensory deficit, and represents a major public health issue with substantial economical and societal costs. Untreated, child hearing loss leads to significant language delay and impaired auditory-verbal communication, while in adults it results in communication difficulties that can lead to social isolation and withdrawal, depression and reduced quality of life [9, 10]. Hearing loss is also associated with an increased risk of dementia, and this is true especially for older adults [11, 12].

So far, it has not been possible to resolve the causes of sensorineural hearing loss, which can only be aided by means of sound amplification. Gene therapy, consisting of direct administration of genes regenerating the sensory epithelium, or stem cells differentiating into mature cells of the organ of Corti have no clinical application at the moment [13]. Although causal therapy of sensorineural hearing loss is not to be expected for the near future, there are currently several possibilities of hearing aid amplification that can compensate it.

Shared indications to hearing aid application include the following conditions [14]:

- surgical hearing improvement is not possible
- pure tone audiometric hearing loss in the better ear ≥ 30 dB in at least one of the test frequencies in the 500-4000 Hz range
- speech recognition in the better ear (tested with headphones at 65 dB) ≤ 80%
- sufficient cooperation by the patient

FUNCTIONAL PRINCIPLES AND ESSENTIAL COMPONENTS OF HEARING AIDS

Modern hearing aids rely on a completely digital signal processing. The sound is first received by a microphone, which converts it into an electric signal. Then, the electric signal is transformed into a discreet pulse sequence by an analogue-to-digital transducer. Finally, the digital sound is again transduced into an electric sound, which is picked up by the receiver that converts it into sound waves for the patient's ear.

The microphone includes a diaphragm that is set into vibration by the pressure variation of sound waves that enter the opening of the microphone itself. The motion of the diaphragm transduces the acoustical energy to electrical energy.

The Digital Sound Processor (DSP) represents the sound by analyzing it at discrete intervals and converting it to a series of numbers according to specific algorithms. Typically, the sampling rate of modern hearing aids is around 20 kHz. Therefore, a theoretical limit of 10 kHz is determined for further signal representation and processing. After digital conversion, the discrete signals are separated in the hearing device into several frequency bands, corresponding to 4–20 channels. Each channel performs the signal processing, including frequency-specific amplification, independent of other channels. The number of channels, which sets the number of independently adjustable frequency ranges. This number plays a central role in sensorineural hearing losses where only a part of the frequency range is affected, such as high-frequency hearing loss. Since typically only 10 different frequency values are tested in tone audiometry, the number of channels is no longer a challenge from a technical point of view.

Finally, the separately processed signals are merged, amplified, converted back to analogue signals (digital-to-analogue transduction) that are delivered to the ear via a receiver.

The receiver is also a transducer, transforming electrical signals into acoustic sound waves. Like the microphone, it has a diaphragm that is set into vibration, but its movement creates the sound waves that travel through the tubing connecting the receiver to the outside.

CLASSIFICATION OF HEARING AIDS

According to manner of placement, hearing aids can be classified into:
- *Custom-molded hearing aids*, made from an impression of the user's ear. The electronics of these aids are housed in hard plastic, although soft materials are sometimes used for the portion located in the auditory canal. Although they offer the potential for better quality control, they generally suffer from size and shape limitations that adversely impact cosmetics and the functional integration of the hearing aid and earmold.
- *Completely-in-the-canal (CIC) hearing aids*, the most cosmetically appealing and smallest contemporary hearing aid styles, they often have their electronics completely within the cartilaginous segment of the external auditory canal, although some extend into the bony portion of the canal, terminating close to the

tympanic membrane. Despite gain and output of these hearing aids are limited because of small transducers, they allow the patient to benefit from improved cosmetics, greater overall sound pressure level especially for the high frequencies, reduced occlusion effect and feedback and normal telephone use.

- *In-the-canal (ITC)* hearing aids, sized between the CIC and the in-the-ear (ITE) hearing aid, they fit within the concha and the cartilaginous portion of the external auditory canal, with the microphone opening located at the outer portion of the concha. Because of vents, "feedback control" trimmers may be needed, which attenuate the high frequencies. Owing to deeper insertion than ITE aids, they often require lower gains and provide a better high-frequency response, while size limits the number or dimension of circuits and trimmer controls, together with use of the large vents that could suppress the occlusion effect. For users, telephone use is much easier with this hearing aid type than with a larger ITE device thanks to reduced feedback, more favorable microphone locations and larger air volume under the telephone receiver.
- *In-the-ear (ITE)* hearing aids include "full concha," "low profile" and "half concha" instruments. Full concha ITE aids are the most common, allowing the entire concha volume to be filled with electronics and therefore enabling the implementation of complex circuit designs, venting and performance control.
- *Behind the Ear (BTE)*: the hearing device is above the auricle and the processed sound is conducted into the auditory canal either electrically or via a sound tube. BTE hearing aids can be divided into the traditional ones, with a receiver within the case of the hearing aid, and those with a receiver removed from the case and instead located at the end of the tubing and placed inside the auditory canal (receiver-in-the-canal or RIC). BTE aids can be worn in an "open" configuration, where the coupling consists of a tube to the ear and the ear domes do not completely occlude the ear. Open fitting is particularly good for subjects with normal hearing in the low frequencies and hearing loss in the high frequencies, because the low-frequency sound can exit the ear canal as it does for normal-hearing listeners.

TYPES OF AMPLIFICATION

The most common ways to provide amplification in a hearing aid are linear and non-linear amplification. In the context of linear amplification, all input levels are amplified to the same extent until the hearing aid reaches output sound pressure level 90. This way, a sound entering the hearing aid is increased of a constant decibel value. This type of amplification is suitable for low-grade sensory hearing losses or conductive hearing losses. In cases of higher-grade hearing losses with defined recruitment a lower amplification has to be set for higher input levels in order to consider the discomfort limit. This goal is achieved by means of amplitude compression. In amplitude compression systems, a linear amplification is typically applied up to a certain input level, whereas it is reduced for higher levels. The non-linearity can be described by the knee point, i.e., the point where the output curve deviates from linear, and the compression ratio, i.e., the degree of such a deviation. There are several compression variants that function in a similar way.

Another type of special, non-linear of amplification is achieved by frequency lowering or reduction [15], a function that changes the spectral representation of sound signals and can be obtained both as frequency transposition and as frequency compression. The rationale behind frequency reduction is that most sensorineural hearing losses are characterized by a descending auditory threshold for high-frequencies, for which an amplification is neither useful nor possible. By taking high-frequency input signals and presenting these sounds to lower-frequency regions, the hearing aid allows the patient to hear otherwise inaudible and not amplifiable sounds. Frequency reduction is possible either via frequency transposition, whereby the signal is lowered by a fixed frequency value with no alteration of the overall bandwidth, or via frequency compression, whereby both frequency and bandwidth are reduced by a preset ratio. These procedures are associated with unavoidable signal distortions. In many cases, however, a better hearing perception can be achieved after some months of acclimatization. It is important to remind that frequency reduction does not so much lead primarily to a better speech understanding than mainly improve sound impression [16]. Since frequency reduction algorithms are initially disturbing, the possibilities to implement them in commercially available hearing aids are rather limited.

Up to now, there is no possibility to identify particular subjects who might benefit from frequency reduction. In contrast to earlier analogue aids, not only the hardware but also the quality of technical components in digital hearing devices is essential. The function of a hearing aid is determined by the signal processing defined in the software. Thus, there are today technically identical hearing aids that are only different regarding their technical features (and price). The software determines for example the feedback suppression, wind noise suppression, directional microphones etc.

FITTING OF HEARING AIDS

The fitting of a hearing aid is a process of several weeks and months in which the most suitable hearing aid is identified and the optimal settings for daily life are established. First, the audiological profile is determined by measuring the severity and the type of hearing loss and the individual needs are assessed. It is clarified which hearing conditions appear frequently and are especially relevant. Patient needs or request to be taken into account at this stage are: speech understanding in quiet compared to in noise, telephone use, frequent lecture situations (e.g., school children or students), or specific requests for directionality (e.g., taxi drivers), or special requirements regarding dirt and water repellency (e.g., pool attendants). Additional settings must also be considered: are highly different settings constellations necessary? Does switching have to be automatized or at the touch of a button? Those and other similar questions lead to a selection of the possible hearing aid. The initial setting of the hearing aid is generally performed by means of a software according to audiometric parameters such as hearing (air and bone conduction) and discomfort thresholds, even loudness scaling if needed. Because of the approximation of measurements, most hearing aid fittings are performed only based on tone audiograms and the discomfort thresholds are directly estimated by the fitting programs.

The objective of compensation in cases of sensory hearing losses is never the complete amplification of an existing hearing loss, whereas the target amplification is rather at half of the hearing loss dynamic range. Most fitting formulas such as the National Acoustics Laboratories of Australia (NAL) [17], the Prescription of Gain and Output (POGO) [18] generally correct the values, adjusting them downwards for higher frequencies and upwards for lower frequencies. Other procedures such as the Desired Sensation Level (DSL) [19] try to restore the loudness sensation via the dynamic range and thus require the measurement of individual loudness scaling over several frequencies.

In the practice, hearing aid fitting is completely performed by the software provided by the hearing aid manufacturer. Based on the audiometric data, the prescription is calculated and the hearing aid is programmed. Additional information such as having to do with an inexperienced or with an experienced hearing aid user lead to further automatic adjustments. Furthermore, other modifications of the hearing aid settings can be performed after testing the device in daily routine. Finally, fine tuning must take into account the hearing environment and include algorithms to optimize sound quality.

TECHNOLOGICAL ADVANCEMENTS AND FUTURE DEVELOPMENTS

Modern hearing aids are miniaturized high-power computers that have to function with little energy for a possibly long duration. While formerly hearing aids were limited by the components (microphone, amplifier, receiver), the quality of a modern hearing device is rather defined by the immanent software. Even if there are permanent improvements of the hearing aid technology, exaggerated advertising measures often lead to disappointments owing to the fact that the effectiveness of the single improvements is not always noticeable. Nonetheless, several improvements could be observed over the past years.

Directional microphones are useful when the speech signal comes from the front and the background noise from other directions. Nowadays, directional microphones cannot only be implemented as a fixed part but they can also be digitally added. Adaptive directional microphones only switch on when a speech signal is recognized as coming from the front. This is possible due to the evaluation of the time delay of the sound input at two different microphones.

Wind noise elimination: the wind reaching a normal hearing ear is mostly well eliminated and only rarely leads to noticeable hearing deterioration. Since most of the hearing aid microphones are located above the auricle, this natural protection is missing. Furthermore, most microphones have a directional effect set to the front. Thus, also low wind velocities lead to significant deterioration of the signal quality. In the past, this fact led to dissatisfaction in nearly half the hearing aid users [20]. Several algorithms for wind noise reduction were thus developed, with the aim to increase the wearing comfort and also to improve speech understanding in challenging acoustical environments.

Binaural coupling: coupling two hearing aids of the same user became possible after the development of an appropriate wireless protocol. Initially, binaural coupling was limited to the (wireless) transmission of parameter settings of one hearing aid to another. In this context, for example, the change of loudness in one hearing aid was also effective in the contralateral one. Later, this feature was extended by real time transmission of audiodata. This way, a very important directional effect of the microphones can be achieved. Additionally, the hearing aid can recognize on which side the speech signal is presented and amplify it. During phone calls, such devices can transmit the telephone signal to both ears. It is highly efficient to use binaural coupling also to suppress wind noise when they only occur in one ear.

HEARING AIDS FOR UNILATERAL HEARING LOSS IN CHILDREN

Although a hearing aid may be a useful intervention option for children with unilateral hearing loss (UHL) who have usable residual hearing in the impaired ear, clinicians do not appear to be making this recommendation consistently. Only 26% of children with UHL received an initial recommendation for amplification [21], whereas across studies 48% of children with UHL received a conventional hearing aid [22, 23]. A parental survey indicates similar findings: 42% of families of children with UHL were told that hearing aids would not help, although only 8% of the children had no residual hearing [24]. However, evidence indicates that a conventional hearing a does provide benefits: 20 parents of children with mild to moderate UHL surveyed via a questionnaire reported improved hearing and better performance in academic and social situations with a hearing aid and many parents indicated that they wished their child had received a hearing aid sooner [25]. Children with UHL who used a hearing aid have also reported greater ease of listening in quiet and noise [22]. Even with no measurable change in speech perception, subjective reports from parents, teachers, and children showed significant aided benefits at home, school and quality of life [26]. Younger children with mild to severe UHL have also shown significantly improved localization, although children who were fit later showed bilateral interference [27]. Yet only about 26% of children with UHL use their hearing aid full-time; compared to 72% of children with a moderate bilateral hearing loss. This reduced compliance in children with UHL may be because they are often fit with hearing aids later than children with bilateral hearing loss, and wearing compliance is typically poorer when children are fitted later [28]. One limitation in fitting a hearing aid to children with UHL concerns the prescriptive method used: there is no evidence to date to indicate whether children with UHL prefer the gain from prescriptive methods designed for bilateral hearing loss [29]. A possible solution to this problem has been suggested [30], which is to use a technique to achieve binaural fusion in individuals with asymmetric hearing losses [31-32]. However, this method requires patient participation and therefore is not useful in fitting infants and young children with UHL.

Overall, the evidence indicates that children with UHL who have usable residual hearing in the affected ear can receive benefits from conventional digital amplification including greater ease of listening, better performance in academic and social situations, and improved localization if fitted early.

HEARING AIDS FOR UNILATERAL HEARING LOSS IN ADULTS

Adults with UHL also have positive outcomes with conventional hearing aid use. Of 119 adults with UHL who were fit with a conventional hearing aid, 68% continued use 6 months post-fitting and the primary predictors for successful hearing aid use were social/work activities and digital signal processing [33], suggesting that although individual demands on communication may affect use, advanced technology devices may be more appropriate for individuals with UHL.

In adults, unilateral hearing loss is often acquired suddenly and accompanied by tinnitus [34-36]. Positive outcomes of hearing aid use in the adult population are reported as well. Of 119 adults with UHL who were fit with a conventional hearing aid, 68% continued use 6 months post-fitting and the primary predictors for successful hearing aid use were social/work activities and digital signal processing [37], suggesting that although individual demands on communication may affect use, advanced technology devices may be more appropriate for individuals with UHL.

Unfortunately, there are only few studies that examine the effectiveness of hearing aids on tinnitus alone. With hearing aids, many patients experience effective relief of their tinnitus, but studies on hearing aids as solitary therapy do not exist because they are always embedded in an audio-therapeutic concept. Nonetheless, hearing aids are essential in the tinnitus therapy because they nearly always include and compensate the existing hearing loss. In a retrospective tinnitus analysis [38-39], 58 tinnitus patients with hearing loss were followed-up; 29 used hearing aids, 29 did not – both groups had nearly identical audiograms, the same duration of tinnitus, and the same age on the average. Only in the group of hearing aid users, a significant improvement of the tinnitus could be achieved based on the Tinnitus Handicap Questionnaire.

Another work reported about 74 tinnitus patients who received hearing aids with a linear frequency transposition [40-41]. Those hearing aids are especially active in the high frequencies and very suitable for patients with a steep drop of the hearing curve. In 60 patients, the tinnitus could be permanently eliminated. In this study, patients whose hearing loss was related to noise exposure had permanent tinnitus suppression a few days after starting hearing aid use. A review study from the Netherlands reviewed 10 articles, showing improvement 25–72% of the patients and complete tinnitus suppression in 8–45% of the patients. Up to 25%, however, even mentioned deterioration, new additional tinnitus developed in up to 10% [41].

REFERENCES

[1] Heller, A. J. (2003) Classification and epidemiology of tinnitus. *Otoryngol Clin North Am,* 36:2390-2489.

[2] Eggermont, J. J., Roberts, L. E. (2004) The neuroscience of tinnitus. *Trends Neurosci*, 27:676-682.

[3] Salvago, P., Rizzo, S., Bianco, A., Martines, F. (2017) Sudden sensorineural hearing loss: is there a relationship between routine haematological parameters and audiogram shapes? *International Journal of Audiology,* 56(3): 148-153.

[4] Ballacchino, A., Salvago, P., Cannizzaro, E., Costanzo, R., Di Marzo, M., Ferrara, S., La Mattina, E., Messina, G., Mucia, M., Mulè, A., Plescia, F., Sireci, F., Rizzo, S., Martines, F. (2015) Association between sleep-disordered breathing and hearing disorders: Clinical observation in Sicilian patients. *Acta Medica Mediterranea,* 31(3): 607-614.

[5] Martines, F., Maira, E., Ferrara, S. (2011) Age-related hearing impairment (ARHI): A common sensory deficit in the elderly. *Acta Medica Mediterranea,* 27 (1):47-52.

[6] Martines, F., Salvago, P., Bartolotta, C., Cocuzza, S., Fabiano, C., Ferrara, S. et al. (2015) A genotype-phenotype correlation in Sicilian patients with GJB2 biallelic mutations. *Eur Arch Otorhinolaryngol,* 272:1857–1865.

[7] Bartolotta, C., Salvago, P., Cocuzza, S., Fabiano, C., Sammarco, P., Martines, F. (2014) Identification of D179H, a novel missense GJB2 mutation in a Western

Sicily family. *European Archives of Oto-Rhino-Laryngology,* 271 (6), pp. 1457-1461.

[8] Salvago, P., Martines, E., La Mattina, E., Mucia, M., Sammarco, P., Sireci, F., Martines, F. (2014) Distribution and phenotype of GJB2 mutations in 102 Sicilian patients with congenital non syndromic sensorineural hearing loss. *International Journal of Audiology,* 53 (8), pp. 558-563.

[9] Thomas, E., Martines, F., Bianco, A., Messina, G., Giustino, V., Zangla, D., Iovane, A., Palma, A. (2018) *Decreased postural control in people with moderate hearing loss.* Medicine (Baltimore); 97(14): e0244.

[10] Mathers, C., Smith, A., Concha, M. (2000) Global burden of hearing loss in the year 2000. *Global Burden of Disease,* 18:1–30.

[11] Davis, A., Smith, P., Ferguson, M., Stephens, D., Gianopoulos, I. (2007) Acceptability, benefit and costs of early screening for hearing disability: a study of potential screening tests and models. *Health Technology Assessment*, 11:1–294.

[12] Lin, F. R., Metter, E. J., O'Brien, R. J., Resnick, S. M., Zonderman, A.B., Ferrucci, L. (2011) Hearing loss and incident dementia. *Arch Neurol*, 68:214–220.

[13] Davies, H. R., Cadar, D., Herbert, A., Orrell, M., Steptoe, A. (2017) Hearing Impairment and Incident Dementia: Findings from the English Longitudinal Study of Ageing. *J Am Geriatr Soc*; 65: 2074–2081.

[14] Ibekwe, T. S., Ramma, L., Chindo, B. A. (2012) Potential roles of stem cells in the management of sensorineural hearing loss. *J Laryngol Otol*, 126:653-657.

[15] Hoppe, U., Hesse, G. (2017) Hearing aids: indications, technology, adaptation, and quality control. *GMS Curr Top Otorhinolaryngol Head Neck Surg*, 18:1-24.

[16] Simpson, A. (2009) Frequency-lowering devices for managing highfrequency hearing loss: a review. *Trends Amplif,* 13:87-106.

[17] Miller, C. W., Bates, E., Brennan, M. (2016) The effects of frequency lowering on speech perception in noise with adult hearing-aid users. *Int J Audiol*, 55:305-312.

[18] Byrne, D., Dillon, H. (1986) The National Acoustic Laboratories' (NAL) new procedure for selecting the gain and frequency response of a hearing aid. *Ear Hear*, 7:257-265.

[19] McCandless, G., Lyregaard, P. E. (1983) Prescription of gain/output (POGO) for hearing aids. *Hearing Instruments*, 34:16-21.

[20] Cornelisse, L. E., Seewald, R. C., Jamieson, D. G. (1995) The input/output formula: a theoretical approach to the fitting of personal amplification devices. *J Acoust Soc Am*, 97:1854-1864.

[21] Kochkin, S., MarkeTrak VII: Customer satisfaction with hearing instruments in the digital age. *Hearing Journal* 2005; 58: 30, 32-34, 38-40, 42-43.

[22] Fitzpatrick, E. M., Whittingham, J., Durieux-Smith, A. (2014) Mild bilateral and unilateral hearing loss in childhood: a 20-year view of hearing characteristics, and

audiologic practices before and after newborn hearing screening. *Ear Hear*, 35:10-18.

[23] Davis, A., Reeve, K., Hind, S., Bamford, J. (2001) Children with mild and unilateral hearing loss, in: R. C. Seewald, J. S. Gravel (Eds.), *A Sound Foundation through Early Amplification: Proceedings of the Second International Conference*, 2001, 179-186.

[24] English, K., Church, G. (1999) Unilateral hearing loss in children: an update for the 1990s. *Lang Speech Hear Serv Sch.*, 30:26-31.

[25] Kochkin, S. K., Luxford, W., Northern, J. L., Mason, P., Tharpe, A. M., MarkeTrak, VII. (2007) Are 1 million dependents with hearing loss in America being left behind? *Hear Rev*, 14, 1-10.

[26] McKay, S. *To aid or not to aid: children with unilateral hearing loss*, Audiol. Online. Retrieved from, http://www.audiologyonline.com/articles/to-aid-or-not-children. 2002.

[27] Briggs, L., Davidson, L., Lieu, J. E. (2011) Outcomes of conventional amplification for pediatric unilateral hearing loss. *Ann Otol Rhinol Laryngol*, 120:448-454.

[28] Johnstone, P. M., Nabelek, A. K., Robertson, V. S. (2010) Sound localization acuity in children with unilateral hearing loss who wear a hearing aid in the impaired ear. *J Am Acad Audiol*, 21:522-534.

[29] Reeve, K. (2005) Amplification and family factors for children with mild and unilateral hearing impairment. In: *National Workshop on Mild and Unilateral Hearing Loss: Workshop Proceedings, Centers for Disease Control and Prevention*, Breckenridge, CO, pp. 20-21.

[30] McKay, S., Gravel, J. S., Tharpe, A. M. (2008) Amplification considerations for children with minimal or mild bilateral hearing loss and unilateral hearing loss. *Trends Amplif*, 12:43-54.

[31] Cui, T. (2014) Monaural hearing aid fitting considerations for Patients with unilateral hearing loss: who should receive unilateral fittings, and how should you fit them? *Hear Rev*, 21:32-34.

[32] McSpaden, J. B., Brethower, L. D. (2007) Achieving binaural fusion in asymmetric losses. *Hear Rev*, 14:5-40.

[33] Lee, D. H., Noh, H. (2015) Prediction of the use of conventional hearing aids in Korean adults with unilateral hearing impairment. *Int J Audiol*, 54:613-619.

[34] Rizzo, S., Bentivegna, D., Thomas, E., La Mattina, E., Mucia, M., Salvago, P. et al. (2016) Sudden sensorineural hearing loss, an invisible male: State of the art. *Hearing loss: etiology, management and societal implications*, 75-86.

[35] Dispenza, F., De Stefano, A., Costantino, C., Marchese, D., Riggio, F. (2013) Sudden Sensorineural Hearing Loss: results of intratympanic steroids as salvage treatment. *Am J Otolaryngol,* 34:296-300.

[36] Gagliardo, C., Martines, F., Bencivinni, F., Latona, G., Lo Casto, A., Midiri, M. (2013) Intratumoral Haemorrhage Causing an Unusual Clinical Presentation of a Vestibular Schwannoma. *Neurualradiology Journal,* 26: 30-34.

[37] Moffat, G., Adjout, K., Gallego, S., Thai-Van, H., Collet, L., Noreña, A. J. (2009) Effects of hearing aid fitting on the perceptual characteristics of tinnitus. *Hear Res*, 254:82-91.

[38] Dispenza, F., Cappello, F., Kulamarva, G., De Stefano, A. (2013) The discovery of the stapes. *Acta Otorhinolaryngol Ital.* 33(5): 357-359.

[39] Peltier, E., Peltier, C., Tahar, S., Alliot-Lugaz, E., Cazals, Y. (2012) Long-term tinnitus suppression with linear octave frequency transposition hearing aids. *PLoS ONE*, 7:e51915.

[40] Dispenza, F., Mazzucco, W., Bianchini, S., Mazzola, S., Bennici, E. (2015) Management of labyrinthine fistula in chronic otitis with cholesteatoma: case series. *Euro Mediterranean Biomedical Journal* 10(21): 255-261.

[41] Ramakers, G. G., van Zon, A., Stegeman, I., Grolman, W. (2015) The effect of cochlear implantation on tinnitus in patients with bilateral hearing loss: A systematic review. *Laryngoscope*, 125:2584-2492.

In: Sensorineural Hearing Loss
Editors: F. Dispenza and F. Martines
ISBN: 978-1-53615-048-3
© 2019 Nova Science Publishers, Inc.

Chapter 16

COCHLEAR IMPLANT OF SNHL PATIENTS

*Pasquale Marsella, MD, Sara Giannantonio, MD, PhD
and Alessandro Scorpecci, MD, PhD*

Audiology and Otosurgery Unit, Cochlear Implant Referral Center,
"Bambino Gesù" Children's Hospital and Research Institute, Rome, Italy

ABSTRACT

Sensorineural hearing loss (SNHL) is the most common type of hearing loss. The key to the optimal management of congenital SHL is early diagnosis (achieved through the diffusion of Newborn Hearing Screening programs) and early intervention. Treatment for SNHL varies, depending on the severity of the loss itself. Although hearing aids can help most people with mild to moderate SNHL, they are often not sufficient for spoken language development in more severe hearing losses, where cochlear implants represent the gold standard of the treatment. A cochlear implant is a surgically implanted electronic device. Unlike hearing aids, which simply amplify sound, cochlear implants pick up sound and digitize it, convert that digitized sound into electrical signals, and transmit those signals to electrodes embedded in the cochlea. The electrodes electrically stimulate the cochlear nerve, causing it to send signals to the brain. There are several systems available, but generally they have similar external (speech processor, transmitter, microphones) and internal (receiver-stimulator, electrode array) components. The ideal timing for cochlear implantation is between 12 and 18 months of age, and it can be done simultaneously or sequentially. Results vary from person to person. The main factors that can affect the outcomes of cochlear implantation include the age when hearing was lost, the length of time between hearing loss and cochlear implantation (hearing deprivation), and the timely inclusion in an appropriate speech therapy rehabilitation program. Research indicates that children who undergo bilateral (either early sequential or simultaneous) cochlear implant surgery at young age develop better hearing and speech than similar children with hearing aids or who received one cochlear implant or two cochlear implants after longer hearing deprivation. The benefit of cochlear implantation in children with single sided deafness is currently under investigation.

INTRODUCTION

Sensorineural hearing loss (SNHL) affects 1 to 3 of every 1000 children born in developed countries [1, 2]; the rate is probably higher in the developing world [3]. In most cases, the hearing loss is nonsyndromic (i.e., it is not associated with other congenital features) and the child is otherwise healthy. The lack of auditory input during the child's development has a minimal effect on his or her motor and social development during infancy. Thus, if infant hearing screening is not performed, the deafness is often unnoticed during this period, resulting in a late diagnosis (at ≥1 year of age) [4]. The deaf child receives little or no access to environmental sounds and speech; this lack of access arrests or disrupts normal auditory development [5-9]. As the child grows older, auditory deprivation results in cortical reorganization, including an expansion of visually driven inputs into the secondary areas of the auditory cortex. The duration of deafness before diagnosis and intervention is negatively correlated with the child's ability to perceive and use spoken language after being fitted for an auditory prosthesis [10]. Universal newborn hearing screening, which is now available in most countries, has markedly improved the early diagnosis of sensorineural hearing loss.

Effects of Hearing Loss

It is well documented that childhood deafness can have a severe impact on speech and language development, which can result its emotional, social, educational, and vocational disruption as the child matures [11]. In our society, oral language is the primary means through which socialization and learning occur. Development of speech and language occurs rapidly in the first few years of life, primarily through normal family interaction. If the communication interaction between child and family is disrupted during these early critical years, serious delays are likely to occur. If the deprivation goes on for too long, the child may never make up the lost learning, even with extensive rehabilitation. Supporting this claim, the average reading level of deaf 18 year old persons is just below the third grade level [12]. Adults who have been deaf since childhood tend to be undereducated and earn less money, compared with their hearing peers [13]. Severe to profound hearing loss has the potential to adversely affect many aspects of development, including social, cognitive, and academic abilities, primarily because of language delay [14]. In the long term, deficits in these areas can limit vocational and economic potential. Unlike many clinical conditions, the management and treatment of SNHL largely involves the social welfare and educational systems rather than the medical care system. For a child with congenital severe to profound SNHL, the total lifetime cost of hearing loss exceeds US$1000000. Special education costs amount to over half of this total, and medical expenses and the purchase of assistive devices add another US$100000 [15].

Cochlear implants are electronic devices which have been approved as method of treating profound, bilateral, sensorineural hearing loss for persons since the mid-1980s [16]. Although the original cochlear implants were single channel devices, there are now several commercially available, multichannel cochlear implant systems. Additionally, over the course of the last two decades, technological developments in cochlear implant design have yielded substantial gains in spoken word recognition for the average multichannel cochlear implant user. Along with advances in engineering and speech processor design have come changes in the criteria for cochlear implant candidacy. For example, initially only adults with postlingual profound deafness were considered suitable candidates for cochlear implantation; now, audiometric thresholds are no longer a primary determinant of cochlear implant candidacy for postlingually deafened adults. Similarly, congenitally deaf children initially were not considered suitable candidates for multichannel cochlear implantation. When implantation of children was approved by the FDA it was limited to children 2 years of age and up; now, the FDA has approved the use of multichannel cochlear implants in prelingually deafened children as young as 12 months of age, and many children younger than 12 months of age have been implanted off protocol.

CANDIDACY CRITERIA FOR COCHLEAR IMPLANTATION

FDA Guidelines

The FDA has approved cochlear implants for children with severe-to-profound bilateral sensorineural hearing loss (hearing threshold, ≥90 dB in the better ear) who are at least 1 year of age and who have not benefited from an adequate trial (typically 4 to 6 months) of hearing-aid amplification. A similar position was taken in 2000 in a statement of the Joint Committee on Infant Hearing [17], which noted that "cochlear implants may be an option for certain children age 12 months and older with profound hearing loss who show limited benefit from conventional amplification." Currently, clinical practice in recent years has expanded beyond these criteria. Guidelines for cochlear implant candidacy have changed substantially over time. For instance, in the 1980's cochlear implants were recommended for post-linguistically deafened adults with hearing losses greater than 100 dB and no discernable communication benefit from a hearing aid. By the year 2000, FDA approval had extended the implantable age down to 12 months and broadened the general hearing criteria. Current guidelines permit cochlear implantation in persons age 2 years and older with severe-to-profound deafness (i.e., pure tone average thresholds of 70 dB HL or greater), and in children 12 to 23 months of age with profound deafness (i.e., pure tone average thresholds of 90 dB HL or greater.) Whenever possible, outcomes from word and sentence recognition testing are also used to determine candidacy. Current guidelines permit implantation in adults with open-set sentence recognition scores of approximately 50% to 60% words correct. As cochlear implant devices continue to improve, the criteria regarding the degree of hearing loss and the performance with a hearing aid that warrants consideration of a cochlear implant also will continue to evolve.

Medical Evaluation

The medical evaluation examines the status of the patient's overall health, the history and etiology of the patient's hearing loss, and the physical condition of the ear and cochlea. The general health of the patient impacts his fitness for general anesthesia and surgery, and his ability to complete the necessary post-operative programming of the device. Although general health status is rarely a contraindication for implantation, it may affect the timing and preparation for implantation.

Etiology

At present, the etiology and history of a patient's hearing loss cannot accurately predict a patient's performance with the cochlear implant. However, some general relationships have been reported that can moderate the patient's expectations. For example, persons with deafness subsequent to meningitis commonly develop cochlear ossification that can impede the insertion of the electrode array. The degree of cochlear ossification may affect the prognosis for implant performance and increase the possibility of facial nerve stimulation. Individuals with partial insertion of the electrode array perform similarly to those with complete insertion as long as a sufficient number of electrodes can be activated to program the device [18-20]. Individuals with complete cochlear ossification who require a "drill-out" of the bone to provide a space to lay the electrode do not achieve as high a level of auditory perception with their implant [20]. They also are more prone to complications of facial nerve stimulation and pain associated with implant activation [21]. The possibility of less than average performance and a higher incidence of stimulation complications in cases of complete ossification needs to be discussed frankly with a patient and can sometimes affect the patient's decision to proceed with implantation.

History of Hearing Loss

Postlingually deafened adults with a history of progressive hearing loss and a shorter duration of deafness tend to achieve higher speech perception scores than those who have been deaf for a long period of time prior to implantation [22-25]. Adults with prelingual hearing loss generally are not considered good candidates for cochlear implantation, especially if they do not use oral/aural communication [26]. Similar relationships exist between the history of hearing loss in children and performance with an implant, although they are moderated by a child's development. The origins of deafness in children are manifold. The difference must be made between congenital and acquired causes as well as the time of deafness (pre-, peri-, or postlingual). If the onset is observed before language acquisition, the term of pre-lingual deafness is applied, after final language acquisition (around the 10th year of life) it is called post-lingual deafness. If hearing loss is detected during the phase of language acquisition, it is the case of a peri-lingual deafness. The impact of hearing loss on the language development is well-known [27]. It is crucial for the therapeutic success of a cochlea implant to possibly early detect, diagnose, and treat hearing loss in order to keep the consequences of the auditory deprivation for hearing and language development as well as the general mental development on a low level [28]. Hereby, also the development of a binaural hearing system as base of directional hearing and speech understanding in noise must be mentioned. In cases of congenital deafness, the newborn hearing screening is essential for early detection. In contrast to adults, both pre- and postlingually deafened children are candidates for cochlear implantation as long as they receive little or no benefit from conventional amplification. In some instances, better hearing sensitivity before implantation and the use of spoken language in a child's communication and educational setting have been associated with better speech perception [29, 30].

Radiological Examination

High-resolution imaging (Computerized Tomography, CT and Magnetic Resonance Imaging, MRI) is used to estimate the patency of the cochlea and to identify any abnormal anatomical variations that may affect insertion of the electrode. Although imaging may miss some obstructions preventing electrode insertion, this is rare [31, 32]. Some obstructions can be anticipated on the basis of the clinical history of hearing loss. As noted above, clinical histories of otosclerosis or meningitis commonly are associated with cochlear ossification.

Genetic Diagnostics

One relevant pillar of the etiological clarification is the genetic diagnosis. About 50–60% of pediatric hearing impairment are due to a genetic predisposition. They are classified into non-syndromic and syndromic types of hearing loss, i.e., generally the hearing loss is a symptom in the context of a syndrome. Currently, more than 200 so-called deafness genes are known [33]. The most frequent expression is the mutation on the gene locus GJB2 that leads to a disorder of the connexin molecule (Connexin 26), a gap junction protein. The consequences are disorders of the ionic homeostasis of the hair cells that are irreversibly damaged by a potassium intoxication. The difference is made between autosomal recessive, autosomal dominant, X-linked, and mitochondrial, genetically caused hearing losses. Autosomal recessive types often reveal deafness already at birth and are entitled DFNB (e.g., DFNB1 with connexin 26 disorders). Autosomal dominant types often have a postnatal onset and are progressive (DFNA) [33]. X-linked hearing losses are located on the X chromosome and only appear in males (DFN). Mitochondrial hereditary hearing impairment is passed on by maternal genes.

Audiologic Evaluation

The purpose of the audiological evaluation is to quantify the candidate's preoperative hearing, communicative status, and use of prosthetic devices. The results are useful in determining candidacy by comparing the current communicative status to the expected outcome of using a cochlear implant. Results also are important as pre-outcome measures to quantify the benefit of the cochlear implant after implantation. To this end, the audiologic evaluation comprises of a pure-tone audiogram including air and bone-conducted thresholds, tests of speech perception such as word and sentence recognition, an evaluation of current amplification, and, if appropriate, a trial use of amplification. Speech perception tests are most decisive in determining the appropriateness of cochlear implantation. Candidates who demonstrate open-set word or sentence recognition performance that is below the average scores seen for cochlear implant recipients should be considered for implantation. Indications in children – Cochlear implantation in children should be performed immediately after indication. Bilateral implantation should be performed in cases of bilateral profound deafness, if possible simultaneously or otherwise as sequential implantation with a short time interval in order to use the sensitive phase for the development of binaural hearing [34, 35]. Hearing aid fitting beside unilateral cochlear implantation is indicated in cases of asymmetric hearing with unilateral sensory hearing loss and useable hearing ability in the contralateral ear. Narrow controls of the residual hearing as well as the hearing success in this ear must be performed so that progressive hearing loss or development failure of bilateral hearing are detected in time and the point of then necessary sequential cochlear implantation of the second ear may be correctly chosen [28-36]. If maturation is delayed, as it may be expected in cases of increased hearing thresholds and prolonged inter-peak latencies in brainstem audiometry, control examinations in narrow intervals and probatory hearing aid fitting seems to be appropriate.

Often hearing improvement is observed due to maturation of the peripheral auditory system and the central hearing pathway so that a repetition of the examination of the residual hearing after some weeks or months is indicated. If no significant improvement of hearing is observed, cochlear implantation should be performed in the second year of life at the latest. In this context, the so-called perisynaptic audiopathy must be mentioned summarizing disorders of the inner hair cells, the synapsis to the afferent nerve fibers as well as true auditory neuropathy with damage of the afferent neuron (auditory neuropathy spectrum disorder). This term encompasses different pathophysiological disorders of stimulus transmission and stimulus forwarding in the peripheral auditory system. Only in the context of true auditory neuropathy a relative contraindication for a cochlear implant system exists. In cases of particular urgency such as for example threatening cochlear obliteration by labyrinthitis and meningitis require immediate, early implantation.

Performance Measures in Children

The audiological evaluation of young children for cochlear implantation assesses the ear's sensitivity to sound, and, if possible, includes measures of auditory perception. As the age of implantation decreases, visual reinforcement audiometry and auditory evoked response audiometry are the primary methods of measuring hearing sensitivity. Speech/auditory perception testing depends upon the age and linguistic ability of the child. Again, a large number of pediatric perception tests exist which vary from open-set word and sentence recognition, to closed-set measures of prosodic features, word identification, and speech feature identification [37]. For the youngest children, parental reporting scales of auditory listening behavior, such as the Infant-Toddler Meaningful Auditory Integration Scale [38] frequently have been used to assess auditory skill development. For older children, open-set word and sentence tests are employed to determine candidacy. Less difficult tests that include closed-set measures of performance, such as the Early Speech Perception Test [39] can be included if open-set word recognition is not possible. By using tests appropriate for the age and language level of the child, one can scale the child's ability along a continuum and chart a child's progress over time. As the age of implantation decreases, candidacy criteria are generally determined by a lack of progress noted on parental scales of auditory skill development over a given period of time (such as three to six months). In very young children, candidacy also may be determined by the child's progress in developing spoken language with amplification, based on studies of spoken language acquisition in children with cochlear implants versus children with different severity of hearing losses and hearing aids [40, 41].

Psychological/Rehabilitation Evaluation

An important aspect of cochlear implant candidacy that is much harder to define than the audiological or medical evaluation is the assessment of whether the candidate's overall life situation is one that will integrate and promote the use of a cochlear implant. The anticipation of cochlear implant surgery and the hope for a positive outcome introduces stress into the lives of the candidate and his or her family. Evaluation of a patient's family's expectations for life after implantation can be beneficial in tempering unrealistic expectations and anticipating alternative pathways if the postimplant performance is not as expected. In children, the psychosocial evaluation is more extensive and includes developmental and educational evaluations as well as family assessments. In the pediatric population, the choice of a cochlear implant is usually associated with the choice of spoken language as the primary communication mode of the deaf child and family. Establishing a plan of rehabilitation and education before implantation makes the integration of the implant smoother and reduces the likelihood that progress will be hindered by poor follow-through or gaps in rehabilitative services.

Patient Counseling and Expectations

Candidates for cochlear implantation come for evaluation with all levels of knowledge about cochlear implants and need to be informed of the potential risks and benefits of cochlear implantation and the impact it may have on their life. The surgical procedure and its risks should be described along with a physical description and, preferably demonstration, of the internal and external portions of the device. The various cochlear implant systems available at the center also should be shown and described to the candidate. The post-surgical programming commitment should be described and planned. In addition, potential cochlear implant candidates need to be aware of what day-to-day living with the device entails. This is best done by contacting other cochlear implant wearers and their families. The most important, yet sometimes difficult, aspect of patient counseling is generating realistic expectations regarding performance outcome with the implant. Almost all candidates (or their families) seek the implant because they want to improve their ability to hear and understand speech. Although the mean and range of performance with implants can be described, most people will naturally hope for the best of outcomes. Redundantly reviewing the range of performance, including the bottom of the range, during the course of the candidacy evaluation and discussing post-implant plans in case performance with an implant is poorer than anticipated can assist those recipients who obtain minimal postimplant benefit.

THE CI TEAM

Minimally, the role of a cochlear implant team is to determine candidacy for cochlear implantation, to help prospective recipients make informed decisions about cochlear implant surgery and device options, to provide necessary medical care, to carry out the surgical implantation, and to provide postimplant device setting and monitoring. Aural rehabilitation specialists, speech-language pathologists and educators play an important role in the preimplant evaluation and/or postimplant management of children with cochlear implants. Prelingually deafened children must learn to use the sound provided by an implant to organize and access spoken language and to produce speech that can be understood by others. Aural rehabilitation specialists and speech-language pathologists are members of some cochlear implant teams. Other teams may not have these professionals on staff; in that case, aural rehabilitation and speech-language pathology may be provided by private therapists or by school personnel. Because many children with cochlear implants require special classroom placement and educational support services, at least during the early years of cochlear implant use, it is important for cochlear implant professionals to work closely with educators in developing and coordinating appropriate intervention strategies. Larger cochlear implant teams may routinely include representatives of multiple disciplines; others may bring in additional specialists or refer to outside specialists as needed. Either way, it is important to have access to the disciplines required to provide quality health care. Hearing loss impacts not only communication and educational development, but also a child's emotional and social development. A number of cochlear implant programs have access to the expertise of psychologists or social workers who can assist families as needed. Close communication among the cochlear implant team and other professionals working with the child is essential for children to receive maximum benefit from a cochlear implant.

Otologist/Otosurgeon

The core personnel required to carry out these responsibilities include the surgeon (otologist/otolaryngologist) and the audiologist. Prior to implantation, the focus of care is determining medical and audiological suitability for cochlear implant surgery and managing any medical conditions that may prevent surgery. Following cochlear implant surgery and postimplant healing, the focus shifts from primarily medical management to primarily audiological management. Although the surgeon and audiologist have the principal roles in providing services to cochlear implant candidates and recipients, the needs of different populations may require the services and expertise of additional professionals, not all of whom need be involved with each potential candidate or implantee.

Aural Rehabilitation Specialists

The type of intervention provided by an aural rehabilitation specialist depends on his or her philosophy of communication development and on the needs of the child. A variety of philosophies exist concerning the appropriate communication methods for children with hearing impairment or deafness. One philosophy, oralism, promotes the development of speaking and listening skills for communication. There are several different approaches within this philosophy. For example, some oral therapists use both lip-reading and listening as a means of learning to speak whereas others follow a more unisensory approach emphasizing listening alone without visual cues. An alternative philosophy promotes the use of sign language to develop communication skills, either alone or in conjunction with spoken language. Signing and speech used together is defined as total communication. In total communication, reception of language occurs through listening to speech and watching the signs. Expressive language is conveyed via speech and sign. The speech-language pathologist may be called upon to carry out evaluations of the child's spoken or signed communication abilities and to make recommendations for intervention. Some teams have speech-language pathologists who provide ongoing postimplant speech-language therapy to cochlear implant recipients.

Psychologist

The psychologist provides input related to the level of functioning and mental status of the child. The psychologist can also provide intervention when necessary or appropriate. For example, if family dynamics or behavioral problems present potential obstacles to success with a cochlear implant, the patient and family may be referred for counseling before and/or after cochlear implantation.

Neuropsychologist

Cochlear implant candidates may be referred for a neuropsychological evaluation if there is some concern about their ability to understand and actively participate in the preimplant and postimplant processes.

Educational Specialists

School personnel such as teachers of the deaf, itinerant teachers of the hearing impaired, and mainstream classroom teachers often work closely with the implant team during the evaluation and postimplant periods. They provide important information about how the child is functioning in his or her daily environment, and implement suggestions given by the team for maximizing communication. Sometimes a cochlear implant team includes an educator who assists in the planning of the educational placement and protocol. This individual can act as a formal liaison between the implant center and the school system.

Social Worker

The social worker can provide guidance and support to the child and the family in all areas, including financial planning. Social workers also may help to coordinate necessary appointments and services and provide counseling for families.

CI COMPONENTS

Cochlear implants are electrical prostheses that trigger auditory sensations via a direct electrical stimulation of the hearing nerve. They replace the function of the inner hair cells that have the role of biological microphone. Hereby, a technical simulation of the natural hearing process is performed with tonotopic presentation of the frequencies along the basilar membrane on different parts of the hearing nerve. In comparison to the natural hearing process, only a low number of electrically separated channels is available for signal transmission. This bottleneck of the electrode-nerve interface becomes especially obvious when listening to music or understanding speech in noise.

The cochlear implant systems of today are generally conceived as two component systems. The external speech processor is used for sound recording, sound preprocessing, and transformation of the acoustic information into a logical sequence of electrical impulses (so called speech processing) and it is the sender of the FM signal for a transcutaneous transmission and power supply of the implant per induction by a sending coil. The implant that is located under the skin, contains the receiver coil for reception of the FM signal, a demodulator for extraction of the electrical pulses, an electrode carrier with different intracochlear electrode contacts for transmission of the electrical impulses to the hearing nerve and telemetric measurement systems. Current cochlear implant systems dispose of a broad spectrum of signal pre-processing including directional microphones, beam former, noise elimination, and acoustic scene analysis, and of a mostly wireless interaural connection of the systems in cases of bilateral and bimodal treatment. In this way, both speech processors can be synchronized. Telemetric measurement systems record electrophysiological data with the implant itself such as electrode impedances, measurement of acoustically and electrically evoked potentials. Some systems may assess the intracochlear components of electrocochleography with Cochlear Microphonics, compound action potential of the hearing nerve and summation potential. Additionally, electrically triggered stapedius reflexes can be measured. Those objective measurements allow the intra and postoperative functional control of the implants and provide support for adjustment, which is a great advantage in children. They also allow an indirect control of the position of the implant electrodes. Different electrode systems are available for the individual cochlear implantation. Generally, a sufficient cochlear coverage should be achieved in order to stimulate possibly all spiral ganglia cells. For this purpose, insertion depths of 360° and more are needed. Some manufacturers postulate a higher cochlear coverage to reach apical neuronal elements. For cochlear implant surgery with hearing preservation, specially designed thin electrodes are used that are most frequently placed on the lateral wall and advanced depending on the hearing loss. To achieve a possibly selective stimulation with low stimulation current, preformed, perimodiolar electrodes are inserted, but generally it is less probable to preserve the hearing ability. Special electrodes are available for malformations and for ossified cochleas (double or split array. Those arrays distribute the electrode contacts on 2 electrode carriers that are inserted into the first and second turns via 2 cochleostomies. Compressed arrays are shortened electrode carriers with a normal number of stimulus contacts that are placed into the drilled initial part of the basal turn. Both procedures aim at approaching the number of intracochlear stimulus contacts as near as possible to the normal cochlear anatomy. To achieve a secure watertight closure of the cochlea in cases of malformations, special electrodes with thickened basal end are applied.

THE CI SURGERY

As with many surgical procedures, different surgeons employ different techniques and hold different opinions related to cochlear implant surgery. However, there are some basic principles that underlie all cochlear implant surgical procedures. The major goals are: (1) to insert the electrode array as atraumatically as possible into the scala tympani, (2) to place the device on the side of the head in a manner that most protects it from trauma and (3) to ensure that the device and electrode array are secure enough to prevent movement. The intent is to accomplish these goals without damaging the surrounding tissue, device, and electrode array or causing infection and with an acceptable cosmetic result. Modifications in surgical technique often are determined by the physical and structural properties of a given device. Although the surgical technique is basically the same for both children and adults, some modifications may be required due to head size; no increased surgical risks or complications have been found in very young children (12 months). Alterations and/or adjustments to the surgical technique also may be required for special cases such as a Mondini deformity (malformed cochlea) or a hearing loss secondary to meningitis accompanied by ossification. Depending on the amount of ossification, the surgeon has choices of technique to maximize the possibility of obtaining a full insertion of the electrode array or of using a specially designed electrode array for the more heavily ossified cochleas [42]. Cochlear implant surgery is performed under general anesthesia, and typically lasts between one and four hours. Because of the immaturity of the organs, the implantation should be performed generally from the 12h month of age in cases of congenital deafness. Only in cases of particular urgency such as the risk of obliteration in the context of labyrinthitis, the implantation should be performed earlier. The implantation should include both sides to allow the development of binaural hearing with the ability of directional hearing and improved speech understanding in noise. Hereby, the simultaneous implantation should be preferred if it is possible from an anesthesiologic point of view. Compared to sequential implantation, the following advantages should be mentioned: only one hospital stay; only one anesthesia for surgery; simultaneous activation of the hearing system for the development of binaural hearing. The disadvantage is the prolonged anesthesia and the duration of surgery with the associated risk for example of increased blood loss. If sequential bilateral cochlear implantation is performed, the interval should be rather short in order to keep the auditive deprivation of the second ear as low as possible and thus to achieve a similar hearing ability for both ears. If the intervals are longer, poorer hearing results in the later implanted ear and poorer bilateral and binaural hearing performance are observed [43].

Standard Surgical Technique

The surgical technique is largely standardized and may be applied in all age groups and special cases. Generally a transmastoid surgical approach with posterior tympanostomy is performed comprising the following steps [44]:

- Retroauricular incision
- Creation of a periostal pouch in occipital direction to insert the receiving part of the implant
- Partial mastoidectomy with exposure of the posterior wall of the auditory canal, the antrum with the incus, the mastoid course of the facial nerve, and the canal of

the chorda tympani, the labyrinthine block with the 3 semicircular canals, the sigmoid sinus, and the cortex to the middle and posterior cranial fossa as well as the sinus-dura angle
- Creation of a bone bed to insert the implant at 1 cm behind and above the sinus-dura angle. Hereby, advancing sometimes onto the dura is necessary, especially in very young children. Afterwards careful coagulation is performed
- Creation of a connecting canal or tunnel to the mastoid in projection on the sinus-dura angle to securely insert and fix the electrode
- Performance of the posterior tympanostomy by removal of the bone between the bone-covered facial nerve and the chorda tympani, in order to visualize the middle ear and the relevant structures of the inner ear. Those are the promontory, the round and oval windows with stapes and stapedius tendon. In children, revisions, and malformations generally intraoperative monitoring of the facial nerve should be performed to avoid neural damages and facilitate identification of the nerve
- Opening of the cochlea by incision of the round window membrane or cochleostomy
- Insertion of the electrode carrier. Generally this should be performed in an atraumatic and slow procedure. The selected insertion depths depend on the size of the cochlea as well as the dimension of residual hearing. The insertion is performed down to the calculated depth. Depending on the electrode type, different insertion techniques, possibly using special instruments, are required. Lateral wall electrodes may be easily inserted by means of a specially developed insertion forceps in one-hand technique. Preformed electrodes require special insertion techniques. In the context of advanced-off stylet technique, the electrode is advanced into the cochlea by the stylet after partial insertion.
- Closure of the cochlea: to avoid perilymph fistula, a secure closure of the cochlea is essential. Either a fascia collar may be used that had been created before insertion, or muscle pieces that are positioned carefully around the electrode opening
- Positioning of the electrode carrier. The electrode carrier has to be securely positioned in the mastoid in order to avoid the contact with the covering skin. Although there is no absolute indication in children, in some cases a fixation of the receiver-stimulator in indicated.
- Intraoperative electrophysiology is obligatory for the intraoperative functional control of the implant as well as for measuring the stimulus response of the nerve. Via an attached coil system the implant can be activated. Then the following measurements can be performed: electrode impedances; electrically triggered stapedius reflex with determination of the threshold; electrically triggered compound action potential of the hearing nerve (NRT, neural response

telemetry); cochlear monitoring. During insertion of the electrode, residual hearing can be monitored by measuring cochlear microphone potentials outside and inside the cochlea. Critical changes of the Cochlear Microphonics amplitude indicate an impairment of the inner ear function. By repositioning the electrode, a permanent hearing loss might be avoided [45].
- Appropriate wound closure in several layers to securely cover the implant.
- The intraoperative control of the electrode position by radiography or cone beam tomography is the standard in order to identify insertion failures in time and to correct them in the same session. Furthermore, the insertion depth has to be critically verified and to be corrected, if necessary. Radiography provides important information for the postoperative fitting [46]. The chosen surgical technique is associated with a very low complication rate.
- Compressive dressing

CI COMPLICATIONS

Device Failure (Technical Complications)

Device failure occurs in about 2–4% of the cases. In children they are more frequently observed than in adults which is mainly due to a higher incidence of external forces. The continuous technical improvement of the implant, in particular since the introduction of titanium cases by nearly all manufacturers, a clear reduction of the cumulative failure rate (percentage of all implant defects over a defined observation time) could be achieved. Beside complete, also partial technical failures may occur, as for example the breakdown of an electrode contact. Re-implantation is indicated when the hearing performance is significantly impaired. Intermitting failures are difficult to assess technically as well as soft failure, i.e., the patient reports convincingly about hearing deterioration but a defect cannot be verified with the available technical means. When a device failure is observed and confirmed, re-implantation should be performed as soon as possible. This is especially true for children with implant in only one ear [47].

Medical Complications

Although the rate of complications associated with cochlear implant surgery is very small and thus postimplant complications are rare, there are certain risks involved in both the surgical procedure and postoperative period.

- Intraoperative complications – Intraoperative complications mainly occur as damage of the facial nerve, the sigmoid sinus, the internal carotid artery, or the ossicular chain. Further complications are injuries of the external wall of the auditory canal, the tympanic membrane, and the dura. The risk of facial nerve damage is somewhat greater in those individuals with anatomic malformation of the inner ear such as are found with a Mondini deformity. In general, they can be avoided by an adequate surgical technique. A low complication rate reflects a high quality standard of cochlear implantation and sufficient training due an adequate minimum number of surgeries performed per year [48, 49].
- Postoperative complications – The difference is made between severe and mild complications. In general, those are either acute complications such as infections, postoperative bleedings, vertigo, or inner ear damage in the context of cochlear implantation with hearing preservation. In cases of late complications, usually long-term complications are observed. Those are among others the migration of the implant or the electrode when they are insufficiently fixed, e.g., without bone bed or without fixation of the electrode, thinning out of the skin covering the implant sometimes with perforation of the skin and infection, irritation of the facial nerve in the context of advanced ossification, obliteration of the cochlea in the context of labyrinthitis, or meningitis occurring after implantation [50]. Mild complications can mostly be treated conservatively. Those are also hearing deterioration with increased impedance and increased stimulus threshold, e.g., as consequence of labyrinthitis. Interestingly, those changes may also be observed in the context of overstimulation of the hearing nerve, e.g., with a very short pulse width and high rate of stimuli sequences. Hereby, the interruption of stimulation, the administration of corticosteroids as well as a careful reactivation of the stimulation are usually suitable measures to restore the stimulation capacity. Severe complications require surgical revision, for example for re-fixation of the implant and the electrode, dislocation of the implant in cases of skin defect and according plastic measures in the sense of e.g., local rotation of the temporal muscle. Meningitis is a rare though potentially serious complication in those people with inner ear deformities. Leakage of cerebrospinal fluid into the ear should be controlled if and when it occurs in order to prevent the onset of meningitis. The vestibular portion of the ear, which controls the balance mechanism, may have remaining function even when there is little or no residual hearing. When this occurs, opening the inner ear to the electrode could cause a temporary imbalance. For meningitis prophylaxis, vaccination against Pneumococci and Haemophilus influenza is recommended since CI users have an increased risk. In children, specific risks must be considered that may have severe consequences. Complications require an adequate management that must be controlled by the cochlear implant surgeon. Continuous improvement of the

surgical technique led to a relevant reduction of the complication rates. With 6.9%, the percentage of inflammatory complications is clearly higher than in adults as well as the rate of electrode migration, which occurs in particular in atraumatic lateral wall electrodes. It becomes obvious by hearing loss as well as missing NRT responses to the electrode contacts that have left the cochlea. In general, surgical revision with re-insertion of the electrode and adequate fixation is required.

SETTING THE COCHLEAR IMPLANT SPEECH PROCESSOR

Approximately three to five weeks following surgery, recipients return to the cochlear implant center to receive their external equipment and to have their speech processor programmed. Device programming involves selecting and individually fitting the speech processing strategy or strategies the patient will use. Processing strategies are used to translate incoming acoustic stimuli into electrical pulses that stimulate auditory nerve fibers. Despite the numerous speech encoding strategies implemented in the various cochlear prostheses, the basic parameters of programming are neither device nor strategy dependent: the audiologist needs to obtain basic psychophysical measures i.e., thresholds and comfort levels on all electrodes. Although the basic parameters are the same, the techniques used to obtain these measures do depend on individual characteristics such as age, cognitive skills, length of deafness, and other potential factors affecting responses the use of both subjective and objective techniques. If the recipient is an adult or an older child, the subjective method can be used to set the threshold at the lowest level where the patient responds 100% of the time. The implant users also can report the level at which the loudness of the stimuli is most comfortable. After the thresholds and comfort levels are obtained for all electrodes, the computer simulates this information and translates it into an operating program that is transferred to the speech processor; live voice stimulation then can begin. Many parameters, including global increases in loudness, frequency allocation to electrodes, and speed of transmission to name a few, can be manipulated to improve the quality of sound and increase open-set speech understanding for a given patient. The precise characteristics that can be regulated are dependent on the speech processing strategy used and the manifestation of that strategy in a given cochlear implant system. Whether the patient is a child or an adult, accurate electrical thresholds and comfort levels are critical contributors to postoperative performance. Because of this, it is essential that a comprehensive schedule of programming sessions be established. The number of visits required to adequately program and maintain the speech processor depends on a number of factors including but not limited to patient age, previous auditory experience, and ability to actively participate in the device programming tasks. Furthermore, because responses to auditory stimulation from a cochlear implant can change over time, long-term audiological follow-up is required. It is recommended that cochlear implant recipients contact their cochlear implant center for speech processor programming if they or their family notices a decrease in auditory responsiveness, perception, discrimination, speech production, or a change in vocal quality in between regularly scheduled audiological appointments.

Postoperative Fitting and Hearing-Speech Training

In adults and older children, the fitting is performed psycho-acoustically with assessment of the co-called T and C levels (threshold and current of comfortable loudness) for every single electrode contact. Then the loudness between the contacts is balanced, the dynamic range is defined, and the speech processing strategy is selected. The strategy is an algorithm according to which the acoustic signal is transformed – completely or partially – into a defined sequence of electrical pulses that are then transmitted to the hearing nerve via the electrode. The aim is a possibly physiological activation pattern of the hearing nerve. The single electrode contacts are allotted to different frequency ranges in the form of frequency bands. The allocation is made according to the subjective hearing impression and should follow the tonotopic order, i.e., high frequencies should be transmitted to the basal electrodes, low frequencies to the apical electrode contacts. An anatomically correct depictions is generally not possible because the presented frequencies and the position of the electrode contact are usually not congruent with the physiological representation on the cochlea (so called Greenwood function). In an intraoperative process, an optimized fitting may be achieved until the patient reaches an open speech understanding. After longer intervals of hearing habituation, further optimizations may follow. Already during fitting, a hearing and speech training take place. First, the focus is placed on the recognition of basic auditive categories such as loud, quiet/soft, high, low, the recognition of single syllables, of vowels and consonants, later it is speech understanding [51]. In children, fitting is performed based on objectively assessed parameters. So called NRT based maps allow an approximation of the profile over the complete electrode carrier as soon as a T and C level can be psycho-acoustically determined on an electrode contact. Additionally, electrically evoked brainstem potentials and EEG signals are applied [52]. In order to control the usage by means of a so-called datalogging, the implant registers several parameters such as the daily time of usage. This information can be used to support rehabilitation [53]. It is imperative that audiologists involved in device programming take the training courses offered by individual device manufacturers and avail themselves of the support personnel at each company in order to provide the highest quality care to the patient. Because cochlear implant speech processor technology and speech programming software constantly evolve, continuing education is a necessity.

The Use of Objective Measures in Speech Processor Programming

Over the course of the past decade there has been a trend toward implanting children at progressively younger ages. Programming the speech processor of the cochlear implant can be challenging if the recipient is either very young or has limited response capabilities. It such cases, programming techniques that are less dependent on the ability of the child to give a behavioral response can prove helpful. While there are several different types of electrically evoked potentials that could be used to assist with device programming, most of the attention in the literature has focused on the electrically evoked auditory brainstem response (EABR), the electrically evoked compound action potential (ECAP) and the electrically evoked acoustic reflex threshold (EART). All three measures have acoustic analogs, have been well studied and can be recorded in young children. When cochlear implant recipients can actively participate in the speech processor programming process, these techniques typically will not result in speech processor programs that are superior to those constructed using traditional behavioral programming techniques. Additionally, few clinics will use these tools routinely. They are typically incorporated into clinical practice in cases where the audiologist has reason to question the validity of the behavioral measures that were obtained. However, with the decrease in age of implantation and the increase in our understanding about how these tools can be used in the clinical management of cochlear implant recipients, the need for supplemental, non-behaviorally based measures of sensitivity to electrical stimulation increasingly has become evident.

Electrically Evoked Auditory Brainstem Response (EABR)

The EABR is a recording of the synchronous neural activity in the brainstem that results when the auditory nerve is stimulated. It is recorded using commercial evoked potential equipment and surface recording electrodes positioned on the head. The EABR can be recorded either in the operating room at the time of surgery or during the postoperative period. However, obtaining a successful recording does require a very quiet or sleeping subject. The stimulus used to evoke the EABR is a biphasic current pulse that is generated by the software used to program the speech processor. Studies have shown that the EABR can be successfully measured using a variety of different implant types both in congenitally deaf children and postlingually deafened adults [54-59]. The EABR is similar in form to the acoustically evoked ABR [60] and EABR thresholds have been shown to correlate well with behavioral thresholds for the electrical stimulus used to elicit the EABR [54, 61, 62]. From a clinical perspective, however, the comparison of interest is between EABR thresholds and the levels needed to program the speech processor of the cochlear implant. Research has shown that this correlation is significant but not strong [54, 62, 63]. In general, EABR thresholds are recorded at levels where the stimulus used to program the speech processor is audible but below the maximum level of stimulation that is comfortable for a congenitally deaf child [54, 62]. This information can be useful in cases where the child is showing little or no reaction to electrical stimulation at the initial device stimulation and there is question about whether or not he/she hears the programming stimulus. The EABR threshold can provide a point to begin conditioning the child to respond to electrical stimulation. EABR thresholds tend to be relatively stable over time [64], and therefore this response provides a baseline measure of neural responsiveness to electrical stimulation that can be valuable if problems develop at any point following the initial device programming session, or hookup [65]. Additionally, in children with extremely limited response capabilities, the EABR can allow the audiologist to approximate the levels needed to program the speech processor. Few clinics routinely record the EABR. The primary reason for this is that recording this particular response requires that the subject be sedated or very still during the recording period and the process of establishing threshold on an individual electrode is time consuming. Additionally, in most cases, the relationship between the EABR threshold and the levels used to program the speech processor are not strong enough to warrant routine postoperative sedation. Some clinics do record the EABR in the operating room at the end of the surgical procedure to implant the device. Unfortunately, time is very limited during surgery and there are data suggesting that the threshold measures made in the OR immediately following insertion may change during the immediate postoperative period [54]. Nevertheless, the presence of an EABR indicates that the device and the auditory nerve are functioning. It is also possible to identify electrodes that activate the facial nerve. Because facial nerve stimulation can complicate the process of device setting, it can be very helpful to identify electrodes that cause this prior to the initial stimulation of the device. Furthermore, the parents of the child and the surgeon often find intraoperative EABR results reassuring given the necessary delay between surgery and hookup.

Electrically Evoked Compound Action Potential (ECAP)

An alternative auditory evoked potential that can be used in much the same way as the EABR is the electrically evoked compound action potential (ECAP). This is a measure of the synchronized response of the auditory nerve to electrical stimulation. Rather than being measured using surface electrodes like those used to record the EABR, the ECAP typically is recorded from an intracochlear electrode. This requires specialized technology. Cochlear Corporation was the first company to develop this technology.

Since the introduction of the Nucleus CI24M device in 1998, it has been possible to measure electrically evoked intracochlear potentials in all Nucleus cochlear implant users. Cochlear Corporation refers to the software and hardware used to record this response as Neural Response Telemetry (NRT). Recently the other manufacturers have also introduced a cochlear implant with neural telemetry capabilities and is in the process of developing software to drive this system. The ECAP has several advantages over the EABR as a tool for assessing the response of the auditory system to electrical stimulation. The fact that the recording electrode is within the cochlea is advantageous for several reasons. First, it is located close to the auditory nerve, which means that the response has a large amplitude (much larger than the EABR). Second, the intracochlear location of the recording electrode results in a recording that is not adversely affected by muscle artifact, which in turn means that sedation is not necessary. This is a distinct advantage for pediatric applications. The lack of contamination by muscle artifact means that we have an electrophysiologic tool that can be incorporated into the routine post-operative evaluation of an implanted child, rather than being limited to the pre- or intraoperative period. While using an intracochlear electrode to record the ECAP is advantageous in several ways, it also can present some challenges. The primary challenge is that the close proximity of the stimulating and recording electrodes leads to significant levels of electrical stimulus artifact in the recordings. Early publications describing ECAP recordings dealt primarily with the pragmatics involved with obtaining artifact free responses [66-69]. Current research focus has shifted to studies designed to assess the response of the auditory nerve to electrical stimulation and to identify potential clinical applications for this technology [70-75]. One such application for this technology is to assist with the prediction of threshold and maximum comfort levels needed to program the speech processor of the cochlear implant. It has been shown that ECAP thresholds correlate well with behavioral thresholds if the same stimulus is used to evoke both responses [66]. Unfortunately, however, the stimulus that results in an optimal ECAP response is a relatively slow rate pulse train (≤ 80 Hz) while the stimulus used to program the speech processor of the cochlear implant is a considerably higher rate pulse train (≥ 250 Hz). Peripheral neural responses such as the ECAP (or the EABR) will exhibit adaptation effects and decrease in amplitude as the rate of stimulation is increased. Perceptually, however, the loudness of a stimulus will increase as the stimulation rate increases. This is due to the fact that the brain is able to integrate neural information over time. It is not surprising, therefore, that ECAP thresholds for an 80 Hz pulse train will exceed behavioral thresholds for the high rate stimulus used to program the speech processor of the cochlear implant. Additionally, temporal integration can vary across individuals [55]. As a result, the correlation between the evoked potential thresholds and behavioral thresholds used for programming may be expected to weaken as the difference in rate between the two stimuli increases. Like the EABR, research has shown that the ECAP is typically recorded at levels where the programming stimulus is audible to the child [70-75]. Thus, one method of using this technology with very young children is to slowly increase the programming stimulus to the ECAP threshold and begin working on conditioning the child to respond at that level. Additionally, ECAP thresholds can be used to cross check the results of behavioral testing. Very young children may let the stimulus become elevated before responding. ECAP thresholds should not be recorded at levels where the programming stimulus is inaudible. If this occurs, the behavioral thresholds should be rechecked and/or decreased to a level that is just less than the ECAP threshold. Systematic studies comparing ECAP threshold and programming levels have been published only for recipients of the Nucleus cochlear implant. Generally, these studies show correlations between NRT thresholds and the behavioral levels needed to program the speech processor of the cochlear implant that are significant, but only moderately strong [70-73]. For some people, ECAP thresholds can be recorded near the threshold for the stimulus used to program the speech processor. For other people, the electrophysiologic response is only measurable at levels that exceed maximum comfort levels for the stimulus used to program the speech processor. It is possible to use ECAP thresholds recorded on electrodes spaced across the electrode array to get an idea of how the behavioral threshold and maximum comfort levels vary across while recording electrode array. Furthermore, methods for improving the clinical utility of the NRT measures by combining the physiologic data with a limited amount of behavioral data have been proposed [69, 72]. The adequacy of programs constructed using the ECAP data was tested in a small group of Nucleus CI24M cochlear implant users [76]. Speech recognition was measured using sentences in noise for a small group of postlingually deafened adults. Performance using a program that was constructed using traditional behavioral programming techniques was contrasted with programs created based on the ECAP threshold data. The results of this study revealed that on average, individuals tended to perform slightly worse with ECAP-based programs than with programs created using standard behavioral programming techniques but this trend was not statistically significant [76]. If these results can be extrapolated to congenitally deaf children, they suggest that NRT-based speech processor programs, although not ideal, may be adequate to support speech and language development—at least until the child is older and able to be tested more accurately using behavioral techniques. These data should be reassuring to the families of children with developmental delays, who may never be able to be programmed using behavioral techniques. Additionally, future research also may demonstrate how these physiologic measures of the response of the auditory nerve to electrical stimulation may be helpful in selecting the most appropriate programming strategy for a particular cochlear implant recipient or in determining the number of electrodes to use to avoid channel interaction.

Electrically Evoked Acoustic Reflex Threshold (EART)

An alternative "objective" measure that has shown promise for assisting with device programming is the electrically evoked reflex threshold (EART). In children or adults with normal middle ear function, it is possible to elicit a reflexive contraction of the muscles of the middle ear in response to the presentation of a loud sound. Stimulation of one ear, either electrically or acoustically, causes the simultaneous contraction of the middle ear muscles in both ears. Contraction of the middle ear muscles in turn results in stiffening of the eardrum that can be measured using instrumentation available in most audiology clinics. One advantage that the EART has over the ECAP or the EABR is that it can be elicited using the same high-rate stimulus used to program the speech processor. Additionally, recording this response does not require sedation (although it does require that the patient remain still for the time required to perform the test). These facts make the EART an ideal tool for clinical use. Several studies have explored potential clinical applications for the EART [77-81]. Many of these studies have shown relatively good agreement between the EART and the maximum comfort levels used to program the speech processor; however, to date most of the comparisons that have been published have used congenitally deaf adults who wore relatively low rate processors. Additionally, these studies report that they were unable to measure the EART for approximately 20–30% of the individuals tested [77]. This may be due either to middle ear or tympanic membrane abnormalities, inability to maintain a seal for the period of time required for testing or unusually low loudness discomfort levels. From a theoretical perspective, limiting the electrical dynamic range based on the level at which a reflex is elicited does make some sense. Congenitally deaf children often have little concept of loudness and can have unusually wide dynamic ranges. In these cases, limiting the upper levels of stimulation provided by the implant to levels that do not evoke an acoustic reflex may make the speech processor program more comfortable for the child. In children who are not responding behaviorally to electrical stimulation, stimulation levels that evoke an acoustic reflex also could be interpreted as evidence that the device is functioning and the auditory nerve is intact. Additionally, levels that evoke an EART are levels that should be audible for the child and so this may also be used for conditioning during the first stimulation settings. Hodges [77] reported that speech processor programs constructed using EART thresholds to set maximum stimulation levels are tolerated well by both children and adults. More research is needed to determine how EART measures correlate with behavioral levels used to program the speech processor of the cochlear implant for congenitally deaf children and for persons who use high rate processing strategies and to assess more fully the quality of programs created using the EART.

RESULTS

Cochlear implantation in children with congenital or prelingual deafness may have a profound impact on all aspects of communication, and the assessment battery employed for children should be broad enough to reflect these changes [82]. Thus, clinical researchers must have available a wide array of age-appropriate outcome measures that allows them to target different aspects of communication development [83]. The outcome is assessed and documented by means of standardized test procedures. The thresholds with cochlear implant are measured. They should amount to values between 20 dB and 30 dB over the whole frequency spectrum. The consistent amplification over all electrode contacts is important for a good hearing result. For the assessment of speech understanding, age-dependent test procedures are available. They register the speech understanding for numbers and monosyllables as well as the understanding of sentences in quiet and in defined noise. In the context of children, speech development is documented. In order to take into account that the test results depend on the age and to perform comparative evaluations, the scale of the CAPs (categories of auditory performance) was developed [84]. These CAPs describe the hearing performance and its use for communication. The categories range from 0 to 9 and reach from "no auditory sensation" up to "open speech understanding" and "use of the telephone." The majority of children with current cochlear implant devices achieve good levels of open-set word recognition [85-87]. Recognition of isolated words is a very difficult task in that there are no linguistic or contextual cues to aid the listener. When linguistic cues are available, such as in sentence recognition tasks, average performance levels are substantially higher [86]. One of the most consistent findings is that the speech perception abilities of children with cochlear implants improve with increased device experience [88]. The average spoken language processing skills of children with cochlear implants do not plateau over five or more years of device use [87]. This is in contrast to postlingually deafened adults with cochlear implants whose word recognition skills typically plateau within the first few months of device use. Children must use the sound they receive via a cochlear implant to acquire a spoken language. The development rate of children's auditory skills following implantation seems to be increasing as cochlear implant technology improves and as children are implanted at a younger age [89]. The total hearing situation in cases of bimodal and bilateral cochlear implantation can be assessed by free-field testing. Often the patients are either bimodally treated (cochlear implant and hearing aid) or bilaterally (2 cochlear implants) or have a hybrid system for electroacoustic hearing in one ear and a hearing aid in the contralateral ear (so-called combined mode). The various hearing situations have to be assessed separately and the percentage of the different hearing modalities (acoustic, electric, electroacoustic) regarding the total hearing situation must be evaluated. Numerous studies have confirmed that the successful development of language in children with early-onset deafness is strongly correlated with cochlear implantation between 12 and 24 months of age [90]. These findings reflect the importance of minimizing the interval between the onset of bilateral deafness and cochlear implantation, given that auditory development can proceed before the onset of acquired deafness and that the central auditory system is known to undergo reorganization during the period of bilateral auditory deprivation [91]. To further minimize this interval, implantation in infants with early-onset or congenital deafness before 12 months of age has been performed with good results [92, 93]. Implantation in babies as young as 3 months of age has been reported [94]; however, the reliability of the audiometric results at this early stage of development remains questionable, and surgical safety must be viewed in the context of the uncertain, theoretical, physiological advantage [95]. Moreover, there is a risk that unrecognized developmental delays will emerge with age. Nonetheless, interest in early implantation is increasing. Additional input through bilateral cochlear implants provides further benefits for adults who had bilateral hearing before their deafness; these benefits include improved hearing in noisy situations and sound localization with the use of intensity cues [96]. Relatively little has been reported regarding the outcomes of bilateral implantation in children with congenital deafness, although early data indicate better hearing in noisy situations with two implants rather than one [97, 98] an ability to discriminate between sounds at different locations [99] and electrophysiological evidence of binaural processing in the brainstem [100]. Just as the interval between the onset of bilateral deafness and cochlear implantation has implications for the development of oral speech and language, the interval between the implantation in the first and the second ear may affect the development of binaural processing in children [100]; thus, there may be at least two sensitive periods in auditory development. Risks are taken twice for bilateral implantation, with an additional theoretical risk of vestibular or balance dysfunction, or both [101,102]. Bilateral implantation is also associated with a substantially increased cost, since two devices must be purchased and, when not done simultaneously, two procedures must be performed. However, simultaneous bilateral implantation requires less than double the surgical time and eliminates the need for two separate anesthetics, recoveries, and device activations. It may be possible to promote binaural hearing by adding a hearing aid in the ear without the implant, provided that there is sufficient residual hearing. This "bimodal" hearing can successfully supply bilateral auditory cues and access to fine-frequency information that is lost by the constant (and comparatively slow) rate of electrical pulse presentation from the cochlear implant. The decision by the FDA to approve cochlear implants for children in 1990 aroused controversy in the deaf community, with some persons asserting that deaf persons should be considered to be members of a distinct culture rather than patients with a disability, and arguing that parental approval of implants in their children is unethical [103]. More recently, however, this view has undergone some evolution. In 2000, a position paper of the National Association of the Deaf [104] stated that "cochlear implantation is a technology that represents a tool to be used in some forms of communication, and not a cure for deafness." The paper added that "the NAD recognizes the rights of parents to make informed choices for their deaf and hard of hearing children." Usually, early implanted children (1st year of life) achieve very good speech development scores that nearly correspond to those of normally hearing children, especially in quiet environments. In noise, however, poorer scores are observed, which reveals that a cochlear implant does not make a child normally hearing but that it is hearing impaired. Under the aspect of the overall development, it can be summarized that, compared to normally hearing people, deficits remain even in cases of early implantation that impair the cognitive development of the brain. This is mainly due to the close interrelation between the hearing system and other brain areas and functions [28]. In cases of early implantations, about 2/3 of the children may visit regular schools [105]. The professional education is usually also significantly facilitated by cochlear implant. All professions are thus open for implanted children. Usually, however, lower school categories and professional qualifications are observed [51].

Comparison of Sensory Aids in Children

In children, postimplant improvements in communication abilities may result from implant use, from maturation, or from their combined effects. The use of a within-subject design to assess cochlear implant performance does not permit researchers to separate the effects of maturation and cochlear implant use. Osberger and her colleagues were among the first to address this problem [106]. They compared the communication abilities of children with cochlear implants to those of age-matched children with similar hearing thresholds who used other sensory aids, such as hearing aids or vibrotactile aids and demonstrated that the cochlear implant users generally yielded superior results [107]. Similar studies have been carried out by other investigators to examine the effects of pediatric implantation on speech perception, speech production, or the development of language skills in children with prelingual deafness [85, 108]. Although the audiological characteristics of the control groups in these studies evolved over time as persons with more residual hearing were implanted, the vast majority of hearing aid users in these studies were profoundly deaf. Overall, these studies demonstrated that the speech perception abilities of pediatric cochlear implant recipients meet or exceed those of their peers with unaided pure tone average thresholds ≥90 dB HL who use hearing aids [109].

Bilateral Implantation

In normal hearing situations, sound reaching one ear differs from sound reaching the opposite ear in two ways: there is a difference in intensity (loudness) and a difference between the times when the sound reaches each ear. These differences allow the listener to identify the direction from which a sound (and speech) emanates and to separate the speech signal from any background noise. Both of these are critical in professional and social situations because the lack of ability to understand speech in the presence of competing noise reduces an individual's ability to communicate effectively. Traditionally, cochlear implant surgery routinely has been performed in one ear due to the possible loss of residual hearing following cochlear implantation, the belief that one ear should be preserved in order to benefit from future technologies and the cost/benefit issues associated with a second device. However, because of the success of unilateral implantation and the improved functioning of individuals using binaural hearing aids, investigators have demonstrated that bilateral cochlear implantation provide increased speech understanding and localization benefits to cochlear implant users. Compared with unilaterally implanted individuals, bilateral implant recipients show better speech comprehension in noisy conditions, better directional hearing and improvement with regard to binaural mechanisms such as the head shadow and squelch effects, and better binaural summation [110-113]. Children and adolescents who underwent sequential bilateral cochlear implantation show poorer speech comprehension outcomes for the second-implanted ear than for the first side [114, 34] although these children also benefit in terms of binaural listening. In children with unilateral CIs, a modifying influence of unilateral hearing on the auditory system has been shown that induces auditory maturation; however, at an implantation age of 6.5–7.0 years, developmental maturation is less likely to be initiated [115]. Sharma et al. [116] assumed that a second, 'late' implant would stimulate cortical areas and also that there would not be normal connections either within cortical layers or to higher-order auditory and language areas, which may lead to inferior outcomes for the later-implanted ear. Nonetheless, speech recognition improves in children who undergo sequential bilateral cochlear implantation. Systematic studies on the effects of stimulation of the second-implanted ear are rare and include only limited numbers of individuals [9, 117, 118]. Unilateral cochlear implantation reorganizes the brain and generates a "stronger" and a "weaker" ear, resulting in an abnormal "aural preference" of the stronger ear [117, 119]. While this may evoke comparison with presbyopia in the visual system, the condition is significantly different in that the 'representation' of the weak ear in the cortex is preserved [119, 120]; training techniques may, therefore, provide help in overcoming the aural preference. At present, however, the easiest means of preventing abnormal auditory preference may be through simultaneously cochlear implantation or by using hearing aids to take advantage of residual hearing [34, 121]. Inter-implant interval correlates significantly with speech comprehension results obtained with the second-implanted side. To avoid abnormal aural preference in pediatric implantation, this interval should – in children first implanted under the age of 4 – be limited to less than four years. The older the children were at first implantation, the shorter the inter-implant interval needed to be. It is a direct consequence of the inter-implant interval that children for whom this interval was longer were also older.

Cochlear Implants and Cognitive Effort

People who are hard of hearing and use hearing aids or cochlear implants often complain about being tired from straining to hear, especially in the presence of noisy environments or multiple talkers. Self-reports of listening effort and fatigue are very common even among "star" patients who score particularly well in speech recognition tests, both in quiet and in noise, yet at the cost of deploying a great deal of cognitive resources [122]. A frequent consequence of such difficulties is early exhaustion, discouragement and ultimately withdrawal from social life, where the ability to listen in challenging conditions is often required. In children and adolescents with sensorineural hearing loss, the effect of prolonged effortful listening is likely to be even more detrimental, impairing the acquisition of linguistic abilities and being an obstacle to achieving satisfactory academic performance [123]. Given these premises, it is clear that reliable measures of the listening effort experienced by hearing-impaired subjects would enable to investigate an issue of crucial importance, whose assessment is currently beyond the possibility of conventional audiometric tests. If available for clinical use, such measures could have important implications [124]: first, they would help clinicians in decision-making concerning the most appropriate treatment of hearing loss (e.g., hearing aids vs. cochlear implants); secondly, they would allow a more comprehensive assessment of functional outcomes, especially in cases where treatment is aimed at restoring binaural hearing, such as asymmetrical hearing loss or single-sided deafness [125]. Despite the growing importance of this topic, the assessment of effortful listening still represents a challenge for a number of reasons. In the first instance, there is currently no shared general definition of this concept; secondly, and subsequently, there is no agreement as to which outcome measures should be applied; thirdly, very little is known about age-related variations of the proposed outcome measures and, more specifically, about how they should be applied to pediatric subjects. In a recent consensus paper, listening effort was generally defined as "deliberate allocation of mental resources to overcome obstacles in goal pursuit when carrying out a listening task" [126], and in the frame of an established limited-capacity resource model [127]. In this model, a subject's cognitive resources are limited; while listening, a subject deliberately allocates a part of such resources to the task, depending on the inherent demands: when demands increase, due to environmental factors (acoustically unfavorable environment), subject-related factors (e.g., hearing impairment or poor knowledge of a language) or talker-related factors (poorly intelligible accent or timbre), the amount of cognitive load invested in the task will also increase. Therefore in this paper, we will include the listening effort in the more general concept of cognitive load. In a recent paper [128], the authors applied EEG to investigate frontal theta and parietal alpha power levels of EEG in relation to cognitive load during an audiological task. In particular, the study focused on the pre-stimulus phase, i.e., the time interval when noise is on and the subject is waiting for the word to be delivered. The main findings of this research indicate that: 1) frontal theta power did not reveal a significant increase in adverse listening conditions compared to the listening-in-quiet condition; 2) parietal alpha power increased significantly in only some of the more adverse listening conditions compared to the listening-in-quiet condition. Going back to the study hypothesis, we found that only alpha power met expectations that it would be higher in the most difficult listening conditions, whereas theta power showed no significant variations. An increase in theta power is unanimously considered as an electrophysiological marker of engagement in a task [129]. Over the years, it has been studied in relationship to cognitive load, excitation and interest, high attentional demands, task difficulty, cognitive and mental efforts [130, 131]. The finding of non-significant changes for theta power throughout the various listening configurations assessed in this research may seem contradictory to that reported in the existing literature. A possible interpretation would be to assume that the task was not exciting enough for the subjects, and a higher degree of mental effort would have been necessary to elicit significant variations in theta band. Another explanation concerning why theta power levels did not increase could be that in the present study the pre-stimulus interval (i.e., the interval before word onset) was analyzed. In this "pre-word" phase, subjects were only hearing the competing babble noise, anticipating of the test signal but not actively engaged in decoding a test sound signal. In a recent experiment on normal-hearing subjects conducted with an auditory oddball task, Wisniewski et al. [132] found no significant theta variations either before word onset or during "passive" exposure to stimuli, namely as subjects were engaged in another activity. Thus, the pre-stimulus phase of our study may be equivalent to the passive exposure described in Wisniewski's work, where subjects were asked not to pay attention to background noise, but to focus on the incoming word stimuli. However, the significant within-subject correlation found between frontal theta and parietal alpha power levels suggests that theta activity could be a potential indicator of cognitive resource deployment in effortful audiological tasks, providing a higher degree of effort is required or a different epoch (e.g., during or poststimulus) is analyzed. The main finding of the present study was the significant increase of parietal alpha power in two of the three most challenging listening conditions, i.e., binaural noise and noise delivered to the worse hearing ear. This verified the study hypothesis concerning alpha power only partially, since the expected rise in the acoustically most adverse condition, where noise was delivered to the better ear, was not observed. Such results need to be interpreted in the light of the large amount of literature investigating the general relevance of alpha activity and its possible generators, bearing in mind that only a few studies have focused specifically on the impact of various listening tasks. The earliest research investigating the behavior of parietal alpha power in the pre-stimulus phase was conducted using visual stimuli. Parieto-occipital alpha power was shown to increase as tested subjects are required to direct attention to a relevant stimulus while neglecting other task-irrelevant stimuli, such as portions of space containing distractor information [133], colors, or motions [134]. Other studies have even demonstrated that selective increases of alpha activity occur retinotopically over areas of the parietooccipital cortex where distracting visual stimuli are likely to be processed [135, 136]. Also works using a double modality of stimulus presentation (e.g., visual vs auditory) have confirmed that alpha power increases as tested subjects try to suppress one modality in favor of another one [137, 138]. When purely auditory tasks were used, alpha power in the parietal and occipital cortex was once again found to increase as subjects were preparing for expected auditory stimuli [139, 140]. A lateralization of alpha band activity was also observed, whereby alpha power increases over the parietal cortex contralateral to the to-be-ignored stimulus. Our results with the "binaural noise" and "noise to the worse ear" listening conditions seem to fit the model, suggesting that increases in the parietal alpha power can be an indicator of attentional suppression even in a pediatric sample [128]. In that study, words were the relevant auditory stimulus and babble noise was irrelevant to the task and thus a to-be-ignored stimulus or distractor. Overall, this is consistent with recent theories attributing task-related increases of alpha activity to the activation of a supramodal functional inhibition system [141, 142], i.e., a "top-down" gating system where inhibitory neural pathways eliminate task-irrelevant stimuli and constrain potentially erroneous behaviors. To the best of our knowledge, this is the first time that a drop in alpha power has been observed in the most challenging listening condition tested (noise was delivered to the better hearing ear). As stated above, under this circumstance our study hypothesis was not fulfilled, whereby alpha power fell to the level of that observed in the quiet test condition. Possibly, this is the reason why no correlation could be found between alpha power levels and SRT scores: whereas average SRT scores decreased with increasing difficulty of the task (i.e., from Quiet to better ear), alpha power levels increased from Quiet to worse ear, but then decreased again in the better ear condition. This "alpha drop phenomenon" may be explained by subjects mentally withdrawing from the task, when it became exceeding difficult [143]. In their "Framework for Understanding Effortful Listening" model, Pichora Fuller et al. [126] postulate that listening effort increases as task demands increase as long as the subject is motivated toward the task itself, up to a point where task demands exceed the subject's cognitive resources. When this occurs, the subject loses motivation and stops deploying these resources in the task. Specifically, it is likely that the "noise to better ear condition" was too difficult for the subjects selected in the study, whose SRT in that condition was on average 15 dB, that is to say well above the þ10 SNR level at which the EEG recordings took place. In this case, it is plausible that the patients stopped directing their attention selectively toward the presented words and completely lost their overall "engagement" in the task. A support to this interpretation comes from the work by Wizniewski [140], in which alpha power levels were compared in normal-hearing adults during an active listening and a passive exposure experiment: during the passive experiment, alpha power levels dropped to rest values. Thus, it is plausible that in our subjects loss of interest in a too difficult task may have equaled the "passive exposure" condition in Wizniewski's study [140]. Overall, our results suggest that EEG alpha activity derived from the parietal cortex can be used in pediatric subjects with sensorineural hearing loss as an objective measure of cognitive load during effortful listening. In particular, since the pre-stimulus phase was analyzed, sustained attention and selective inhibition seem to be the likeliest behavioral correlates of the observed alpha variations. If confirmed on larger samples, the alpha power drop characterizing the most adverse listening condition suggests that cognitive withdrawal from a task can also be measured objectively. Even if consistent with recent works in the literature, the results of our study should be interpreted with caution and be supported by further investigations in larger cohort datasets. Firstly, our data refer to a pediatric population in whom the brain is notoriously immature and, as a consequence, normative data is age dependent. Most of the literature, on the contrary, reports on adult or elderly subjects. For example, it is known that alpha frequency itself increases in a non-linear way [144], whereas global alpha and theta power increase and decrease, respectively, from childhood to puberty [145]. Secondly, the lack of normative data from normal-hearing subjects makes it impossible, at this point, to use absolute alpha and theta power levels to quantify cognitive load. However, if confirmed by further research on diverse and larger samples, these findings could be used to refine indications for hearing aid or cochlear implant treatment of sensorineural hearing loss, and for a more in-depth assessment of the audiological outcomes of listening devices.

REFERENCES

[1] National Institute on Deafness and Other Communication Disorders. *Statistics about hearing disorders, ear infections, and deafness.* (Accessed November 9, 2007, at http://www.nidcd.nih.gov/health/statistics/ hearing.asp.).

[2] Smith, R. J. H., Bale, J. F., White, K. R. (2005) Sensorineural hearing loss in children. *Lancet,* 365:879-90.

[3] Olusanya, B. O., Newton, V. E. (2007) Global burden of childhood hearing impairment and disease control priorities for developing countries. *Lancet,* 369:1314-7. [Erratum, Lancet 2007;369:1860.

[4] Ballacchino, A., Mucia, M., Cocuzza, S., Ferrara, S., Martines, E., Salvago, P., Sireci, F., Martines, F. (2013) Newborn hearing screening in sicily: Lesson learned. *Acta Medica Mediterranea,* 29 (4), pp. 731-734.

[5] Ponton, C. W. Critical periods for human cortical development: an ERP study in children with cochlear implant. In: Lomber S. G., Eggermont J. J., eds. *Reprogramming the cerebral cortex: plasticity following central and peripheral lesions*. New York: Oxford University Press, 2006:213-28.

[6] Martines, F., Maira, E., Ferrara, S. (2011) Age-related hearing impairment (ARHI): A common sensory deficit in the elderly. *Acta Medica Mediterranea,* 27 (1):47-52.

[7] Sharma, A., Dorman, M. F., Kral, A. (2005) The influence of a sensitive period on central auditory development in children with unilateral and bilateral cochlear implants. *Hear Res,* 203:134-43.

[8] Kral, A., Hartmann, R., Tillein, J., Heid, S., Klinke, R. (2001) Delayed maturation and sensitive periods in the auditory cortex. *Audiol Neurootol*, 6:346-62.

[9] Gordon, K. A., B. C. Papsin. (2009) Benefit of short interimplant delays in children receiving bilateral cochlear implants. *Otol. Neurotol.,* 30, pp. 319-331.

[10] Geers, A. E. (2004) Speech, language, and reading skills after early cochlear implantation. *Arch Otolaryngol Head Neck Surg,* 130:634-8.

[11] Schwab, W. A. Effects of hearing loss on education. In: Jaffee B. E., editor. *Hearing loss in children: a comprehensive text.* Baltimore: University Park Press; 1977;650-4.

[12] Allen, T. (1986). Patterns of academic achievement among hearing impaired students. In S. Schildroth & M. Karchmer (Eds.), *Deaf children in America* (pp. 161–206). San Diego, CA: Little and Brown.

[13] Martines, F., Ballacchino, A., Sireci, F., Mucia, M., La Mattina, E., Rizzo, S., Salvago, P. (2016) Audiologic profile of OSAS and simple snoring patients: the effect of chronic nocturnal intermittent hypoxia on auditory function *European Archives of Oto-Rhino-Laryngology,* 273 (6), pp. 1419-1424.

[14] Klein, L., Huerta, L. E., National Library of Medicine (US). *Early identification of hearing impairment in infants and young children.* Bethesda (MD): US Dept, of Health and Human Services, National Institutes of Health; 1992:1-2.

[15] Mohr, P. E., Feldman, J. J., Dunbar, J. L. (2000) The societal costs of severe to profound hearing loss in the United States. *Int J Technol Assess Health Care,* 16: 1120–35.

[16] House, W. F., & Berliner, K. I. (1991). Cochlear implants: From idea to clinical practice. In H. Cooper (Ed.), *Cochlear implants: A practical guide* (pp. 9–33). San Diego, CA: Singular Publishing.

[17] Joint Committee on Infant Hearing. Year 2000 position statement: principles and guidelines for early hearing detection and intervention programs. *Pediatrics* 2000;106:798-817.

[18] Kemink, J., Zimmerman-Phillips, S., Kileny, P. R., Firszt, J., & Novak, M. (1992). Auditory performance of children with cochlear ossification and partial implant insertion. *Laryngoscope,* 102, 1002–1005.

[19] Kirk, K. I., Sehgal, M., & Miyamoto, R. T. (1997). Speech perception performance of Nucleus multi-channel cochlear implant users with partial electrode insertions. *Ear and Hearing,* 18, 456–471.

[20] Rauch, S., Hermann, B., Davis, L., & Nadol, J. (1997). Nucleus 22 cochlear implantation results in postmenningitic deafness. *Laryngoscope,* 107, 1–4.

[21] Niparko, J. K., Oviatt, D., Coker, N., Sutton, L., Waltzman, S. B., & Cohen, N. (1991). Facial nerve stimulation with cochlear implants. *Otolaryngology - Head and Neck Surgery,* 104, 826–830.

[22] Blamey, P. J., Arndt, P., Bergeron, F., Bredberg, G., Briamacombe, J., Facer, G., Larky, J., Linstrom, B. J. N., Peterson, A., Shipp, D., Staller, S., & Whitford, L. (1996). Factors affecting auditory performance of postlinguistically deaf adults using cochlear implants. *Audiology & Neuro-Otology,* 1, 293–306.

[23] Geir, L., Barker, M., Fisher, L., & Opie, J. (1999). The effect of long-term deafness on speech recognition in postlingually deafened adult Clarion cochlear implant users. *Annals of Otology, Rhinology, & Laryngology,* 108(Suppl. 177), 80–83.

[24] Rizzo, S., Bentivegna, D., Thomas, E., La Mattina, E., Mucia, M., Salvago, P., Sireci, F., Martines, F. Sudden sensorineural hearing loss, an invisible male: State of art. *Hearing loss: etiology, management and societal implications* 2016, 75-86.

[25] Dispenza, F., Cappello, F., Kulamarva, G., De Stefano, A. (2013) The discovery of the stapes. *Acta Otorhinolaryngol Ital.* 33(5): 357-359.

[26] Waltzman, S. B., & Cohen, N. L. (1999). Implantation of patients with prelingual long-term deafness. *Annals of Otology, Rhinology, & Laryngology,* 108, 84–87.

[27] Salvago, P., Martines, E., La Mattina, E., Mucia, M., Sammarco, P., Sireci, F., Martines, F. (2014) Distribution and phenotype of GJB2 mutations in 102 Sicilian patients with congenital non syndromic sensorineural hearing loss. *International Journal of Audiology,* 53 (8), pp. 558-563.

[28] Kral, A., Kronenberger, W. G., Pisoni, D. B., O'Donoghue, G. M. (2016) Neurocognitive factors in sensory restoration of early deafness: a connectome model. *Lancet Neurol.* 15(6):610-21. DOI: 10.1016/S1474-4422(16)00034-X.

[29] Sarant, J. Z., Blamey, P. J., Dowell, R. C., Clark, G. M., & Gibson, W. P. R. (2001). Variation in speech perception scores among children with cochlear implants. *Ear and Hearing,* 22(1), 18–28.

[30] Zwolan, T. A., Zimmerman-Phillips, S., Ashbaugh, C. J., Heiber, S. J., Kileny, P. R., & Telian, S. A. (1997). Cochlear implantation of children with minimal open-set speech recognition. *Ear and Hearing,* 19, 240–251.

[31] Jackler, R., Luxford, W., Schindler, R., & McKerrow, W. (1987). Cochlear patency problems in cochlear implantation. *Laryngoscope,* 97, 801–805.

[32] Martines, F., Bentivegna, D., Maira, E., Marasà, S., Ferrara, S. (2012) Cavernous haemangioma of the external auditory canal: Clinical case and review of the literature *Acta Otorhinolaryngologica Italica,* 32 (1), 54-57.

[33] Martines, F., Salvago, P., Bartolotta, C., Cocuzza, S., Fabiano, C., Ferrara, S., La Mattina, E., Mucia, M., Sammarco, P., Sireci, F., Martines, E. (2015) A genotype–phenotype correlation in Sicilian patients with GJB2 biallelic mutations. *Eur Arch Otorhinolaryngol,* 272(8): 1857-1865.

[34] Illg A., A. Giourgas, A. Kral, A. Büchner, A. Lesinski-Schiedat, T. Lenarz. (2013) Speech comprehension in children and adolescents after sequential bilateral cochlear implantation with long interimplant interval. *Otol. Neurotol.,* 34 682-689.

[35] Ramsden, J. D., Gordon, K, Aschendorff, A., Borucki, L., Bunne, M., Burdo, S., Garabedian, N., Grolman, W., Irving, R., Lesinski-Schiedat, A., Loundon, N., Manrique, M., Martin, J., Raine, C., Wouters, J., Papsin, B. C. (2012) European Bilateral Pediatric Cochlear Implant Forum consensus statement. *Otol Neurotol.* 33(4):561-5. DOI: 10.1097/MAO.0b013e3182536ae2.

[36] Dispenza, F., Mazzucco, W., Bianchini, S., Mazzola, S., Bennici, E. (2015) Management of labyrinthine fistula in chronic otitis with cholesteatoma: case series. *Euro Mediterranean Biomedical Journal* 10(21): 255-261

[37] Zwolan, T. A. (2000). Selection criteria and evaluation. In S. Waltzman & N. Cohen (Eds.), *Cochlear implants* (pp. 63–73). New York: Theime.

[38] Martines, F., Martines, E., Ballacchino, A., Salvago, P. (2013) Speech perception outcomes after cochlear implantation in prelingually deaf infants: The Western Sicily experience. *International Journal of Pediatric Otorhinolaryngology,* 77 (5), pp. 707-713.

[39] Moog, J. S., & Geers, A. E. (1990). *Early Speech Perception Test for profoundly hearing-impaired children.* St. Louis: Central Institute for the Deaf.

[40] Geers, A. E., & Moog, J. (1994). Effectiveness of cochlear implants and tactile aids for deaf children: The sensory aids study at Central Institute for the Deaf. *The Volta Review,* 96.

[41] Svirsky, M. A., & Meyer, T. (1999). Comparison of speech perception in pediatric Clarion cochlear implant and hearing aid users. *Annals of Otology, Rhinology, & Laryngology,* 177, 104–109.

[42] Balkany, T., Hodges, A., & Luntz, M. (1996). Update on cochlear implantation. *Otolaryngological Clinics of North America,* 29, 227–289.

[43] Illg A., Giourgas, A., Kral, A., Büchner, A., Lesinski-Schiedat, A., Lenarz, T. (2013) Speech comprehension in children and adolescents after sequential bilateral cochlear implantation with long interimplant interval. *Otol Neurotol.* 34(4):682-9. DOI: 10.1097/MAO.0b013e31828bb75e.

[44] Lenarz, T. Cochlear implantation. *The Hannover Guideline.* Tuttlingen: Endo Press; 2006.

[45] Choudhury, B., Fitzpatrick, D. C., Buchman, C. A., Wei, B. P., Dillon, M. T., He, S., Adunka, O. F. (2012) Intraoperative round window recordings to acoustic

stimuli from cochlear implant patients. *Otol Neurotol.* 33(9):1507-15. DOI: 10.1097/MAO.0b013e31826dbc80.

[46] Stolle, S. R., Groß, S., Lenarz, T. Lesinski-Schiedat, A. (2014) Postoperative Früh- und Spätkomplikationen bei Kindern und Erwachsenen nach CI-Implantation [Complications in children and adults with cochlear implant]. *Laryngorhinootologie.* 93(9):605- 11. DOI: 10.1055/s-0034-1370924.

[47] Battmer R. D., Backous D. D., Balkany T. J., Briggs R. J., Gantz B. J., van Hasselt A., Kim C. S., Kubo T., Lenarz T., Pillsbury H. C. 3rd, O'Donoghue G. M.; International Consensus Group for Cochlear Implant Reliability Reporting. International classification of reliability for implanted cochlear implant receiver stimulators. *Otol Neurotol.* 2010 Oct;31(8):1190-3. doi: 10.1097/MAO.0b013e3181d2798e.

[48] Miyamoto R. T., Young M., Myres W. A., Kessler K., Wolfert K., Kirk K. I. Complications of pediatric cochlear implantation. *Eur Arch Otorhinolaryngol.* 1996;253(1-2):1-4. DOI: 10.1007/BF00176693.

[49] Cohen N. L., Hoffman R. A., Complications of cochlear implant surgery in adults and children. *Ann Otol Rhinol Laryngol.* 1991 Sep;100(9 Pt 1):708-11.

[50] O'Donoghue G., Balkany T., Cohen N., Lenarz T., Lustig L., Niparko J. Meningitis and cochlear implantation. *Otol Neurotol.* 2002 Nov;23(6):823-4.

[51] Illg A., Haack M., Lesinski-Schiedat A., Büchner A., Lenarz T. Long-Term Outcomes, Education, and Occupational Level in Cochlear Implant Recipients Who Were Implanted in Childhood. *Ear Hear.* 2017 Sep/Oct;38(5):577-587. DOI: 10.1097/AUD.0000000000000423.

[52] Finke M., Billinger M., Büchner A. Toward Automated Cochlear Implant Fitting Procedures Based on Event-Related Potentials. *Ear Hear.* 2017 Mar/Apr;38(2): e118-e127. DOI: 10.1097/AUD.0000000000000377.

[53] Vaerenberg B., Smits C., De Ceulaer G., Zir E, Harman S., Jaspers N., Tam Y., Dillon M., Wesarg T., Martin-Bonniot D., Gärtner L., Cozma S., Kosaner J., Prentiss S., Sasidharan P., Briaire J. J., Bradley J., Debruyne J., Hollow R., Patadia R., Mens L., Veekmans K., Greisiger R., Harboun-Cohen E., Borel S., Tavora-Vieira D., Mancini P., Cullington H., Ng A. H., Walkowiak A., Shapiro W. H., Govaerts P. J. Cochlear implant programming: a global survey on the state of the art. *Scientific World Journal.* 2014;2014:501738. DOI: 10.1155/2014/501738.

[54] Brown, C. J., Abbas, P. J., Fryauf-Bertschy, H., Kelsay, D., & Gantz, B. J. (1994). Intraoperative and postoperative electrically evoked auditory brain stem responses in nucleus cochlear implant users: implications for the fitting process. *Ear and Hearing,* 15(2), 168–176.

[55] Brown, C. J., Hughes, M. L., Lopez, S. M., & Abbas, P. J. (1999). Relationship between EABR thresholds and levels used to program the CLARION speech processor. *Annals of Otology, Rhinology, & Laryngology* (Suppl. 17), 50–57.

[56] Firszt, J. B., Rotz, L. A., Chambers, R. D., & Novak, M. A. (1999). Electrically evoked potentials recorded in adult and pediatric CLARION implant users. *Annals of Otology, Rhinology, & Laryngology* (Suppl. 177), 58–63.

[57] Hodges, A. V., Ruth, R. A., Lambert, P. R., & Balkany, T. J. (1994). Electrical middle ear muscle reflex: Use in cochlear implant programming. *Archives of Otolaryngology - Head & Neck Surgery,* 120(10), 1093–1099.

[58] Plescia, F., Cannizzaro, E., Brancato, A., Martines, F., Di Naro, A., Mucia, M., Plescia, F., Vita, C., Salvago, P., Mulè, A., Rizzo, S., Sireci, F., Cannizzaro, C. (2015) Acetaldehyde effects in the brain. *Acta Medica Mediterranea,* 31 (4), pp. 813-817.

[59] Truy, E., Gallego, S., Chanal, J. M., Collet, L., & Morgon, A. (1998). Correlation between electrical auditory brainstem response and perceptual thresholds in Digisonic cochlear implant users. *Laryngoscope,* 108(4 Pt 1), 554–559.

[60] Abbas, P. J., & Brown, C. J. (1991). Electrically evoked auditory brainstem response: Growth of response with current level. *Hearing Research,* 51, 123–138.

[61] Miller, C. A., Woodruff, K. E., & Pfingst, B. E. (1995). Functional responses from guinea pigs with cochlear implants. *Electrophysiological and psychophysical measures. Hearing Research,* 92, 85–99.

[62] Shallop, J. K., VanDyke, L., Goin, D. W., & Mischke, R. E. (1991). Prediction of behavioral threshold and comfort values for Nucleus 22-channel implant patients from electrical auditory brain stem response test results. *Annals of Otology, Rhinology, & Laryngology,* 100, 896–898.

[63] Mason, S. M., Sheppard, S., Garnham, C. W., Lutman, M. E., O'Donoghue, G. M., & Gibbin, K. P. (1993). Improving the relationship of intraoperative EABR thresholds to T-level in young children receiving the Nucleus cochlear implant. In I. J. Hochmair-Desoyer & E. S. Hochmair (Eds.), *Advances in cochlear implants*. Vienna: Manz.

[64] Brown, C. J., Abbas, P. J., Bertschy, M., Tyler, R. S., Lowder, M., Takahashi, G., Purdy, S., & Gantz, B. J. (1995). Longitudinal assessment of physiological and psychophysical measures in cochlear implant users. *Ear and Hearing,* 16(5), 439–449.

[65] Kileny, P. R., Meiteles, L. Z., Zwolan, T. A., & Telian, S. A. (1995). Cochlear implant device failure: Diagnosis and management. *American Journal of Otology,* 16(2), 164–171.

[66] Abbas, P. J., Brown, C. J., Shallop, J. K., Firszt, J. B., Hughes, M. L., Hong, S. H., & Staller, S. J. (1999). Summary of results using the nucleus CI24M implant to record the electrically evoked compound action potential. *Ear and Hearing,* 20(1), 45–59.

[67] Brown, C. J., Abbas, P. J., & Ganz, B. J. (1990). Electrically evoked whole-nerve action potentials: Data from human cochlear implant users. *Journal of the Acoustical Society of America*, 88, 1385–1391.

[68] Brown, C. J., Abbas, P. J., & Gantz, B. J. (1998). Preliminary experience with neural response telemetry in the nucleus CI24M cochlear implant. *American Journal of Otology*, 19(3), 320–327.

[69] Miller, C. A., Abbas, P. J., & Brown, C. J. (2000). An improved method of reducing stimulus artifact in the electrically evoked whole-nerve potential. *Ear and Hearing*, 21(4), 280–290.

[70] Brown, C. J., Hughes, M. L., Luk, B., Abbas, P. J., Wolaver, A., & Gervais, J. (2000). The relationship between EAP and EABR thresholds and levels used to program the Nucleus 24 speech processor: Data from adults. *Ear and Hearing*, 21(2), 151–163.

[71] Cullington, H. (2000). Preliminary neural response telemetry results. *British Journal of Audiology*, 34(3), 131–140.

[72] Franck, K. H., & Norton, S. J. (2001). Estimation of psychophysical levels using the electrically evoked compound action potential measured with the neural response telemetry capabilities of Cochlear Corporation's CI24M device. *Ear and Hearing*, 22(4), 289–299.

[73] Hughes, M. L., Brown, C. J., Abbas, P. J., Wolaver, A. A., & Gervais, J. P. (2000). Comparison of EAP thresholds with MAP levels in the nucleus 24 cochlear implant: Data from children. *Ear and Hearing*, 21(2), 164–174.

[74] Shallop, J. K., Facer, G. W., & Peterson, A. (1999). Neural response telemetry with the nucleus CI24M cochlear implant. *Laryngoscope*, 109(11), 1755–1759.

[75] Thai-Van, H., Chanal, J. M., Coudert, C., Veuillet, E., Truy, E., & Collet, L. (2001). Relationship between MRT measurements and behavioral levels in children with the Nucleus 24 cochlear implant may change over time: Preliminary report. *International Journal of Pediatric Otorhinolaryngology*, 58(2), 153–162.

[76] Seyle, K., & Brown, C. J. (2002). Speech perception using maps based on Neural Response Telemetry (NRT) measures. *Ear and Hearing*, 23(Supplement), 72S–79S.

[77] Hodges, A. V., Balkany, T. J., Ruth, R. A., Lambert, P. R., Dolan-Ash, S., & Schloffman, J. J. (1997). Electrical middle ear muscle reflex: use in cochlear implant programming. *Otolaryngology - Head and Neck Surgery*, 117(3 Pt 1), 255–261.

[78] Shallop, J. K., & Ash, K. R. (1995). Relationships among comfort levels determined by cochlear implant patient's self-programming, audiologist's programming, and electrical stapedius reflex thresholds. *Annals of Otology, Rhinology, & Laryngology* (Suppl. 166), 175–176.

[79] Spivak, L. G., & Chute, P. M. (1994). The relationship between electrical acoustic reflex thresholds and behavioral comfort levels in children and adult cochlear implant patients. *Ear and Hearing,* 15(2), 184–192.

[80] Stephan, K., & Welzl-Muller, K. (1992). Stapedius reflex in patients with an inner ear prosthesis. *International Journal of Artificial Organs,* 15(7), 436–439.

[81] Van den Borne, B., Mens, L. H., Snik, A. F., Spies, T. H., & Van den Brock, P. (1994). Stapedius reflex and EABR thresholds in experienced users of the Nucleus cochlear implant. *Acta Oto-Laryngologica,* 114(2), 141–143.

[82] Bartolotta, C., Salvago, P., Cocuzza, S., Fabiano, C., Sammarco, P., Martines, F. (2014) Identification of D179H, a novel missense GJB2 mutation in a Western Sicily family. *European Archives of Oto-Rhino-Laryngology,* 271 (6), pp. 1457-1461.

[83] Kirk, K. I., Eisenberg, L. S., Martinez, A. S., & Hay-McCutcheon, M. (1999). The Lexical Neighborhood Test: Test-retest reliability and inter-list equivalency. *Journal of the American Academy of Audiology*, 10, 113–123.

[84] Archbold, S. M., Nikolopoulos, T. P., Nait, M., O'Donoghue, G. M., Lutman, M. E., & Gregory, S. (2000). Approach to communication, speech perception and intelligibility after paediatric cochlear implantation. *British Journal of Audiology,* 34(4), 257–264.

[85] Martines, F., Ballacchino, A. Speech intelligibility and perception after cochlear implant in deaf children with or without associated disabilities: *A review (2014) Cochlear Implants: Technological Advances, Psychological/Social Impacts and Long-Term Effectiveness*, pp. 67-77.

[86] Geers, A. E., Nicholas, J., Tye-Murray, N., Uchanski, R., Brenner, C., Davidson, L., Toretta, D., & Tobey, E. A. (2000). Effects of communication mode on skills of longterm cochlear implant users. *Annals of Otology, Rhinology, & Laryngology,* 109, 89–92.

[87] Papsin, B. K., Gysin, C., Picton, N., Nedzelski, J., & Harrison, R. V. (2000). Speech perception outcome measures in prelingually deaf children up to four years after cochlear implantation. *Annals of Otology, Rhinology, & Laryngology,* 109, 38–42.

[88] Tyler, R. S., Teagle, H. F. B., Kelsay, D. M. R., Gantz, B. J., Woodworth, G. G., & Parkinson, A. J. (2000). Speech perception by prelingually deaf children after six years of cochlear implant use: Effects of age at implantation. *Annals of Otology, Rhinology, & Laryngology*, 109, 82–84.

[89] Allum, J. H., Greisiger, R., Straubhaar, S., & Carpenter, M. G. (2000). Auditory perception and speech identification in children with cochlear implants tested with the EARS protocol. *British Journal of Audiology,* 34, 293–303.

[90] McConkey Robbins, A., Koch, D. B, Osberger, M. J., Zimmerman-Phillips, S., Kishon Rabin, L. (2004) Effect of age at cochlear implantation on auditory skill development in infants and toddlers. *Arch Otolaryngol Head Neck Surg* 130:570-4.

[91] Lee, H. J., Giraud, A. L., Kang, E., et al. (2007) Cortical activity at rest predicts cochlear implantation outcome. *Cereb Cortex* 17:909-17.

[92] Tait, M., De Raeve, L., Nikolopoulos, T. P. (2007) Deaf children with cochlear implants before the age of 1 year: comparison of preverbal communication with normally hearing children. *Int J Pediatr Otorhinolaryngol* 71:1605-11.

[93] Dettman, S. J., Pinder, D., Briggs, R. J., Dowell, R. C., Leigh, J. R. (2007) Communication development in children who receive the cochlear implant younger than 12 months: risks versus benefits. *Ear Hear* 28: Suppl:11S-18S.

[94] Colletti, V., Carner, M., Colletti, L. (2006) Cochlear implant surgery in children under 6 months. In: *Abstracts of the 8th European Symposium on Pediatric Cochlear Implantation,* Venice, Italy, March 25–28, 49. abstract.

[95] James, A. L., Papsin, B. C. (2004) Cochlear implant surgery at 12 months of age or younger. *Laryngoscope* 114:2191-5.

[96] Wackym, P. A., Runge-Samuelson, C. L., Firszt, J. B., Alkaf, F. M., Burg, L. S. (2007) More challenging speech-perception tasks demonstrate binaural benefit in bilateral cochlear implant users. *Ear Hear* 28: Suppl:80S-85S.

[97] Peters, B. R., Litovsky, R., Parkinson, A., Lake, J. (2007) Importance of age and postimplantation experience on speech perception measures in children with sequential bilateral cochlear implants. *Otol Neurotol* 28:649-57.

[98] Wolfe, J., Baker, S., Caraway, T., et al. (2007) 1-Year postactivation results for sequentially implanted bilateral cochlear implant users. *Otol Neurotol* 28:589-96.

[99] Litovsky, R. Y., Johnstone, P. M., Godar, S., et al. (2006) Bilateral cochlear implants in children: localization acuity measured with minimum audible angle. *Ear Hear* 27:43-59.

[100] Gordon, K. A., Valero, J., Papsin, B. C. (2007) Auditory brainstem activity in children with 9-30 months of bilateral cochlear implant use. *Hear Res* 233:97-107.

[101] Buchman, C. A., Joy, J., Hodges, A., Telischi, F. F., Balkany, T. J. (2004) Vestibular effects of cochlear implantation. *Laryngoscope* 114:Suppl 103:1-22.

[102] Thomas, E., Martines, F., Bianco, A., Messina, G., Giustino, V., Zangla, D., Iovane, A., Palma, A. (2018) *Decreased postural control in people with moderate hearing loss. Medicine* (Baltimore); 97(14): e0244.

[103] Balkany T. J., Hodges A. V., Goodman K. W. Ethics of cochlear implantation in young children. *Otolaryngol Head Neck Surg* 1996;114:748-55.

[104] National Association of the Deaf (NAD). *Cochlear implants: NAD position statement.* (Accessed November 9, 2007, at http://www.nad.org/site/pp.asp?c=foINKQMBF &b=138140).

[105] Schulze-Gattermann, H., Illg A., Schoenermark, M., Lenarz, T., Lesinski-Schiedat, A. (2002) Cost-benefit analysis of pediatric cochlear implantation: German experience. *Otol Neurotol.* Sep;23(5):674-81. DOI: 10.1097/00129492-200209000-00013

[106] Osberger, M. J., Maso, M., & Sam, L. K. (1993). Speech intelligibility of children with cochlear implants, tactile aids, or hearing aids. *J Speech Hear Res.* 1993 Feb;36(1):186-203.

[107] Miyamoto, R. T., Kirk, K. I., Robbins, A. M., Todd, S. L., & Riley, A. I. (1996). Speech perception and speech production skills of children with multichannel cochlear implants. *Acta Oto-Laryngologica*, 116(2), 240–243.

[108] Geers, A. E., & Brenner, C. (1994). Speech perception results: Audition and lipreading enhancement. Effectiveness of cochlear implants and tactile aids for deaf children. *The Volta Review*, 95, 97–108.

[109] Meyer, T. A., Svirsky, M. A., Kirk, K. I., & Miyamoto, R. T. (1998). Improvements in speech perception by children with profound prelingual hearing loss: Effects of device, communication mode, and chronological age. *Journal of Speech, Language, and Hearing Research,* 41, 846–858.

[110] Brown, K. D., Balkany. T. J. (2007) Benefits of bilateral cochlear implantation: a review. *Curr. Opin. Otolaryngol. Head Neck Surg.,* 15 (5) 315-318.

[111] Ching, T. Y. C., Van Wanrooy, E., H. Dillon. (2007) Binaural-bimodal fitting or bilateral implantation for managing severe to profound deafness: a review. *Trends Amplif.,* 11 (3) 161-192.

[112] Galvin K. L., M. Mok, R. C. Dowell, R. J. Briggs. Speech detection and localization results and clinical outcomes for children receiving sequential bilateral cochlear implants before four years of age. *Int. J. Audiol.,* 47 (10) (2008), pp. 636-646.

[113] Sparreboom M, A. F. M. Snik, E. A. M. Mylanus Sequential bilateral cochlear implantation in children: development of the primary auditory abilities of bilateral stimulation. *Audiol. Neurotol.,* 16 (4) (2011), pp. 203-213.

[114] Gordon K. A., M. R. Deighton, P. Abbasalipour, B. C. Papsin. Perception of binaural cues develops in children who are deaf through bilateral cochlear implantation *Plos One* (2014).

[115] Kral A., A. Sharma. Developmental neuroplasticity after cochlear implantation. *Trends Neurosci.,* 35 (No 2) (2012), pp. 111-122.

[116] Sharma A., M. F. Dormann, A. Kral. The influence of a sensitive period on central auditory development in children with unilateral and bilateral cochlear implants. *Hear. Res.,* 203 (2005), pp. 134-143.

[117] Gordon K. A., Y. Henkin, A. Kral. Asymmetric hearing during development: the aural preference syndrome and treatment options. *Pediatrics,* 136 (2015), pp. 141-153.

[118] Graham J., D. Vickers, A. M. Ghada, et al. Bilateral sequential cochlear implantation in the congenitally deaf child: evidence to support the concept of a 'critical age' after which the second ear is less likely to provide an adequate level of speech perception on its own. *Cochlear Implant Int.*, 10 (3) (2009), pp. 119-141.

[119] Kral A., P. Hubka, S. Heid, J. Tillein. Single-sided deafness leads to unilateral aural preference within an early sensitive period. *Brain*, 136 (2013), pp. 180-193.

[120] Tillein J., P. Hubka, A. Kral. Monaural congenital deafness affects aural dominance and degrades binaural processing. *Cereb. Cortex*, 26 (2016), pp. 1762-1777.

[121] Wolfe J., S. Baker, T. Caraway, et al. 1-year postactivation results for sequentially implanted bilateral cochlear implant use. *Otol. Neurotol.*, 28 (2007), pp. 589-596.

[122] Zekveld A. A., S. E. Kramer, J. M. Festen, Cognitive load during speech perception in noise: the influence of age, hearing loss, and cognition on the pupil response, *Ear Hear* 32 (2011) 498e510.

[123] Yoshinaga-Itano C., A. L. Sedey, D. K. Coulter, A. L. Mehl, Language of early- and later-identified children with hearing loss, *Pediatrics* 102 (1998) 1161e1171.

[124] McGarrigle R., K. J. Munro, P. Dawes, A. J. Stewart, D. R. Moore, J. G. Barry, S. Amitay, Listening effort and fatigue: what exactly are we measuring? A British society of audiology cognition in hearing special interest group 'white paper', *Int. J. Audiol.* 53 (2014) 433e440.

[125] van Schoonhoven J., M. Schulte, M. Boymans, K. C. Wagener, W. A. Dreschler, B. Kollmeier, Selecting appropriate tests to assess the benefits of bilateral amplification with hearing aids, *Trends Hear* 20 (2016) 1e16.

[126] Pichora-Fuller M. K., S. E. Kramer, M. A. Eckert, B. Edwards, B. W. Hornsby, L. E. Humes, U. Lemke, T. Lunner, M. Matthen, C. L. Mackersie, G. Naylor, N. A. Phillips, M. Richter, M. Rudner, M. S. Sommers, K. L. Tremblay, A. Wingfield, Hearing impairment and cognitive energy: the framework for understanding effortful listening (FUEL), *Ear Hear* 37 (2016) 5Se27S.

[127] Kahneman D., *Attention and Effort*, Prentice-Hall, Englewood Cliffs, NJ, 1973.

[128] Marsella, P., Scorpecci, A., Cartocci, G., Giannantonio, S., Maglione, A. G., Venuti, I., Brizi, A., Babiloni, F. (2017) EEG activity as an objective measure of cognitive load during effortful listening: A study on pediatric subjects with bilateral, asymmetric sensorineural hearing loss. *Int J Pediatr Otorhinolaryngol.* Aug;99:1-7.

[129] Sauseng P., W. Klimesch, What does phase information of oscillatory brain activity tell us about cognitive processes? *Neurosci. Biobehav. Rev.* 32 (2008) 1001e1013.

[130] Onton J., A. Delorme, S. Makeig, Frontal midline EEG dynamics during working memory, *Neuroimage* 27 (2005) 341e356.

[131] Zakrzewska M. Z., A. Brzezicka, Working memory capacity as a moderator of load-related frontal midline theta variability in Sternberg task, *Front. Hum. Neurosci.* 8 (2014) 399.

[132] Wisniewski M. G., E. R. Thompson, N. Iyer, J. R. Estepp, M. N. Goder-Reiser, S. C. Sullivan, Frontal midline q power as an index of listening effort, *Neuroreport* 26 (2015) 94e99.

[133] Kelly S. P., E. C. Lalor, R. B. Reilly, J. J. Foxe, Increases in alpha oscillatory power reflect an active retinotopic mechanism for distracter suppression during sustained visuospatial attention, *J. Neurophysiol.* 95 (2006) 3844e3851.

[134] Snyder A. C., J. J. Foxe, Anticipatory attentional suppression of visual features indexed by oscillaory alpha-band power increases: a high-density electrical mapping study, *J. Neurosci.* 30 (2010) 4024e4032.

[135] Rihs T. A., C. M. Michel, G. Thut. (2007) Mechanisms of selective inhibition in visual spatial attention are indexed by a-band EEG synchronization, *Eur. J. Neurosci.* 25 603e610.

[136] Cosmelli, D., V. Lopez, J. P. Lachaux, J. Lopez-Calder on, B. Renault, J. Martinerie, F. Aboitiz, (2011) Shifting visual attention away from fixation is specifically associated with alpha band activity over ipsilateral parietal regions, *Psychophysiology* 48, 312e322.

[137] Foxe J. J., G. V. Simpson, S. P. Ahlfors, Parieto-occipital approximately 10 Hz activity reflects anticipatory state of visual attention mechanisms, *Neuroreport* 9 (1998) 3929e3933.

[138] Fu MKG, J. J. Foxe, M. M. Murray, B. A. Higgins, D. C. Javitt, C. E. Schroeder, Attention-dependent suppression of distractor visual input can be crossmodally cued as indexed by anticipatory parieto-occipital alpha-band oscillations, *Cogn. Brain Res.* 12 (2001) 145e152.

[139] Banerjee S., A. C. Snyder, S. Molholm, J. J. Foxe, Oscillatory alpha-band mechanisms and the deployment of spatial attention to anticipated auditory and visual target locations: supramodal or sensory-specific control mechanisms? *J. Neurosci.* 31 (2011) 9923e9932.

[140] Wisniewski, M. G. (2016) Indices of effortful listening can be mined from existing electroencephalographic data, *Ear Hear* 38 e69ee73.

[141] Jensen O., J. Gelfand, J. Kounios, J. E. Lisman, Oscillations in the alpha band (9e12 Hz) increase with memory load during retention in a short-term memory task, *Cereb. Cortex* 12 (2002) 877e882.

[142] Strauss A., M. Wostmann, J. Obleser, Cortical alpha oscillations as a tool for auditory selective inhibition, *Front. Hum. Neurosci.* 8 (2014) 1e7.

[143] Cartocci G., A. G. Maglione, G. Vecchiato, G. Di Flumeri, A. Colosimo, A. Scorpecci, P. Marsella, S. Giannantonio, P. Malerba, G. Borghini, P. Arico, F. Babiloni, Mental workload estimations in unilateral deafened children, in:

Engineering in Medicine and Biology Society (EMBC), IEEE, 2015, pp. 1654e1657, 37th Annual International Conference of the IEEE.

[144] Hudspeth W. J., K. H. Pribram, Stag W. J. Hudspeth, K. H. Pribram, Stages of brain and cognitive maturation, *J. Educ. Psychol.* 82 (1990) 881e884.

[145] Somsen, R. J. M., B. J. Van-Klooster, M. W. Van-der-Molen, H. M. Van-Leeuwen, (1997) Growth spurts in brain maturation during middle childhood as indexed by EEG power spectra, *Biol. Psychol.* 44 187e209.

Chapter 17

PRESBYASTASIS: FROM DIAGNOSIS TO MANAGEMENT

Serena Rizzo[1], MD, Valeria Sanfilippo[1], MD, Pietro Terrana[1], MD, Lorenza Lauricella[1], MD, Dalila Scaturro[1], MD, Francesco Martines[2], MD, PhD, and Giulia Letizia Mauro[1], MD

[1]University of Palermo, Di.Chir.On.S. Department,
Section of Physical Medicine and Rehabilitation,
Palermo, Italy
[2]Bio. Ne. C. Department, University of Palermo,
Audiology Section, Palermo, Italy

ABSTRACT

Currently, the elderly population (> 65 years old) is in very growth. In fact, in Italy old age index (number of elderly per 100 persons under the age of 14 years) is estimated to be 157,7 and is projected to increase to 257,9 in the year 2065 [1, 2]. The increase of the elderly population determines the increase of the age-dependent diseases including also impairment of the vestibular function, this problem is defined "presbiastasia". Patient suffering from this condition exhibit disturbances of static and dynamic postural control with far less frequent cases of relapsing objective rotatory vertigo. Occasionally, they also report a feeling of insecurity in new or unknown environments, increasing the risk of falls.

These balance disorders significantly affect patients' private and social life, as they interfere with a large number of daily activities, as transfer into bed, ambulation, car transfers, eating, using of telephone. The number of patients with this disease is expected to increase with the rise in the number of elderly population and this has important implications on the national health system's resources. Thus, the rehabilitation of these balance disorders presents serious difficulties. This explains the great number of techniques, with or without the use of equipment, which have so far been proposed. Some authors suggested to apply actual protocols, more or less modifiable according to patient characteristics; others recommended individual exercises or special equipment-aided techniques.

In these cases, vestibular rehabilitation allows to stimulate the equilibrium system by preventing and slowing down the effects of aging, through the use of "adaptive, substitutive and custom" strategies.

Keywords: dizziness, fall, presbiastasia

INTRODUCTION

"Dizziness is prevalent in all adult populations, causing considerable morbidity and utilization of health services.

In the community, the prevalence of dizziness ranges from 1.8% in young adults to more than 30% in elderly people… Dizziness is one of the most challenging symptoms in Medicine: it is difficult to define, impossible to measure, a challenge to diagnose, and troublesome to treat. …Not the best example of evidence based practice…" [3] the dizziness prevalence in elderly people is very high. Often the dizziness is associated with a poor state of health.

In this chapter is very important the study of global balance function, in fact we have to study vision, hearing, posture and proprioception functions in all of patients. Why? Because in particular hearing function is considered by some authors to be an indispensable element for maintaining equilibrium [4-10].

The aims of rehabilitation in elderly subject are to train them how to control their movements, to teach how to get up after a falling, to walk in harmonious way. Thus, the doctor's purpose is to establish a rehabilitative plan to follow, considering:

- the patient's age
- the cognitive state of the patient
- the social factor
- the education
- vestibular canal and/or otolithic impairment
- muscle pain
- osteo-articular development

This information is essential for the initial assessment of the patient, because this is an individual rehabilitation plan.

PATIENT'S EVALUATION

Falling is the first problem of these patients, therefore is essential to predict the risk to fall and reduce it. The principal tests used are: Tinetti balance assessment tool [11], timed "get up and go" test [12-14], Berg balance test.

TINETTI PERFORMANCE ORIENTED MOBILITY ASSESSMENT (POMA)

It is a qualitative test involving static and dynamic tasks which serves mainly to predict the risk to fall in elderly subjects.

BALANCE SECTION

Patient sitting in hard, armless chair

Sitting Balance	Leans or slides in chair = 0		
	Steady, safe = 1		
Rises from chair	Unable to without help = 0		
	Able, uses arms to help = 0		
	Able without use of arms = 2		
Attempts to rise	Unable to without help = 1		
	Able, requires > 1 attempt = 1		
	Able to rise, 1 attempt = 2		
Immediate standing Balance (first 5 seconds)	Unsteady (staggers, moves feet, trunk sway) = 0		
	Steady but uses walker or other support = 1		
	Steady without walker or other support = 2		
Standing balance	Unsteady = 0		
	Steady but wide stance and uses support = 1		
	Narrow stance without support = 2		
Nudged	Begins to fall = 0		
	Staggers, grabs, catches self = 1		
	Steady = 2		
Eyes closed	Unsteady = 0		
	Steady = 1		
Turning 360 degrees	Discontinuous steps = 0		
	Continuous = 1		
	Unsteady (grabs, staggers) = 0		
	Steady = 1		
Sitting down	Unsafe (misjudged distance, falls into chair) = 0		
	Uses arms or not a smooth motion = 1		
	Safe, smooth motion = 2		
	BALANCE SCORE	/16	/16

GAIT SECTION

Patient standing with therapist, walks across room (+/- aids), first at usual pace, then at rapid pace.

Indication of gait (Immediately after told to 'go'.)	Any hesitancy or multiple attempts= 0 No hesitancy= 1		
Step length and height	Step to = 0 Step through R= 1 Step through L= 1		
Foot clearance	Foot drop= 0 L foot clears floor= 1 R foot clears floor= 1		
Step symmetry	Right and left step length not equal= 0 Right and left step length appear equal= 1		
Step continuità	Stopping or discontinuity between steps= 0 Steps appear continuous = 1		
Path	Marked deviation = 1 Mild/moderate deviation or uses w. aid = 1 Straight without w. aid = 2		
Trunk	Marked sway or uses w. aid = 0 No sway but flex. knees or back or uses arms for stability = 1 No sway, flex., use of arms or w. aid = 2		
Walking time	Heels apart = 0 Heels almost touching while walking = 1		
	GAIT SCORE	/12	/12
	Balance score carried forward	/16	/16
	Total Score = Balance + Gait score	/28	/28

RISK INDICATORS

Tinetti Tool Score	Risk of Falls
≤18	High
19-23	Moderate
≥24	Low

Stands up from a chair, walks 3 meters, turns around, and sits down again. The results are:

- normal mobility: patients who are autonomous for balance and for prehension tasks perform it in less than 10 seconds

- normal limits for weak, elderly and disabled people: patients who are independent for transfers only perform them in less than 20 seconds
- a range higher than 20 seconds means the person needs assistance outside and indicates the necessity of further examinations and interventions [15]
- a score of 30 seconds or more suggests that the person has an severe risk to fall

BERG'S BALANCE SCALE

Berg's Balance Scale (BBS) was developed in 1989 via health personnel and patients' interviews that studied the various methods used to assess balance. Although the Berg Balance Scale was originally developed to measure balance in the elderly people, it has been used to measure balance in a wide variety of patients [16-18]. This test graded items from 0 (bad) to 4 (good):

- Sitting position without back support nor armrests
- Going from standing to sitting position
- Going from sitting to standing position
- Transfer from one seat to another
- Standing upright with closed eyes
- Standing upright with feet together
- Standing upright with feet in tandem position (one foot behind the other along a line)
- Standing on one foot
- Trunk rotation
- Picking up an object from the floor
- Turning around completely (360°)
- Climbing up one step
- Bending forward

REHABILITATION STRATEGY

Proprioceptive training is based on stimulation of the neuromotor system. This training consists of series of exercises designed to re-educate reflexes. The goal is to achieve optimal control of posture and balance. The proprioceptive training must be set on situations that lead the subject to lose balance, in order to activate the muscles quickly and correctly. The improvement of the equilibrium happens both by the maintenance of the position and the ability to quickly correct the imbalances. To achieve the objective of a correct stimulation of proprioceptive reflexes it is necessary that the elderly subject is motivated and considered the protagonist of his own improvement. The training technique is based on controlled stress and it is applied to the joints, using both unloading and natural loading exercises, resting on the ground or on oscillating surfaces of varying difficulties, such as boards, bouncers, skymmi, bosu, trampolines and many others devices. All proprioceptive exercises must be performed avoiding wearing shoes, in order not to divert the proprioceptive sensations from the foot. To further intensify the training, you can perform the exercises with your eyes closed, as the balance is also controlled by the exteroceptors (view and vestibular apparatus), which receive information from the outside world. Information coming from exteroceptors and proprioceptors gives the exact position of one's body.

PROPRIOCEPTIVE TRAINING

Proprioceptive Exercises to Restore a Correct Load

- Step training with scales to re-establish a correct load during the step
- Throw a ball and keep the balance
- Build an obstacle course and cross it

Exercises with Boards

- Sitting with a foot on a board, move the ankle in flexion and extension
- Sitting with a foot on a rectangular board, move the ankle in flexion and extension
- Sitting with a foot on a rectangular board, move the ankle in flexion and extension and foot in inversion and eversion

These exercises must be repeated first in a monopodalic and then bipodalic manner. According to the characteristics of the subject (osteo-articular, muscular and cognitive conditions), these exercises must also be done in orthostatism, using boards or on a stable plane.

Proprioceptive Self-Analysis

The technique is based on the cortical ability to reconstruct postural attitude, relying mainly on proprioceptive inputs. The subject is placed in front of a squared mirror. In this way the patient can assume different positions. The technique consists in getting reconstructing body position, first thanks to the image reflected in the mirror, then the mirror is moved away, the patient must memorize and therefore maintain the correct position. By repeating this exercise many times the subject becomes more aware of his body. This method has many advantages: it activates central mechanisms that are rarely used in rehabilitation, patients can perform the exercises at home, and results are evident to the subject. Moreover, this method helps elderly people to accept their image and coordinate movements.

LEARING TO GET UP AFTER A FALL

Falling does not only represent a trauma itself; it also indicates a general failure of the balancing system, in fact, "Falls are a marker of frailty, immobility, and acute and chronic health impairment in older persons. Falls in turn diminish function by causing injury, activity limitations, fear of falling, and loss of mobility" [19].

The physiotherapist gets the patient quickly to lie down on the back. The patient is shown how to swing a leg after swinging an arm to find himself lying on face down, and then to crouch to get on all limbs in order to draw near to a table or any forniture. He is then shown how to raise a knee, and to stand up progressively by lean on to the piece of forniture. Repeating the exercises helps overcome the problem of falling.

CONCLUSION

The aim of our chapter is to find a personalized rehabilitative project-program that leads the elderly people to achieve a high and autonomous lifestyle. The best tool to employ is a multidisciplinary approach starting from the diagnosis until the treatment of the various disabilities old-age related, without the mindless claim to cure an inexorable physiological process that is old age. The key of the success in achieving this result is the team work involving different professional figures like physiatrist, physiotherapist, neurologist and otolaryngologist. Within this multidisciplinary team, physiatrist plays a managing role. The treatment is based on proprioceptive rehabilitation exercises, on the reduction of auditory [20-23], visual and neurological problems. Certainly the results are always closely related to the motivational support given by the team work to the patient. Furthermore, it is essential for the patient to interact with the surrounding environment in order to overwhelm his anxiety and fear improving, in this way, his quality and length of life [24-27].

REFERENCES

[1] Eurostat Demography Report 2010. *Older, more numerous and diverse Europeans.* ISSN 1831-9440, 2010.

[2] https://www.istat.it/it/anziani/popolazione-e-famiglie.

[3] Sloane, P. D., Coeytaux, R. R., Beck, R. S., Dallara, J. (2001) Dizziness: State of the Scienze. *Ann. Intern. Med.,* 1;134(9 Pt 2):823 - 32.

[4] Thomas, E., Martines, F., Bianco, A., Messina, G., Giustino, V., Zangla, D., Iovane, A., Palma, A. (2018) Decreased postural control in people with moderate hearing loss. *Medicine,* 97, 14, 1 DOI: 10.1097/MD.0000000000010244.

[5] Salvago, P., Rizzo, S., Bianco, A., Martines, F. (2017) Sudden sensorineural hearing loss: is there a relationship between routine haematological parameters and audiogram shapes? *International Journal of Audiology,* 56, 3, 148 - 153.

[6] Thomas, E., Bianco, A., Messina, G., Mucia, M., Rizzo, S., Salvago, P., Sireci, F., Palma, A., Martines, F. (2017) The influence of sounds in postural control. *Hearing Loss: Etiology, Management and Societal Implications,* pp. 1 - 11.

[7] Martines, F., Maira, E., Ferrara, S. (2011) Age-related hearing impairment (ARHI): A common sensory deficit in the elderly. *Acta Medica Mediterranea,* 27 (1), 47 - 52.

[8] Martines, F., Messina, G., Patti, A., Battaglia, G., Bellafiore, M., Messina, A., Rizzo, S., Salvago, P., Sireci, F., Traina, M., Iovane, A. (2015) Effects of tinnitus on postural control and stabilization: A pilot study. *Acta Medica Mediterranea,* 31: 907 - 912.

[9] De Stefano, A., Dispenza, F., Citraro, L., Di Giovanni, P., Petrucci, A. G., Kulamarva, G., Mathur, N., Croce, A. (2011) Are postural restrictions necessary for management of posterior canal benign paroxysmal positional vertigo? *Ann. Otol. Rhinol. Laryngol.,* 120(7); 460 - 464.

[10] De Stefano, A., Kulamarva, G., Dispenza, F., (2012) Malignant Paroxysmal Positional Vertigo. *Auris Nasus Larynx,* 39:378 - 382.

[11] Tinetti, M. E., Williams, T. F., Mayewski, R., (1986) Fall Risk Index for elderly patients based on number of chronic disabilities. *Am. J. Med.,* 80:429 - 434.

[12] Mathias, S., Nayak, U., Isaacs, B., (1986) Balance in elderly patients. The "get and go test". *Arch. Phys. Med. Rehabil.,* 67: 387 - 9.

[13] Podsiadlo, D., Richardson, S. (1991) The timed 'Up & Go': A test of basic functional mobility for frail elderly persons. *Journal of the American Geriatrics Society,* 39 (2): 142 - 8.

[14] Bischoff, H. A., Stähelin, H. B., Monsch, A. U., Iversen, M. D., Weyh, A., von Dechend, M., Akos, R., Conzelmann, M., et al. (2003) Identifying a cut-off point for normal mobility: A comparison of the timed 'up and go' test in community-dwelling and institutionalised elderly women. *Age and Ageing,* 32 (3): 315 - 20.

[15] Timed Up and Go (TUG). *American College of Rheumatology*, Retrieved 2010-02-16.

[16] Berg, K., Wood-Dauphine, S., Williams, J. I. (1995) The balance scale: reliability assessment with elderly residents and patients with an acute stroke. *Scandinavian Journal of Rehabilitation Medicine*, 27: 27 - 36.

[17] Berg, K., Wood-Dauphine, S., Williams J. I., Gayton D. (1989) Measuring balance in the elderly: preliminary development of an instrument. *Physiotherapy Canada,* 41: 304 - 311.

[18] Downs, S., Marquez, J., Chiarelli, P., (2013) The Berg Balance Scale has high intra- and inter-rater reliability but absolute reliability varies across the scale: a systematic review. *J. Physiother.*, 59(2):93-9. doi: 10.1016/S1836-9553(13)70161-9.

[19] Institute of Medicine (US) Division of Health Promotion and Disease Prevention. Berg, R. L., Cassells, J. S., editors. *The Second Fifty Years: Promoting Health and Preventing Disability*. Washington (DC): National Academies Press (US); 1992. 15, *Falls in Older Persons: Risk Factors and Prevention*.

[20] Plescia, F., Cannizzaro, C., Brancato, A., Sireci, F., Salvago, P., Martines, F. (2016) Emerging pharmacological treatments of tinnitus. *Tinnitus: Epidemiology, Causes and Emerging Therapeutic Treatments*, p. 43 - 64.

[21] Martines, F., Agrifoglio, M., Bentivegna, D., Mucia, M., Salvago, P., Sireci, F., Ballacchino, A. (2012) Treatment of tinnitus and dizziness associated vertebrobasilar insufficiency with a fixed combination of cinnarizine and dimenhydrinate. *Acta Medica Mediterranea*, 28 (3), 291 - 296.

[22] Martines, F., Ballacchino, A., Sireci, F., Mucia, M., La Mattina, E., Rizzo, S., Salvago, P. (2016) Audiologic profile of OSAS and simple snoring patients: the effect of chronic nocturnal intermittent hypoxia on auditory function. *European Archives of Oto-Rhino-Laryngology,* 273, 6, 1419 - 1424.

[23] Ballacchino, A., Salvago, P., Cannizzaro, E., Costanzo, R., Di Marzo, M., Ferrara, S., La Mattina, E., Messina, G., Mucia, M., Mulè, A., Plescia, F., Sireci, F., Rizzo, S., Martines, F. (2015) Association between sleep-disordered breathing and hearing disorders: Clinical observation in Sicilian patients, *Acta Medica Mediterranea*, 31 (3), pp. 607 - 614.

[24] Canal switch and re-entry phenomenon in benign paroxysmal positional vertigo: difference between immediate and delayed occurrence. (2015) Dispenza, F., De Stefano, A., Costantino, C., Rando, D., Giglione, M., Stagno, R., Bennici, E. *Acta Otorhinolaryngol. Ital.,* 35: 116 - 120.

[25] Analysis of visually guided eye movements in subjects after whiplash injury. (2011) Dispenza, F., Gargano, R., Mathur, N., Saraniti, C., Gallina, S. *Auris Nasus Larynx*, 38(2):185 - 9.

[26] The discovery of stapes (2103) Dispenza, F., Cappello, F., Kulamarva, G., De Stefano, A. *Acta Otorhinolaryngol. Ital.*, 33:357 - 359.

[27] Dispenza, F., Mazzucco, W., Bianchini, S., Mazzola, S., Bennici, E. (2015) Management of labyrinthine fistula in chronic otitis with cholesteatoma: case series. *Euro Mediterranean Biomedical Journal,* 10(21): 255 - 261.

EDITORS' CONTACT INFORMATION

Francesco Dispenza, MD, PhD
AOUP P. Giaccone Hospital, Palermo, Italy;
Bio. Ne. C. Department, University of Palermo, Palermo, Italy;
Istituto Euro-Mediterraneo della Scienza e Tecnologia (IEMEST), Palermo, Italy
Email: francesco.dispenza@gmail.com

Francesco Martines, MD, PhD
(Bio. Ne. C. Department, University of Palermo, Palermo, Italy;
Istituto Euro-Mediterraneo della Scienza e Tecnologia (IEMEST), Palermo, Italy)
Email: francesco.martines@unipa.it

INDEX

A

acute mastoiditis (AM), 71, 82, 83, 132, 133, 165, 206
acute otitis media (AOM), 81, 82, 132
aditus ad antrum, 78, 143
advanced otosclerosis, vi, 189, 190, 191, 192, 193, 194, 195, 196, 198, 199, 200, 201, 202, 203, 204, 218
age related hearing loss, 148
aneurysms, 104, 107, 121
apical turn cochlea, 143
arachnoid cyst, 107, 108, 109, 137
auditory cortex, 4, 8, 9, 18, 20, 21, 22, 23, 55, 56, 57, 58, 59, 60, 62, 63, 64, 65, 153, 154, 165, 166, 178, 180, 185, 282, 284, 312, 342
autoimmune, vi, 92, 101, 102, 208, 209, 210, 211, 215, 219, 233, 234, 235, 236, 237, 238, 240, 241, 242, 243, 244, 245, 246, 247, 248, 249, 250, 284, 287, 295
autoimmune deafness, 233, 235, 242, 243, 244, 245
autoimmune inner ear disease, vi, 211, 215, 233, 234, 235, 247, 288

B

basal turn cochlea, 143
bilateral hearing, 28, 47, 57, 267, 268, 270, 271, 272, 273, 306, 309, 310, 316, 335
brain, 3, 6, 7, 9, 15, 16, 18, 20, 22, 32, 34, 38, 43, 56, 57, 58, 59, 63, 64, 65, 66, 72, 82, 83, 96, 107, 111, 112, 114, 116, 117, 127, 128, 135, 139, 154, 164, 165, 166, 169, 170, 173, 174, 175, 179, 180, 181, 182, 183, 185, 219, 227, 239, 252, 259, 264, 269, 273, 274, 282, 287, 292, 295, 296, 311, 331, 336, 337, 341, 345, 346, 351, 352, 353

C

C1 (atlas) anterior arch, 143
cerebellopontine angle (CPA), 4, 7, 104, 105, 106, 107, 108, 109, 110, 111, 121, 124, 131, 136, 137, 227
children, vi, vii, 27, 31, 34, 37, 38, 50, 51, 55, 56, 57, 59, 63, 66, 68, 79, 81, 92, 104, 121, 132, 135, 136, 139, 141, 183, 204, 243, 244, 257, 262, 265, 267, 268, 269, 270, 271, 272, 273, 274, 276, 277, 282, 285, 291, 293, 299, 304, 305, 306, 309, 311, 312, 313, 315, 316, 317, 318, 319, 320, 322, 323, 324, 325, 326, 328, 329, 330, 332, 333, 334, 336, 337, 338, 341, 342, 343, 344, 345, 346, 347, 348, 349, 350, 351, 352
cholesteatoma, 68, 72, 76, 80, 81, 84, 85, 86, 87, 88, 89, 90, 91, 121, 126, 128, 129, 130, 131, 133, 134, 139, 163, 186, 216, 248, 277, 310, 344, 364
chordoma(s), 111, 120, 137
chronic otitis media (COM), 81, 84, 85, 86, 89, 90, 91, 133, 219, 221
chronic otitis media with effusion (COME), 84
chronic suppurative otitis media (CSOM), 84, 86, 133
CISS, 72, 81, 101, 102, 104, 105, 109, 110, 124, 125, 129
cochlea, 3, 4, 5, 6, 7, 8, 11, 12, 15, 17, 18, 23, 33, 41, 42, 45, 46, 48, 58, 62, 70, 94, 95, 97, 98, 99, 100, 101, 102, 103, 105, 125, 135, 143, 149, 153, 164,

169, 170, 172, 175, 177, 178, 180, 185, 191, 196, 197, 198, 204, 205, 211, 216, 218, 221, 225, 234, 236, 240, 241, 246, 252, 254, 255, 256, 260, 261, 266, 281, 284, 285, 289, 290, 295, 299, 311, 314, 315, 322, 323, 324, 325, 326, 328, 331
cochlear aplasia, 96, 97, 101
cochlear aqueduct, 143
cochlear hypoplasia, 48, 95, 96, 99
cochlear hypoplasia (CH), 48, 95, 96, 99, 106
cochlear implantation (CI), 29, 38, 50, 59, 61, 62, 63, 66, 94, 95, 96, 99, 102, 104, 129, 135, 136, 141, 160, 167, 170, 179, 180, 183, 186, 189, 191, 194, 195, 196, 197, 198, 199, 200, 201, 202, 203, 204, 205, 268, 274, 299, 310, 311, 313, 315, 316, 317, 318, 319, 320, 321, 322, 323, 325, 326, 334, 337, 342, 343, 344, 345, 348, 349, 350, 351
cochlear implants, vi, 29, 30, 32, 34, 38, 50, 55, 59, 60, 61, 62, 63, 64, 65, 66, 68, 71, 93, 94, 95, 102, 103, 104, 129, 130, 134, 135, 136, 141, 160, 167, 170, 179, 180, 183, 186, 189, 191, 194, 195, 196, 198, 199, 200, 201, 202, 203, 204, 205, 234, 243, 245, 247, 267, 268, 274, 276, 299, 310, 311, 313, 314, 315, 316, 317, 318, 319, 320, 321, 322, 325, 326, 327, 328, 329, 330, 331, 332, 333, 334, 336, 337, 338, 342, 343, 344, 345, 346, 347, 348, 349, 350, 351
Cogan's syndrome, 102, 235, 246, 248, 284
common cavity, 96, 97, 98, 99
complete labyrinthine aplasia (CLA), 96
Computerized Tomography (CT), 68, 69
conductive hearing loss (CHL), 31, 37, 38, 39, 44, 47, 48, 49, 50, 79, 81, 82, 84, 85, 91, 112, 114, 116, 171, 172, 174, 175, 189, 190, 240, 302
condylar process, 143
condyloid process, 143
cone beam CT (CBCT), 68, 94, 130
congenital conductive hearing loss, 79
congenital hearing loss, 29, 30, 38, 40, 41, 42, 45, 47, 50, 96
constructive interference in steady-state, 72
contusio labyrinthi, 115
corticosteroids, 180, 181, 223, 233, 234, 235, 241, 243, 244, 245, 282, 283, 288, 289, 290, 291, 294, 326
cranial nerve, 15, 32, 71, 72, 74, 94, 107, 110, 118, 124, 127, 140, 141, 218, 227, 236, 281

D

deafness, 33, 36, 38, 39, 41, 42, 43, 44, 45, 46, 47, 48, 51, 52, 53, 54, 56, 62, 63, 64, 65, 76, 92, 100, 135, 138, 161, 166, 172, 183, 184, 185, 205, 209, 211, 215, 218, 233, 234, 235, 236, 237, 239, 243, 245, 247, 248, 255, 262, 268, 273, 274, 282, 283, 291, 292, 293, 294, 295, 297, 299, 311, 312, 313, 314, 315, 316, 320, 323, 327, 334, 336, 338, 341, 343, 350, 351
dermoid cyst(s), 110, 111, 121
diffusion weighted imaging (DWI), 72, 73, 83, 88, 89, 90, 91, 108, 109, 127
digital subtraction angiography (DSA), 68, 122
dissection, 117, 220
dizziness, 170, 181, 198, 208, 222, 223, 229, 238, 356, 362, 363
dural venous sinus thrombosis, 83, 117, 118, 138

E

endolymphatic hydrops, vi, 178, 217, 218, 219, 220, 221, 222, 224, 229, 230
enlarged vestibular aqueduct (EVA), 27, 29, 43, 48, 99, 100
epidermoid cyst, 108, 109, 139
Eustachian tube entrance, 143
exostosis, 76
external auditory channel (EAC), 76, 77, 86, 87, 124, 125, 128, 129, 143, 171, 174
external ear, 4, 32, 76, 79, 91, 131, 174, 284, 285

F

facial nerve (labyrinthine segment), 95, 96, 129, 140, 143
facial nerve (mastoid segment), 79, 125, 126, 128, 129, 143
facial nerve (tympanic segment), 79, 86, 87, 89, 92, 129, 141, 143
facial nerve injury, 113, 114, 116
facial palsy, 116, 126, 127, 140, 141, 174
fall, 151, 156, 185, 202, 356, 357, 359, 361, 362
fenestral otosclerosis, 92, 93, 189, 190
fibrous dysplasia, 76, 120

G

genetic hearing loss, 25, 32, 37, 38, 41
genetics, v, vii, 25, 26, 27, 29, 35, 54, 139, 149, 262
geniculate ganglion, 81, 89, 125, 126, 127, 128, 143, 198
glioma, 112
glucocorticoids, 213, 257, 282, 287, 289

H

hearing aids, vi, 29, 30, 31, 55, 61, 62, 64, 95, 155, 159, 160, 189, 194, 199, 200, 205, 268, 270, 271, 272, 273, 274, 275, 276, 299, 300, 301, 302, 303, 304, 305, 306, 307, 308, 309, 310, 311, 318, 336, 337, 338, 350, 351
hearing impairment, vii, 29, 38, 41, 42, 44, 46, 52, 53, 54, 57, 60, 64, 135, 147, 148, 149, 154, 157, 161, 162, 164, 166, 205, 208, 213, 215, 230, 240, 241, 251, 252, 259, 260, 263, 265, 268, 269, 274, 281, 282, 283, 284, 285, 286, 300, 307, 308, 309, 316, 320, 338, 341, 342, 362
hypo tympanum, 143
hypoglossal canal, 143

I

immunology, 234
incomplete partition, 96, 99, 100
incomplete partition (IP), 96, 98, 99, 100, 103
incudomalleolar joint, 143
incus, 3, 5, 10, 78, 79, 80, 85, 86, 87, 95, 115, 138, 143, 175, 176, 323
incus (short process), 143
infections, 39, 71, 72, 78, 81, 84, 101, 104, 119, 120, 128, 208, 220, 237, 255, 281, 284, 291, 299, 326, 341
inner ear, 3, 5, 6, 7, 10, 11, 14, 17, 29, 30, 31, 33, 42, 43, 44, 46, 52, 76, 78, 79, 82, 93, 94, 96, 97, 98, 100, 101, 102, 113, 115, 116, 118, 123, 129, 131, 134, 135, 137, 149, 150, 152, 159, 169, 172, 173, 174, 175, 177, 179, 180, 182, 185, 191, 195, 198, 205,209, 210, 211, 214, 215, 216, 218, 219, 220, 221, 223, 224, 225, 227, 228, 229, 233, 234, 235, 237, 238, 239, 241, 242, 243, 246, 247, 248, 249, 253, 254, 256, 258, 259, 260, 261, 266, 281, 282, 284, 285, 286, 288, 294, 295, 296, 324, 325, 326, 348

inner ear malformations (IEMs), 29, 31, 94, 96, 99, 100, 135
internal auditory canal, 93, 104, 106, 116, 135, 136, 171, 172, 180, 185, 209, 226, 227
internal auditory channels (IACs), 72, 74, 81, 82, 95, 97, 98, 100, 101, 103, 104, 105, 106, 107, 109, 110, 122, 124, 125, 128, 129, 143, 226, 227
internal carotid artery (ICA), 117, 118, 121, 143, 326

J

jugular bulb, 117, 122, 143, 220, 227
jugular foramen, 122, 139, 143, 171

K

keratosis obturans, 77

L

labyrinthine concussion, 115, 116, 170, 172, 173, 175, 177, 180, 182, 183
labyrinthitis, 92, 93, 94, 101, 102, 179, 180, 185, 255, 284, 289, 317, 323, 326
lateral semicircular canal (LSCC), 86, 87, 90, 95, 100, 101, 125, 143
lipomas, 104, 110, 128

M

magnetic resonance imaging (MRI), 21, 27, 68, 71, 72, 73, 76, 77, 78, 82, 83, 86, 88, 89, 90, 92, 93, 94, 96, 100, 101, 103, 104, 105, 106, 107, 109, 110, 115, 116, 117, 118, 120, 123, 124, 126, 127, 128, 129, 132, 133, 134, 136, 138, 139, 141, 154, 169, 174, 175, 177, 178, 180, 183, 184, 185, 192, 203, 243, 286, 287, 294, 315
malleus, 3, 5, 10, 11, 78, 79, 80, 86, 87, 115, 143, 176
mastoid cells, 83, 114, 143
Meniere's disease, 218
meningioma, 106, 107, 124, 136
methylprednisone, 244
Michel deformity, 96, 97, 101, 104
middle ear, 3, 5, 6, 10, 11, 68, 72, 77, 78, 79, 80, 81, 82, 83, 84, 85, 86, 87, 88, 90, 91, 92, 95, 97, 100, 104, 114, 115, 128, 129, 132, 133, 139, 150, 158,

170, 171, 173, 174, 175, 176, 177, 183, 198, 211, 218, 222, 225, 228, 230, 240, 241, 284, 285, 289, 324, 333, 346, 347
middle turn cochlea, 143
mixed hearing loss (MHL), 67, 91, 93, 116, 171, 172, 174, 189, 190, 194, 195, 198, 199, 205, 284
modiolus, 95, 98, 99, 100, 105, 143
multi-detector CT (MDCT), 69, 70, 71, 76, 77, 78, 82, 83, 85, 88, 93, 97, 98, 99, 103, 113, 117, 119
multiplanar reconstructions (MPR), 69, 70, 71, 72, 74, 76, 83, 88, 93, 94, 114, 115, 116, 123, 127

N

neural pathway, 56, 59, 166, 282, 284, 340
neural plasticity, 56, 62, 154
neuroplasticity, v, 55, 56, 57, 61, 64, 350
noise induced hearing loss, 251, 252, 253, 261

O

occupational hearing loss, vi, 251, 252, 253, 263
ossicles, 3, 5, 6, 10, 78, 79, 80, 87, 176, 285
otic capsule sparing, 112, 113, 137, 171, 176, 180, 181, 184
otic capsule violating, 112, 113, 116, 137, 176, 181
otosclerosis, 68, 90, 91, 92, 93, 94, 104, 121, 130, 134, 139, 189, 190, 191, 192, 193, 195, 196, 197, 198, 199, 200, 201, 202, 203, 204, 205, 206, 218, 219, 220, 231, 315

P

pinna, 4, 10, 124, 143
plain film radiographs, 68
polyarteritis nodosa, 221, 241, 250
Positron Emission Tomography (PET), 68, 122, 154
posterior semicircular canal (PSCC), 65, 95, 143, 225, 226, 229
pre-lingual, 41, 44, 46, 57, 315
presbiastasia, 355, 356
presbyacusis, 148, 162
prostaglandine E1, 282, 290
pseudoaneurysm, 117
pseudofractures, 114

R

retrofenestral (or cochlear) otosclerosis, 93, 94, 189, 190, 199
rheumatoid arthritis (RA), 240, 246, 247, 263
round window niche, 92, 143, 197

S

scutum, 143
sensorineural hearing loss (SNHL), v, vi, 1, 25, 28, 30, 32, 36, 37, 47, 48, 49, 50, 51, 52, 54, 55, 57, 61, 66, 71, 91, 93, 94, 95, 97, 99, 101, 102, 104, 116, 131, 135, 136, 145, 162, 163, 164, 166, 169, 170, 171, 172, 174, 175, 176, 178, 179, 180, 181, 182, 183, 184, 186, 189, 190, 191, 192, 195, 199, 200, 204, 206, 207, 208, 213, 214, 215, 218, 231, 234, 235, 237, 238, 239, 240, 242, 248, 249, 252, 255, 262, 274, 275, 279, 281, 285, 291, 292, 293, 294, 299, 300, 301, 303, 307, 308, 309, 311, 312, 313, 338, 343, 351, 362
single side deafness, vi, 267, 268, 269
sinus tympani, 87, 143
Sjögren Syndrome, 240
stapedectomy, 92, 189, 194, 195, 196, 199, 200, 201, 202, 205, 209
stapes, 3, 5, 10, 11, 15, 35, 78, 79, 80, 85, 86, 91, 92, 95, 100, 115, 125, 132, 143, 175, 176, 178, 185, 189, 190, 194, 195, 196, 200, 201, 202, 203, 216, 229, 248, 258, 266, 275, 310, 324, 343, 364
stapes surgery, 189, 194, 195, 196, 200, 201, 203, 258, 266
styloid process, 143
sudden hearing loss, 60, 207, 208, 210, 211, 213, 215, 216, 241, 283, 284, 285, 287, 292, 293, 294, 295, 296
sudden sensorineural hearing loss, vi, 35, 169, 186, 207, 216, 229, 241, 248, 262, 277, 281, 282, 283, 291, 292, 293, 294, 295, 296, 297, 309
superior semicircular canal (SSCC), 70, 71, 113, 143
syndromic hearing loss, 26, 28, 31, 37, 39, 53, 149
systemic lupus erythematosus, 102, 241, 247, 249

T

tegmen tympani, 78, 86, 87, 88, 143, 171, 174

temporal bone fractures, 112, 113, 114, 115, 116, 137, 138, 169, 170, 171, 172, 173, 174, 176, 177, 178, 179, 180, 181, 182, 183, 184, 185, 186, 187
tensor tympani muscle, 143
tensor tympani tendon, 143
transection, 116, 117
trauma, 76, 93, 101, 112, 113, 114, 115, 116, 117, 137, 138, 169, 170, 171, 172, 173, 174, 175, 178, 179, 180, 181, 182, 183, 184, 208, 219, 230, 259, 260, 261, 284, 322, 361
traumatic sensorineural hearing loss, v, 169, 170
treatment of Meniere's disease, 222, 224

tympanic membrane, 3, 5, 6, 10, 77, 78, 79, 80, 81, 82, 84, 85, 86, 87, 89, 100, 125, 143, 159, 174, 176, 187, 245, 277, 285, 302, 326, 333

V

vestibular aqueduct, 95, 98, 99, 124, 130, 143, 218, 220, 221, 230, 231, 284
vestibular schwannoma (VS), 104, 105, 106, 107, 136, 214, 310
vestibule, 6, 93, 95, 97, 98, 99, 100, 105, 143, 173, 176, 177, 178, 183, 223, 225, 234, 237
vestibulo-cochlear nerve, 101
Vogt-Koyanagi-Harada (VKH) syndrome, 238, 239

Related Nova Publications

CRUSH OTOLARYNGOLOGY BOARDS. VOLUME 1

EDITOR: Mohamad R. Chaaban, M.D.

SERIES: Otolaryngology Research Advances

BOOK DESCRIPTION: This book is intended as a study guide for students, residents and practicing otolaryngologists. The book style is in bullet points and tables to highlight high yield information that can be used while preparing for the exam.

HARDCOVER ISBN: 978-1-53614-781-0
RETAIL PRICE: $230

CRUSH OTOLARYNGOLOGY BOARDS. VOLUME 2

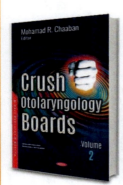

EDITOR: Mohamad R. Chaaban, M.D.

SERIES: Otolaryngology Research Advances

BOOK DESCRIPTION: Two includes the following sections: Otology – topics related to audiology, benign and malignant otologic lesions, conductive and sensorineural hearing loss, facial nerve paralysis, diagnosis and management of vestibular disorders and Facial Plastics and Reconstructive Surgery – topics related to facial analysis, blepharoplasty, brow lift, rhinoplasty, rhytidectomy, local and free flaps for reconstruction, mentoplasty and chin augmentation.

HARDCOVER ISBN: 978-1-53614-801-5
RETAIL PRICE: $230

To see complete list of Nova publications, please visit our website at www.novapublishers.com